Praise f[...]

'A searing account of the r[...]ing
some humanitarian values [...]
A tale for our times . . . written with huge passion.'

Kate Adie, *Mail on Sunday*

'A fascinating discussion of . . . the great modern industry of delivering aid to the poor parts of the world.'

Daily Mail

'Essential for our dire times . . . Orbinski plunges into the heart-break, maelstrom, the moral dilemmas of the genocide territories of the world – Rwanda, Kosovo, Sudan – and finds there enough courage and redemption for us all to feel there is hope for our sad humanity.'

Ariel Dorfman, novelist, playwright and human rights activist.

'James Orbinski has lived for years in the middle of the worst that humans can be, and somehow emerged with both his compassion and his desire to understand us intact . . . The stories he has to tell are some of the most powerful I have ever read.'

Stephanie Nolen, author of 28: *Stories of AIDS in Africa*

'In a narrative of grace and power, [Orbinski] displays the intense components of his remarkable life: integrity, compassion and principle.'

Stephen Lewis, former UN Special Envoy for HIV/AIDS in Africa and author of *Race Against Time*

'Orbinski captures exactly the horror of the surgeon overwhelmed by casualties . . . It is his sheer, human, stick-at-your-post courage that is most estimable.'

Financial Times

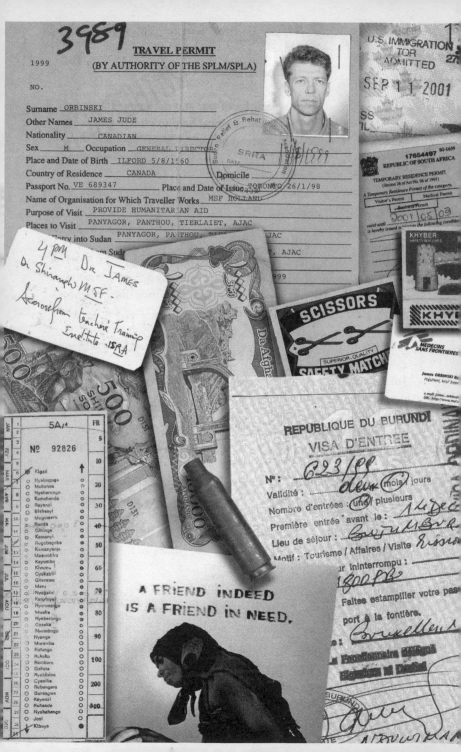

JAMES ORBINSKI

AN
IMPERFECT
OFFERING

DISPATCHES FROM
THE MEDICAL FRONTLINE

RIDER

LONDON · SYDNEY · AUCKLAND · JOHANNESBURG

1 3 5 7 9 10 8 6 4 2

First published in the UK in 2008 by Rider, an imprint of Ebury Publishing

This edition published by Rider in 2009
First published in Canada by Doubleday Canada, a division of Random House of
Canada Limited, in 2008

Ebury Publishing is a Random House Group company

The Random House Group Limited Reg. No. 954009

Addresses for companies within the Random House Group can be found at
www.rbooks.co.uk

A CIP catalogue record for this book is available from the British Library

The Random House Group Limited supports The Forest Stewardship Council
(FSC), the leading international forest certification organisation. All our
titles that are printed on Greenpeace approved FSC certified paper carry
the FSC logo. Our paper procurement policy can be found at
www.rbooks.co.uk/environment

Printed in the UK by CPI Cox & Wyman, Reading, RG1 8EX

ISBN 9781846041020

Copies are available at special rates for bulk orders. Contact the sales
development team on 020 7840 8487 for more information.

To buy books by your favourite authors and register for offers, visit
www.rbooks.co.uk

FOR MY FATHER, STAN
FOR MY MOTHER, MADGE
FOR VEDANAND AND UMA
FOR BENEDICT
FOR MICHAEL
FOR MY CHILDREN
AND FOR ROLIE

We have not yet discovered what it means to be human. And it seems that this *ordinary* discovery is the most epiphanic that can be made—for when we have learnt what it is to be human, when we have *suffered* it, and loved it, we will know our true estate, we will know what gulf separates us from the gods, we will know what it means to be free, and we will know that freedom is really the *beginning* of our mutual destinies.

BEN OKRI, *A Way of Being Free*

CONTENTS

Author's Note   XI

PART ONE

1. Stories Are All We Have   3
2. His Beautiful Eyes and My New Shoes   17
3. In Rwanda, We Danced   37
4. Searching for Humanitarian Space: 67
   MSF in Somalia
5. Afghanistan: No Scars, No Story, No Life   135

PART TWO

6. An Undoing   163

PART THREE

7. Refugees in Zaire: Fear of What They Know,   257
   Fear of What We Cannot See
8. The Politics of Being Apolitical: 301
   Humanitarian Action in North Korea,
   Kosovo and the Sudan
9. Creating a World of Possibility: 351
   The Fight for Essential Medicines
10. Ummera: Always We Begin Again   381

Epilogue: What You Can Do   397

Notes and Sources   400
Photo Credits and Captions   414
Index   415
Acknowledgements   429

AUTHOR'S NOTE

The stories told in this book are recounted from incomplete diaries, failed efforts at writing from the past, other records and publications, and from memory. Though I have tried within my means to check facts as carefully as I can, some of the dates and sequences may be wrong. I apologize for any errors or omissions. Where these occur, I hope I don't add too much uncertainty. Because I have chosen to write the book as a series of stories, I have, in some cases, recreated dialogue for the sake of narrative flow. I have only sometimes changed the names of people to protect their identity, or to respect their privacy. The views and opinions expressed in this book are my own. They are not the official views of any organization, university or hospital with which I have been or am affiliated.

JAMES ORBINSKI
Toronto, 2008

AN IMPERFECT OFFERING

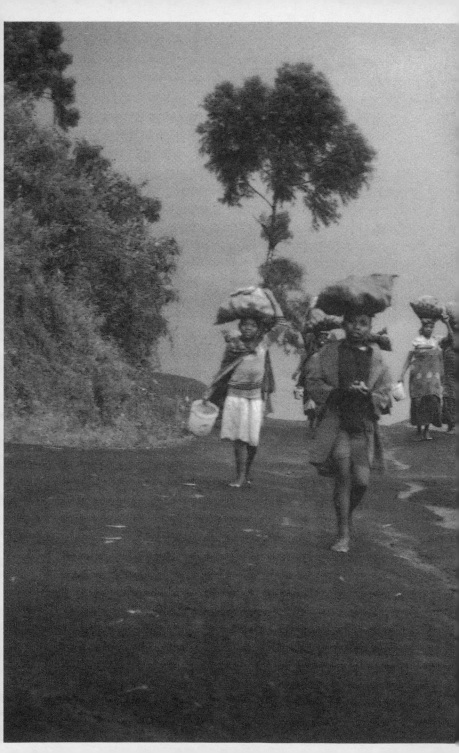

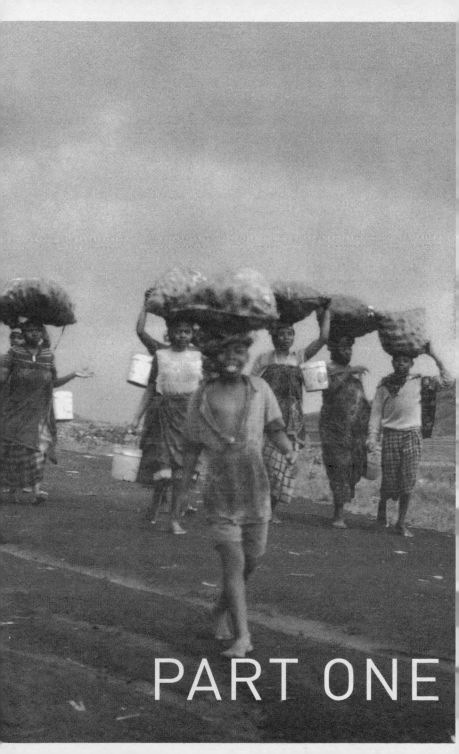

PART ONE

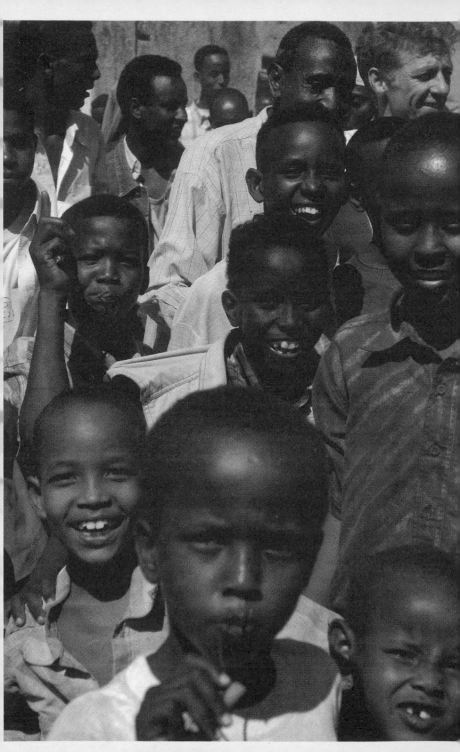

STORIES ARE ALL WE HAVE

I was having a coffee with Austen Davis, a smart, happy man and the general director of Médecins Sans Frontières, or Doctors Without Borders, in Holland. It was the year 2000, and I had just returned from the Sudan, where I had met with the foreign minister to protest government bombings of MSF feeding centres in the south of the country. Austen and I were at an outdoor café beside the main door to the MSF office in Amsterdam. The office is in a refurbished old prison complex, its former courtyard converted to an open-air "paradiso" with cafés, newsstands and a good number of public art installations. A neoclassical archway leads to the courtyard and to the entrance of MSF. On one of its pillars is a plaque with a glass tear, commemorating the Jews of Holland who were lost during the Holocaust. Overhead, engraved on the arch, is the phrase: "Homo sapiens non urinat in ventum"—Man should not piss into the wind. The MSF office belongs here.

"Tears and piss. Is that all we have?" I asked Austen.

"Maybe. But we can refuse to simply cry. I say scream as

3

loud as you can and piss as often as you can. Who knows, maybe the wind will shift!"

That's my man, I thought. The pissing phrase was once graffiti scratched onto the wall of the old prison. During the refurbishment, someone made sure it was transcribed into the arch. Or so the story goes.

Stories, we all have stories. Nature does not tell stories, we do. We find ourselves in them, make ourselves in them, choose ourselves in them. If we are the stories we tell ourselves, we had better choose them well. This book is a series of stories. I ask again and again, "How am I to be, how are we to be in relation to the suffering of others?" It is a question that has preoccupied me for much of my life. This book is a personal narrative about the political journey I have taken over the last twenty years as a humanitarian doctor, as a citizen and as a man. I have witnessed famine, epidemics of preventable diseases, war and its crimes, and genocide. I have witnessed politics fail and I have witnessed the struggle to be fully human when it does. I have witnessed an endless catalogue of terrors, and in them I saw myself, knowing that I might be merely a spectator to these, that I might suffer these, collaborate with these or inflict them on others. It is not a dispassionate story. I do not pretend to be outside of the events and circumstances I describe. I have lived and live in them, between them and through them. For me, these moments have been bigger than the smallness of time itself. They are personal moments, political moments or moments when there is no difference. Nor is this a sentimental story that meets victims with pity and paternalism or worthy of aid only so long as they are not a source of fear. It is about a way of seeing that requires humility, so that one can recognize the sameness of self in the other. It is about the mutuality that can exist between us, if we so choose.

It was my first act as a humanitarian doctor. And there wasn't anything medical about it. It was October 1992. I had been assigned as MSF's medical coordinator to Baidoa, Somalia, a city that had become known around the world as the "City of Death." There, and throughout the country, MSF had set up feeding centres, clinics and hospitals to give assistance to people suffering from starvation and a civil war that was becoming more brutal by the day. By the time the United Nations and various non-governmental organizations flooded in, hundreds of thousands were already dead. I landed in an American military C-130 Hercules on the airstrip just outside of town. An hour later, I was stunned into silence at a feeding centre, looking out over some three thousand people, an island of human hunger in the desert.

They sat in rows on the hard soil, emaciated and waiting. They were mostly silent, mostly beyond exhaustion. The wind was hot against my face. I couldn't help breathing in the fine dust it carried. I watched one woman with her infant in her lap. With a small stick, she was drawing something in the dust. She dropped the stick and poked her child. He didn't cry, and he didn't wake. Maybe he was asleep, or maybe he was comatose—I couldn't tell. She picked up the stick and continued drawing. As I watched her, my knees weakened. I sat on a crate of medical supplies.

In a corner of the feeding centre was a single white tent that had been designated the medical tent. Beside it were three others designated as the morgue. They were full—bodies piled as small imperfect pyramids, each at least three feet high. From the corner of my eye, I saw a movement on top of one of the piles. I turned away. I didn't want to know what it could mean. I looked to see if the wind was strong enough to cause a tent flap to move, or a piece of cardboard to fly though the air. It was.

Then I saw his eyes flutter. The wind caught his long shirt and ballooned it over his body. He lay among the dead, skin stretched taut over his exposed ribs and pelvic bones. One of his hands grasped at something, anything, whatever the wind might hold. I carried him to the medical tent. He weighed less than 70 pounds, and I thought him light as I tried to catch his arm from falling. I did this without thinking. I acted not as I thought I should but as I had no choice but to do.

All the beds inside the medical tent were taken, so I laid him on the ground. A helper put a blanket over him. She was irritated and told me impatiently that he had been moved to the morgue because there was not enough time or people to look after all of the patients, and in any case, he was going to die anyway. At that moment, I felt rage at the efficiency of placing the living among the dead. And I felt despair—for him, for myself. I could be him, dependent on the actions of a stranger for the hope of at least dignity in death.

His eyes opened and closed. He shivered under the blanket, and soon he was dead. This was the last violated remnant of a fuller life. I didn't even know his name, but I knew he had been someone's son, someone's friend and possibly someone's husband, someone's father. What choices led to civil war and famine, leaving hundreds of thousands of people like this man to suffer in this way, at this time, in the last decade of the twentieth century?

When I began working with MSF, I naively accepted the cloak of the apolitical doctor. I believed humanitarianism—with its principles of neutrality, impartiality and independence—to be outside of politics, in some ways even superior to it, and a way of avoiding its messy business. But I would come to see humanitarianism not as separate from politics but in relation to it, and as a challenge to political choices that too often kill or allow others to be killed.

In Somalia, I witnessed the carnage of the political anarchy that came with the end of the Cold War. Here aid was not only a lifeline to those who suffered. For warlords and profiteers, it was the most valuable commodity in the country. Aid was looted, and extortion and protection rackets became part of its delivery. Aid workers were kidnapped, beaten and some-times killed. Even as our compounds came under attack by warlords and looters, we struggled to continue to work. Some called for a UN intervention to impose order, if only to allow humanitarian action to continue. Shortly after my arrival, Somalia would see a US-led and UN-mandated military inter-vention under a humanitarian flag. And within a few months the humanitarian intervention would use force in a clumsy effort at state craft. Between six and ten thousand Somalis were then beaten, tortured and killed by Italian, Belgian, Canadian and American "humanitarian" troops. UN forces knowingly shelled hospitals, and Somali public opinion turned against the UN mission. On October 5, 1993, over a thousand Somalis and eighteen U.S. Rangers were killed in Mogadishu. The image of a ranger being dragged naked and dead through the streets of the capital city changed the for-eign policy of the world's only remaining superpower. In turn, that changed the politics of the United Nations and sealed the fate of Somalia. People were again abandoned into political anarchy, and the possibility and practice of humanitarianism there lay in tatters. I learned that even for the neutral and impartial humanitarian, politics matters, and matters a lot.

In Somalia I worked to apply medical knowledge to the treatment of patients, and to organize clinics, hospitals and feeding centres. But I am first a man, and I struggled to bring my whole person to bear for people like the man who had been on the pile of bodies. Humanitarianism is about more than medical efficiency or technical competence. In its first moment, in its sacred present, humanitarianism seeks to relieve the immediacy of suffering, and most especially of suffering alone.

In our choice to be with those who suffer, compassion leads not simply to pity but to solidarity. Through pity, we respond to the other as a kind of object, and can assume a kind of apolitical stance on the causes of and the conditions that create such suffering, as though these lie somehow outside the responsibility of politics, and as though charity and philanthropy are adequate responses. In being with the victim, one refuses to accept what is an unacceptable assault on the dignity of the other, and thus on the self. Humanitarianism involves an insistence that international humanitarian law be applied and a call to others to act as citizens to demand that governments respect basic human dignity. Solidarity implies a willingness to confront the causes and conditions of suffering that persist in destroying dignity, and to demand a minimum respect for human life. Solidarity also means recognizing the dignity and autonomy of others, and asserting the right of others to make choices about their own destiny. Humanitarianism is about the struggle to create the space to be fully human.

In the winter of 1993–94 I worked in Afghanistan while the Taliban were fighting for political power. The Soviets and the CIA had pulled out not long before, and Kabul and other cities were under siege. In January, 120,000 people walked some 250 kilometres from the capital city to the Pakistan border. They were turned back and had to take refuge in the mountains of the Khyber Pass. The morning after I arrived, I watched one woman who sat on a rock outside an MSF clinic tent. Three of her children huddled around her crying in the cold, and she held her dead infant in her arms. Her lips quivered as she looked at me. I didn't know whether she was cold, afraid or both. My translator, Abdullah, said to me, "Listen. Do you hear that?" I listened around me, and after a while I said, "I don't hear anything. Everyone is so quiet. There is nothing but silence." He paused before answering me. "Exactly."

People come to clinics and hospitals not to be heard but to be treated. And so often they wait in silence. It isn't simply that people speak a different language, or that I am the doctor and they the patients. Their silence is a practised and all but unbearable habit, one learned by suffering in their communities, in their families, in their bodies and with their children. For some, such suffering has been years in the making; for others, their suffering is compressed into the last few weeks of a war or a turmoil that forces a family to leave its home and go elsewhere—anywhere that might be safer. And yet for most—as for this mother in Afghanistan with her children huddled around her—the thought of giving up is inconceivable.

The silence of the people in the clinics, the whispered single syllables acknowledging that the doctor has found the source of their pain—these sounds and the empty spaces between mark where suffering is borne not by those who choose but by those who must endure what is imposed on them.

Simone Weil in her commentary on Homer's *Iliad*—a commentary written in the summer of 1940 after the fall of France to the Nazis—remarked that a "trembling" marks those who "now feel a nothingness in their own presence." It is a trembling, a quivering, of those who are reduced to a bare life that is no longer inherently sacred. It is into this silent place that the humanitarian acts, and in speaking from this place, the voice of outrage is raised. It is a voice that bears witness to the plight of the victim, and one that demands for the victim both assistance and protection, so that the silence does not go unheard. Speaking is the first political act. It is the first act of liberty, and it always implicitly involves another. In speaking, one recognizes, "I am and I am not alone."

At its best, politics is an imperfect human project. It is at its worst when we delude ourselves into thinking it can be perfect. In Rwanda in 1994, I was MSF's head of mission in Kigali, the country's capital city. It was a place with a very particular delusional politics, the criminal politics of genocide. It was a brutal, horrible time, a time of rational, systematic and state-planned evil. More than a million people—virtually all Tutsis—were butchered in fourteen weeks. Bodies filled the streets of the capital, and the gutters alongside a hospital that we managed to keep open ran red with blood.

One night, after many long hours of surgery, a girl of about nine told me how she had escaped murder at the hands of the killing squads. The squads were part of an organized government plan to erase the existence of the Tutsi people from Rwanda. Through an interpreter, the little girl told me, "My mother hid me in the latrines. I saw through the hole. I watched them hit her with machetes. I watched my mother's arm fall into my father's blood on the floor, and I cried without noise in the toilet."

The genocide was life as we *can* choose to live it. For years before the genocide, the French government trained and armed the Rwandan soldiers. And all the way through the genocide, the French supplied them with arms, mercenaries and intelligence. MSF and other NGOs repeatedly called for UN intervention, but Belgium, France and the United States paralyzed the UN, and each knowingly pursued their foreign policies through genocide. The eventual UN/French-led military intervention was too little too late, and barely more than a deception that allowed those who committed the genocide to escape into Zaire.

Many have described genocide and similar human cruelties as unspeakable. But they are as unspeakable as they are undoable. As human beings, we do genocide. Doctors cannot stop this crime. But the little girl in the latrine had no voice, and as doctors we had a responsibility to speak out against what we knew. And we did not speak into the wind. We spoke with a clear intent to rouse the outrage of public consciousness around the world, and to demand a UN intervention to stop this criminal politics.

An Imperfect Offering is about finding a way to confront unjust human suffering in the world as it is. Today one of the greatest challenges facing humanitarianism is the blurring of boundaries between humanitarian assistance and the political objectives of military intervention. In the post–Cold War world, we have seen selective military humanitarian interventions in Somalia, East Timor, Kosovo, Haiti and Sierra Leone. But we have not seen the same actions taken in Angola, Chechnya, Nepal or North Korea. In these and many other countries, egregious violations of human rights and the laws of war have occurred or are occurring, causing profound and widespread human suffering.

I flew to New York City in the early morning of September 11, 2001. From my taxi on the way to a meeting at the United Nations, I watched the twin towers of the World Trade Center burn. As I volunteered at a triage site for victims, I knew that the world had changed. Terrorism and the United States–led Global War on Terror have replaced the Cold War as the overriding geopolitical context in which organized humanitarianism seeks to operate. The selectivity of intervention continues. In Darfur, Sudan, crimes against humanity, if not a slow-motion genocide, are taking place. Yet little more than political rhetoric has been offered for the people of Darfur, where more than 400,000 have died since 2003. Accusations of Western imperialism in Afghanistan and Iraq have made humanitarian practice even more difficult. In both countries, where enormous needs exist, humanitarianism is little more than a wolf in sheep's clothing as the United States and its allies use humanitarian assistance as a political tool to win hearts and minds in their military campaigns. In June 2004, five MSF aid workers were assassinated in Afghanistan. So unsafe are the conditions in both countries that MSF and many other organizations have been forced to withdraw or remain on the sidelines as millions suffer. In a post–9/11 context, the moral waters for a humanitarianism rooted in human dignity are muddied further by those same Western powers that use torture and so-called extraordinary renditions, who openly rewrite the laws of war, and who suspend an increasing number of civil liberties at home—all in the name of George Bush's "Age of Liberty," supposedly an age of freedom, democracy and human rights.

We must confront injustice and hold our own governments accountable for what is done in our name. Catherine Lu, a political philosopher at McGill University, has written that "justice is the hallmark of human society. . . . Like all virtues and vices, [it] is particular to humanity. While we may metaphorically use the language of justice to define acts of the gods, or fate or nature, in the end, it is only human beings who can be just or unjust. . . . Justice is an ideal which requires no superhuman efforts for its attainment, but cannot be effected without human will or effort, and these are most lacking when injustice is done."

The first act of justice is recognizing the victim. In January of 2000, I was in South Africa at an MSF AIDS clinic. In a public act of civil disobedience, MSF was about to illegally import HIV/AIDS drugs into South Africa. Why? AIDS is a fully treatable disease—as treatable as diabetes. Yet today, worldwide, 30 million people have died of the disease, 33 million live with HIV infection, and upwards of 100 million may be infected by 2020. And almost all those infected live in the developing world. In 1996, patented drugs were available in the Western world. But at a cost of more than $15,000 a year for one person (all figures in this book are in U.S. dollars), there wasn't a hope in hell that anyone in the developing world would get them.

At the clinic, I examined a twenty-year-old man. If he were virtually anywhere in the Western world, he would have been just starting his life. But in South Africa his life was nearly over. He weighed less than a hundred pounds. He was so weak that his mother and grandmother had to help him onto the examining table. As he sat gasping for air, he asked me some very simple questions: "Why do you come here with only kindness when what I need is medicine? Your kindness is good, but it will not help this AIDS. They have such medicine in your countries, why not here in South Africa for people like me?"

It was in hearing these kinds of questions that MSF began its Access to Essential Medicines Campaign. We began by gathering information and mobilizing a coalition of citizen groups from around the world. We publicly shamed pharmaceutical companies and governments that supported the privilege of profit over people's right to exist. We pooled our purchasing power and bought generic versions of drugs. And we brought the price for the treatment of AIDS down from over $15,000 for patented drugs to less than $200 for generic versions of the same drugs. From Seattle to Doha, we challenged, pushed and cajoled the World Trade Organization, the WHO, the UN and national governments. We have achieved many victories, and we have failed. And we have had imperfect outcomes, like Canada's Bill C-9 that in theory allows for export of generic drugs to the developing world but in reality is a bureaucratic quagmire. AIDS was the issue at the thin edge of the wedge. But other diseases—symptoms of a politics that has too long neglected millions of people—are at the other end of that wedge. How we approach diseases like African sleeping sickness, malaria and tuberculosis, for example, has been radically changed by the Access to Essential Medicines Campaign.

In 2001, when my term as president of MSF was finished, I worked as chair of MSF's Neglected Diseases Working Group. We focused on why there was so little drug research for diseases that affect primarily poor people in the developing world. Returns on investment are simply not big enough for a global pharmaceutical industry entirely and rapaciously driven by profit, and governments have failed to ensure that the wealth created by patent monopolies is directed towards priority global health needs. Instead of waiting for others to act, MSF created the not-for-profit Drugs for Neglected Diseases initiative. Launched in July of 2003, it now has over seventeen drugs under development, and in March of 2007 it released its first drug, an antimalarial that targets the specific needs of people in the developing world. We acted not to assume responsibility for the problem but to practically demonstrate that effective change and just alternatives are possible.

The campaign acted as social movements have done for centuries. The campaigns for women's rights and labour rights, the movement against slavery, the environmental movement—all have refused to accept the unacceptable, and all have struggled to put human dignity at the centre of their political project. Ideas can be a profound force, more powerful than militaries or economies. Their power is rooted not in weapons or money but in people acting in concert.

In 2004 I travelled with James Fraser of MSF to Malawi. Malawi is a country devastated by AIDS but unable to treat the 14 percent of its population that is HIV-positive, because even with medicines that are now affordable, its health care system is more a fantasy than a reality. I visited the hospital in Zomba where 20 percent of people in the district are HIV-positive. It was a living hell, and just as in my first moment in Somalia in 1992, my knees weakened as I looked around. The hospital was overrun with desperately sick patients. A hundred and fifty people were crammed into a ward that had only thirty beds. Sick people were lying under the trees outside. Ninety percent of the sick were HIV-positive. It was not a hospital but a morgue. There was one nurse, Alice, and no doctor. I spoke with Alice, and she wept when I asked simple questions about how she had seen the disease spread. In a feeble effort to console her, I said, "There is always hope." She wiped away her tears and said, "Yes, Dr. James, there is hope, but it's a long way from here."

James Fraser and I decided at that moment to leave MSF and start a new organization, one that would actively help communities face the crisis on their own terms. We called it

Dignitas International, and it is committed to community-based care for people living with HIV in the developing world. Working with village health workers, doctors, nurses and officials from Malawi's Ministry of Health, and in alliance with a team of international researchers, we have developed a prevention and treatment program at the hospital and in the villages of Zomba. We have ten thousand HIV-positive patients under our care and bring to them the best tools and treatment that medical science has to offer. And with Malawi's Ministry of Health working with us, there will be more who get treatment. Thousands want it, and they will get it. In creating a world of practical possibility, there is hope.

Today I am forty-seven, a husband, a father of two young boys, a doctor, a citizen, a sometimes humanitarian, and always, at the end of the day, a man. Over the last twenty years, I have struggled to understand how to respond to the suffering of others. I have come to know perhaps too well that only humans can be rationally cruel. Only humans can choose to sacrifice life in the name of some political end, and only humans can call such sacrifices into question. As a physician I am given virtually unhindered access to some of the most intimate experiences in people's lives, usually through suffering, but not always. I can see a person, a family or a community grow into health. I have witnessed the good of which we as human beings are capable: the good that calls a mother to feed her child, regardless of how unbearable her own suffering may be; the good of a mother and a grandmother who carry their sick boy to a clinic in South Africa. The good of those who refuse to remain silent as another is violated, and who act to right a wrong. It is the good we can be if we so choose.

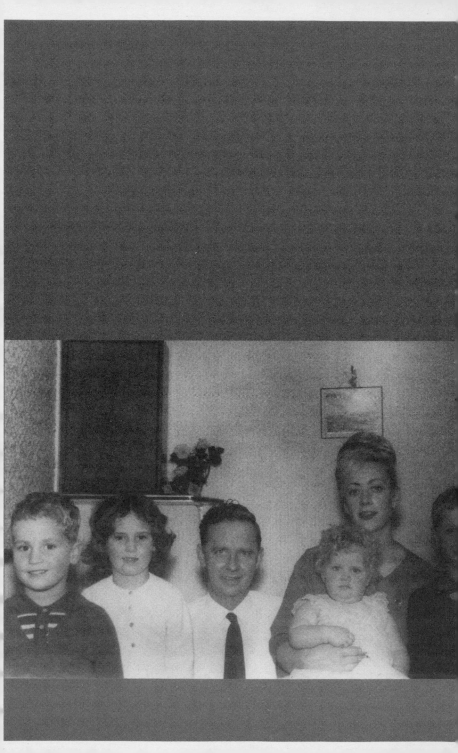

HIS BEAUTIFUL EYES
AND MY NEW SHOES

A man in Afghanistan once said to me, "No scars, no story, no life." Sometimes, the best story is in the space between the words—a space that is a window onto a different way of seeing. And when there are no easy answers, stories are all we have.

I was born in England in 1960 and remember playing as a young boy in the bombed-out rubble of rowhouses near Coventry Cathedral, just outside London. The war was long over, but some of the shelled remnants of people's homes had not yet been cleared. I remember smashing with delight pieces of china—someone else's dinner plates from another time—against a shattered white bathroom sink that had a single broken four-pronged tap handle. I remember jumping from one pile of bricks to another and peeing with my younger brother Kevin into a weathered, laceless boot. I remember looking up at what was left of the bombed-out main wall of the cathedral, to a circular window where some jagged pieces of the original stained glass remained.

I grew up in Montreal. I was ten years old when, in the midst of the 1970 October Crisis, the War Measures Act was invoked. After a bombing campaign of almost ten years directed at federal buildings and symbols of the British monarchy in Quebec, le Front de Libération du Québec, the FLQ, had kidnapped the British trade commissioner James Cross and the Quebec minister of labour, Pierre Laporte. At the request of the Quebec government, Ottawa declared martial law. The Canadian army rolled out of its Quebec City barracks with reinforcements from across the Quebec–Ontario border. The American army mobilized on the Quebec border. Thousands of Canadian troops secured airports and federal installations.

I was fascinated by the soldiers in green uniforms who patrolled the streets and with the way the treads on the tanks tore holes in the asphalt roads. Young men with fear on their pimpled faces and guns at the ready were everywhere—on street corners, in jeeps, in tanks and in trucks that I had only ever seen in the movies. Older men with moustaches, serious eyes and radios were in charge, and everyone did what they said. Troops escorted school buses—particularly those taking children to English schools—and dealt with bomb scares. Soldiers came into our apartment, the door opened to them by my five-year-old sister. We were immigrants, new to the country and to the city, and thus suspect. To this day, my mother recounts this visit with a sense of bewilderment and chides my sister for having "let the soldiers in."

We had come to Canada from England in 1967. I was seven years old as we travelled by ocean liner. I remember seeing whales in the St. Lawrence Seaway off the coast of Canada. My father and mother had both been born and raised in Ireland, but their four children were all born in England. We left for Canada because my parents imagined a better life for us, one free of the anti-Irish sentiments that were still prevalent in England at the time. Racism was not limited to the Irish, of course. My mother often tells of the ship's porter asking her whether she minded if a black man was assigned to our family table. Apparently many other passengers did. "As long as he doesn't mind my children" was her reply.

We settled in Notre Dame de Grace, then the English ghetto of Montreal. NDG was a place replete with the smells and sounds of things different and fresh. One neighbour—he claimed to be a retired police detective—always wore a black hat and a long black winter coat and every morning smoked a fat cigar as he walked his small dog up and down our street. He was like a heavy train never quite getting up to full speed as he held both the leash and his walking cane in one hand, his cigar in the other, chugging his thick blue smoke up the street. He had lived his life on that street, and there was never any mistake about his anglophone allegiance as he taught us songs and poems like "French pea soup and johnnycake makes the French man's belly ache." My Italian friend Frankie lived across the street, and we thought his family fabulously rich because they had an old piano. We played baseball in the park in the summer and hockey on our street in the winter. The man with Tourette's syndrome in the basement apartment downstairs from us greeted my father every morning with a face-twisting "F-f-f-f-fucking shit-fuck-fuck . . . g'morning, Stan." Each morning my father would nod and then look up the circular wrought iron stairs to our duplex apartment to see if any of the children had heard this.

Most who lived in NDG were immigrants and the working poor. Everyone wanted to get out to something better. The radical tide that swept across Paris and most of Europe in 1968, as well as the United States throughout the 1960s, was felt in Montreal too. John Lennon and Yoko Ono held their "Bed-in" against the Vietnam War in a Montreal hotel, and students at Sir George Williams University—a few city blocks from where we lived—rioted, throwing millions of dollars' worth of new computers through faculty windows onto the streets below. I remember being kept home from school one day, sick with a migraine headache. I was eight years old and curled up in our big comfortable green chair, peering through a fold I had made in the blanket my mother had covered me in. I was watching the black-and-white images on TV, replayed again and again, of the assassination of Robert Kennedy. Martin Luther King—"A good man," my mother would often say, to which my father would reply, "A great man"—had been assassinated just a few months earlier. I had no idea who they were or what their deaths meant, only that they were "good and great men."

It was a time of bold ideas in Canada. In the early 1960s, Tommy Douglas, the leader of the first socialist government elected in North America, had created the continent's first publicly funded health system in his province of Saskatchewan. He now brought the challenge to the national stage. Of course none of the meaning of nor struggle for universal access to health care was known to me then, but the fear that fuelled these would be.

I woke up one night to my brother Kevin screaming in the bunk above mine. We had been in Canada only a few months. My parents had very little money and no car, could not afford an ambulance and were afraid to go to the hospital. My mother ran down the hallway of our apartment building to a neighbour, a young doctor who was training in pediatrics at a downtown hospital. The doctor came to our bedroom. My brother had measles and pneumonia and was having a seizure induced by a high fever. The young doctor opened the window, and I remember my goosebumps as the nighttime air flooded in. As he gave my brother a sponge bath to bring down the fever, the big plastic cow over the entrance to the Sealtest ice-cream factory across the street stared back at us through the open window, her face flashing on and off in the dark. I remember my mother crying and my father trying not to cry. And I remember thinking that Kevin would be allowed into heaven because the priest at school had told us that's what happened in most cases. Still, I prayed to remind Jesus of the "in most cases" clause. The doctor left for his hospital and returned a few hours later with medicine. He phoned every few hours and came to see my brother each day for about a week. With every visit, my mother gave him cake and tea—it was all the thanks she could offer. I watched my brother heal, and when he stole my most coveted hockey card, I knew he had recovered.

Each August we would take the bus to the Jewish quarter of Montreal, the home of the rag trade, to buy new shoes for school. It was the last week of August 1969, I was nine years old, and the night before my parents had argued, as they did every year, about the money for four new pairs of shoes, for me and my brother and two sisters. Could another year be put into the old ones? my father asked. "They're growing all the time, Stan," my mother said, and my father countered, "But, Jesus, the money, that's not growing every year, is it?" I knew we'd get our new shoes and I was excited thinking about climbing on the No. 69 bus with my mother to go downtown.

The night before our shopping trip, I saw a television special about the Holocaust. Though I barely understood what I was watching, my attention was held by the voice of the narrator and the images on the screen: yellow-starred people being loaded into cattle cars, children holding dolls in one hand and clutching their mothers' hands in the other, the separate piles of spectacles, shoes and suitcases outside the crematoria, the lampshades made of human skin, the piles of gold from human teeth, people lying dead in pits at Auschwitz covered over by a white blanket of lime, stick-people walking dazed around barbed-wire fences as British and Canadian forces liberated Bergen-Belsen.

My father wanted to change the channel, but I wanted to see. "Is that real?" I asked.

He paused a long time and then said in a slow, careful way, "Yes, but it happened a long time ago . . . a long time ago, James."

"When?"

"During the war, James, during the war."

"Who are those people?"

"They're Jews, James. Jews." In his Irish way, my father would repeat the things he didn't like to say but had reluctantly been drawn into saying. He would say your name as though something precise was being offered, to be fully appreciated by a very particular person at a very particular time.

"Was that the same war when you were a boy?"

"It was. It was, James."

"The one with the Nazis?"

"Yes, that's the one." The camera zoomed in on a woman's arm. She lifted her sleeve to show a row of numbers tattooed onto her forearm. She was very thin and her eyes seemed to swell from deep in her face.

"What are those numbers?" I asked.

My father paused again, and said, "The Nazis tattooed them there."

"Why?"

"It's a lot to understand. I am not sure I understand myself. That's enough. It's time for bed."

Before that day, I had a different knowing of death. I remember the park near our home in England where we played every day. A few weeks before we left for Canada, one of my friends had been killed by a drunk driver who was speeding alongside the park. My mother tried to avoid the accident scene, at least until the blood on the road had washed away, but she overestimated the cleansing power of the rain. My brother and I knew something was wrong because she held our hands in a vise-like grip even after we had crossed the road and were well into the park. We saw the spot, not far from the church where we went every Sunday for Mass. I was captivated by the bloodstain—a streak stretching about 40 feet from where my friend had been struck as he crossed into the park. It seemed to disappear into the road as if some giant pencil had just stopped writing, and I remember wondering if my friend was hiding under the asphalt where the streak passed from sight. Now, with the Nazis and the yellow-starred people on television, death was something we could do to each other. That night I dreamt of bulging eyes from stick people and tattoos on people's arms.

The following day I stood behind my mother as she pulled on the metal handle of the shoe store's front door. "That window needs a good wash," she said. The door caught in its wooden frame warped by many long Montreal winters. My mother announced to the old man behind the counter that we were there to get a decent pair of shoes for school. Boxes were piled one on top of the other almost to the ceiling. A few pairs of shoes were set out in the window for display, and there were plenty of opened boxes on the floor. The man's wife, as old as but more agile than her husband, seemed to be in charge of the boxes. I remember wondering how they knew what was in each box, and how such old people could get to the top of each pile. I tried to work out how they could get one box out from the middle without being buried in an avalanche of shoes.

He moved gently. Even in his frailty, there was a slow sureness to his movements. His clothes hung on his frame like a suit left too long on a hanger too small. He coughed a lot, but couldn't quite produce what he was trying to expel. He looked at me with sharp blue eyes that didn't seem as old as the rest of him. They were beautiful eyes.

The old man and the old woman gave a terse set of complicated orders to each other. I thought they were fighting, and my mother looked at me, then shook her head, her eyes closed, her lips pursed, the sign to pretend you didn't notice. By now two stepladders had appeared. It seemed to take forever as the old woman climbed up one and the old man climbed the other. She lifted a stack of boxes and he steadied the ones on each side and then withdrew the designated shoebox, placing it on the platform of his ladder, then descending and bringing the box over to us.

The old man touched my head with his hand and rubbed my neck. I was surprised at how strong he was for such an old man and I remember liking him then and feeling shy that someone outside my family was being so warm to me. "Here, a good pair of shoes for a good boy," he said. As he took the shoes from the box, his sleeve lifted, and I saw the blue tattooed numbers on his forearm. They weren't straight, and the numbers got smaller towards his elbow. I tried to add them up as he put one of the shoes on my foot. Nazis. Bulging eyes. My mother looked at me and shook her head again, saying silently with a prolonged blink of her eyes, "Don't ask."

That night I wore my new shoes to the dinner table. I could feel blisters starting on my heels. "Is the old man in the store a Jew?" I asked.

"Yes," my father said. "He came here a long time ago, after the war."

"Your uncle Joe married a Jewess, Amy, a lovely woman," my mother said. "He met her in Berlin just after the war. She was in one of the concentration camps, and he was a prisoner of war. That was a long time ago. They're in Australia now. I still have Joe's letters from after the war. There's one from Amy too. Joe was never the same after the war." I asked my mother where Berlin was. "Germany. They're the ones who caused all the trouble." I thought it strange how there was a different name for Jewish women and asked my mother why we didn't call Catholic women Catholicesses. My mother said she didn't know why, but that we just didn't and that was all. She then remarked how she missed her brother Joe and how she always wanted to go to Australia but probably never would.

"Why did the Nazis want to kill the Jews?" I asked.

"Well." My father paused, looking down at his plate. "Because they were Jews."

"Just because they were Jews? Why?" I asked.

"Because they hated Jews."

"Why?"

"Because they were Jews."

"Is it because they killed Jesus?"

"It's more complicated than that," my father said.

"How?"

"Well, it's hard to explain." There was a long pause as I waited for the explanation to come. "Sometimes we can be terrible things," he said, looking first to my mother and then out the window. The room was silent.

After a long pause my mother said, "Eat your potatoes."

That night I woke up in tears. My mother held me to her chest, rubbing my back and saying, "*Whisht, whisht, whisht* . . . now what's the matter? It's just a dream. Ah now, *whisht, whisht, whisht.*" I couldn't explain what was wrong. The Holocaust was now about the man who sold us my new shoes. I didn't have the words for what I knew of a world where people could become lampshades. I couldn't stop crying. By then my father had come into the room, reassured me that school would be okay, that no doubt my new teacher would be very firm but also quite kind.

My mother held the side of my face to her chest. "It's not school, Stan. I don't know what's wrong with him." I remember the warmth of my father's hands and the warmth of the old man's hands. They were the same.

My mother stayed with me, and eventually I fell asleep. That night I dreamt of my mother, my uncle Joe, Amy the Jewess and the old man with the beautiful eyes, and me, all taking off our new shoes for the Nazis.

———

My parents talked fondly but always, at first, reluctantly about their own childhoods—my mother's in Dublin and my father's in Tipperary. Their families were poor, and poverty was embarrassing. They told of the black market in food during the war, of the German bombing of Dublin's Strand district, of my father and his brother's collecting firewood for cooking from a nearby forest, of an uncle who had TB, of skin boils most likely a consequence of malnutrition, of my father's serving Mass as an altar boy twice on Sundays so that he could eat eggs with the priest, of an aunt who died of meningitis.

On rare occasions during such storytelling, the Great Hunger—the Irish famine of 1846–49, when over a million died of starvation and its associated diseases—would be mentioned, almost in passing. Inevitably, we would ask questions, and more often than not only silence heavy with resentment would be offered in response. Full stories were never told, only remnants of stories that could be pieced together over the years. Shared in the space between the words was an indignation at what people had been reduced to and a disgust at what some had become. We were told of the "soupers," who in their hunger converted from Catholicism to Protestantism to feed their children in charity soup kitchens. There were bitter references to the "Gregory Clause" of 1847, a law that declared that any family owning more than a quarter acre of land could not be granted relief, either in or out of the workhouse, unless they gave over their land to British landlords. "What would you do, Daddy?" my brother asked on more than one occasion. We listened carefully as the answer came in silence.

We were a deeply Catholic family. We attended Catholic schools, practised fish-only Fridays, had pictures of the Pope and religious icons in every room, and received the sacraments. We said the rosary every night, atoning for sins done, preparing for sins yet to come. As a young boy I didn't understand much of what this ritual was supposed to mean, and I remember more than the odd cuff to the ears from my father as we children laughed at some joke between us while on our knees saying seemingly endless Hail Marys.

I remember too, as a boy of thirteen, watching television reports of the 1974 Ethiopian famine. I can still recall the face of a tired, listless girl, walking to her mother with stick-like legs that attached to fatless buttocks with sagging skin. I remember crying in my bed that night. I still didn't have words, but this time my mother knew why. "We'll pray for them," she said, and for the last time she comforted me with "Whisht, whisht."

At thirteen, I got a job at a kennel and was quickly introduced to the world of adults outside my family. The bitterness of Mrs. Black, the old woman who owned the small kennel, was pervasive. Her husband had committed suicide, and her only son sent her money but visited infrequently. The dog world was full of characters that passed through the house attached to the kennel. There were gay and lesbian couples who visited frequently and who "slept in separate rooms," but not really. There was the young American pothead who lived upstairs and worked in the kennel and who complained constantly about Mrs. Black—"the old bitch"—over pay and days off, but who needed her to sign his immigration papers. There was the excessive comfort afforded to some dogs because their owners were important, and the neglect of others. There was the breeding of Corgis for their beauty, and the putting down of puppies for their lack of it. Mrs. Black scratched constantly at her psoriasis, made worse by her allergy to dogs. She buried and forgot cash in so many places that hundreds of dollars could sometimes be found between a bag of stale dog food and a bag of laundry. It was a dirty place that smelled of dog shit and bleach. Dog hair was everywhere, even in the jam that I would reluctantly spread over the burnt toast Mrs. Black made for me every Sunday morning. It was a place that felt tired, defeated, covered in a blanket of lies that everyone knew everyone else was telling but everyone took comfort in. I worked there for two years, and Mrs. Black loved me in a strange kind of way. I loved her too, but I didn't know why.

I found another job as a short-order cook and waiter at a small family-run hotel near the airport, not far from our home. The small basement bar was the local for night-shift workers from the airport, who would arrive just after I started my 7 a.m. weekend shifts. Steve was one of many morning alcoholics at the bar whose two hands shook as he cupped his triple gin and tonic to his lips. One morning as I served him his daily fried-egg sandwich with mayonnaise he said, "You're a good kid. What the fuck are you doing here in this shithole?" Lee, the chef, would arrive around nineish and begin his futile efforts to bed Carrie. By two he would be drunk, and Carrie, the most beautiful and oldest of the barmaids who didn't like the day-light in the restaurant kitchen, would have coaxed a lunch of shrimp cocktail and steak out of him.

The hotel had a contract with the Department of Immigration to provide hotel services to immigrants and refugees detained at the airport or being held for deportation hearings. Several floors of the small hotel and a back building known to us as the Annex had been converted into a secure holding facility with guards who kept the detainees in and everyone else out. I would cook and deliver the food for the detainees on weekends.

It was sometimes a violent place, with some attempted escapes thwarted, and some not. I remember a young Salvadoran woman who was detained for several months. I brought her books. She told me her husband had been killed by the regime and that she feared for her life if she was forced to return. The detainees were there because officials doubted their stories, but I could not doubt, only listen to what was told privately and with no possibility that this telling would change the out-come of the hearings. The Salvadoran woman gave me a gold neck chain the night before her final hearing. She was granted refugee status, and I still have the chain.

My brother and I were altar boys well into our teens. Like many a Catholic boy, I toyed with the idea of becoming a priest but gave up on it when I caught sight of two priests embracing in the vestry—though they tried to make it seem so, it was more than a greeting of friends. I decided, with the absolute certainty that only a fifteen-year-old can have, that I would become not a priest but a monk. Michael Leiberman, my favourite high-school teacher, had a longstanding friendship with a monk, Brother Benedict, at the Oka Monastery just outside Montreal. Benedict had helped the Catholic mother of a friend of Michael's who had been living with breast cancer. Over the years, she had had a double mastectomy, an arm amputated because of metastatic cancer, and endless rounds of chemotherapy that left her bald, in constant pain and without faith. For years, she was a bitter woman, wanting and waiting to die. Michael and his friend credited Benedict with helping her find at least an inkling of peace in her last years of life. They told me that when they took her to Benedict, he had simply listened and walked with her. Pushing her wheelchair before him, he had said very little, but prayed silently with her. A few days after this meeting, she was a different, happier woman.

Michael took me to meet Benedict. A tall, thin man with tightly cropped greying hair, his black and white Benedictine robes made him seem taller still. The imposing sense I had of him from a distance was dispelled by the warmth of his two hands as he shook mine. As we walked alone through the forest around the monastery, Benedict listened more carefully than I had ever been listened to before, and as with the stories my parents had told us as children, it was what was not said that he heard. Benedict carefully explored not my conclusion to become a monk but the questions that had led me to this uncertain answer. At first I spoke tentatively, and then less so. I was preoccupied by questions about suffering, the struggle to escape it or the living of lies in it. I tried to describe how confused I was by what we were capable of, by the pain we inflicted on one another. As he listened, he remarked on the sunlight falling differently on the layers of coloured leaves on the branches above us. I watched the bright sun coming through the leaves and making shadows on my suede jacket, and I remember feeling safe and unafraid.

"There is no escape, James. There is only what you do." I wrote down what he said, though I had little idea what his words meant. It was the end of my short-lived monastic fantasy and the beginning of learning how to live in the world. While I was not certain what I would do, it was as though a knot of unanswered questions was relaxed and I could breathe more fully. A few days later, Michael, who is Jewish, gave me a pendant of a mezuzah, offering it as a constant reminder that God is present, even if we cannot understand.

I finished high school and travelled Canada for a year before going to university. I mostly worked construction, but at one point I had a job travelling in small-town Quebec and Ontario selling encyclopedias door to door. I quit after several weeks, having sold only two sets—one to my parents and the other to a farm family that probably couldn't afford them.

I studied Arts and Science at Trent University in Ontario and worked several part-time jobs to pay for my education. When I finished university I got a job as a youth worker at a juvenile detention centre, a lock-up facility for adolescents in Calgary. It was a tough place, but on some nights we would watch a video, and the kids would sprawl together in the lounge on couches or on the floor and eat popcorn. During sentimental Hollywood moments, the kids would be silent and some cried in the dark. Steve, first raped by his stepfather, was an addict and hustler on Calgary's "chicken patch"; Martin was a "well-adjusted teen" who for no apparent reason had walked into his parents' bedroom one morning and allegedly shot them both as they slept; Mark, a farm boy known to the other kids as the "horse fucker," was unusually cruel to animals; and Mary, also raped repeatedly by her father, and a hooker famous among her peers for her blow jobs, was ordered into care after she attacked a john with a broken bottle.

It was a violent place. In the two years that I worked there, I had surgery on a knee blown out during an attack and saw many kids leave the centre only to come back again. There was a certain inevitability to their return, and yet there remained the faint possibility that, however imperfectly, they could see and choose something different. I had helped some to see different paths but could not choose for them.

After a year at the centre, I went again to see Benedict at Oka. We walked through the forest surrounding the monastery, and he remarked on the rabbit tracks in the mud. He commented on the crispness of the cold morning air that would be warm by midday. As we walked, I experienced the freshness of the forest, its smells, the sounds of leaves in the wind, of branches rubbing against each other. I watched my feet breaking small branches as we walked, finding an easy rhythm together. He asked me about violence at the centre. He had been a boxer in his youth. He told me that he had not been very good, but that his reach had been his advantage. He did not have much visible physical power. He had long arms though, and I could see this as an edge over his opponents. I was surprised that such a gentle man could have boxed. He knew the adrenalin of giving or taking a punch and the sting of your own sweat in your eyes. He knew the gauging of your opponent's skill and weakness and something of the measured use of force and the thin line past which force can become violence.

I asked Benedict how he knew the way to right living. He laughed and said, "Well, like everyone else, James, I get out of bed and put one shoe on at a time. I walk around this log and I break these small branches as I step. I am acting and being acted upon. Meaning is in the living, not simply in the thinking or feeling. And it seems to me that living well is mostly about loving well." As we walked, he remarked, "Correct answers can rarely be given. We can, though, be conscious of the questions so that we can live ourselves into the answers, into what in retrospect can be right living." Puzzled, but lacking other options, I decided to take Benedict's advice.

I wanted to be able to live in the world so that I could live with myself. I wanted to do something practical to relieve the suffering of others, while at the same time striving to understand the circumstances of such suffering. I applied to the McMaster University School of Medicine in Ontario and was accepted.

Within a few days at McMaster, I knew there would be no turning back. In my first week I fell in love with immunology, a dancing world of microscopic precisions and unfolding magic among proteins, cells and pathogens. My gateway was a five-year-old boy with meningitis who had been taken to his doctor a few days earlier with an ear infection. The boy—presented as a hypothetical problem drawn from real experience—had died. So little was known about immunology in the mid-eighties, a relatively new field then, and research was a way that I could pose questions that mattered and perhaps help find some answers.

In learning about science and medicine, I also learned something of their limitations. My first tutor, Jack Rosenfeld, an immunologist, insisted that the findings of science themselves were not to be deified or held as immutable truths. Over endless pints of Kingfisher beer, I listened to another tutor, Brian Sealy, a British cardiologist, tell of working with traditional healers in Africa and India. "Whatever works for the patient works for me, as long as it really works" was one of his favourite retorts. Thomas Muckle, a bearded Scottish sheep farmer and pathologist, emphasized the limits of scientific evidence, saying to me one morning as I struggled with the meaning of a negative lab report in a very sick patient that "the absence of evidence is not always evidence of absence. In other words, just because you can't find it doesn't mean it's not there. Step back from the haystack and figure out where!"

Vic Neufeld, my supervisor, introduced me to the art of being a physician. In my first year of medical school, while I was doing an elective in infectious diseases, a boy of sixteen was brought to the emergency room after collapsing on the basketball court after school. He had had a headache and a rash that had spread through the morning and early afternoon. His parents and the teacher that accompanied him were frantic. Inadvertently, I became their conduit to the medical team that looked after their son in the intensive care unit. I knew more about life outside the hospital—about life before disease—than I knew about medicine. As I sat with his family in the ICU waiting room I learned about the boy. He wanted to be an engineer, he had a girlfriend, he was the only child of older parents and he was very funny. I remember the last time I saw him comatose in the ICU, his muscular arms laid limp, his face calm, covered in sweat and a tangle of tubes and fluids entering and exiting his body. I left the hospital late that night and returned the following morning to learn that he was in the morgue. He had died of meningitis within twelve hours of admission.

I never saw his family again, but I saw him. I went down to the morgue in the hospital basement. The boy's face had been surgically peeled back off a skull sawed open so that the pathologist could determine the cause of death. I was shocked into silence as the pathologist listened to classical music as he worked. The boy I had come to know though never talked with was now an object whose carefully opened corpse could yield the secrets of his death. I couldn't get the boy and his family out of my mind. For weeks, I was silent on ward rounds. Vic asked me what was wrong. I broke down in tears as I told him.

He listened as he poured cream in my coffee, then began to tell me about the first patient of his who had died. He remembered her in detail and told me that if ever I doubted why I wanted to become a doctor, to remember the boy that was mine.

In December 1986 I made the long drive to Oka. Benedict and I walked into the woods over a lightly powdered layer of crusted snow that cracked sound back to us as our heavy boots broke through to the wetter layers beneath. A penetrating cold, the kind that freezes the exposed jaw within minutes, made talking difficult. I could see Benedict's eyes and hear his voice from the end of the tunnel-like hood of his goosedown parka. He commented on the ice that wrapped like insulation on a wire around the twigs and small branches at the base of the trees and bushes. We talked about medical school, and I told him about the boy. Benedict listened carefully. The next day as we walked through a different part of the forest we continued our conversation, and he warned of becoming simply a user of what I knew. "The knowledge is one thing. Who you are and what you do with it is quite another," he remarked. "It may be that you are struggling with the choice of meeting the world with your whole person. And it is the right struggle—and a good one at that."

As I continued my training, I was open in an entirely new way to the question of "how to be as a doctor." Many of my professors explored this question deeply. One gave a series of lectures on whether the data from medical experiments conducted in the Nazi concentration camps should be available as "none-the-less" objective contributions to science. An unequivocal no was his answer. I remember others too, like José Venturelli, a heavyset, gregarious man with a warmth and seriousness of purpose. He was a Chilean doctor, a refugee to Canada who had escaped torture and had retrained as a pediatric intensive care specialist. Of the many teaching sessions with him, one in particular stays with me. He showed slide after slide of bruises, broken bones, shattered feet, electrical burns to genitals—injuries inflicted on people in a manner designed to torture but not to kill. Doctors had been present at many such torture sessions or had trained others to determine whether the subject could endure more. José talked dispassionately—clinically—about the medical details of how such assessments are made, and then described the betrayal, the human failure that torture is. I remember his mane of carefully coiffed hair, the jiggling of his generous belly and his dark brown eyes as he said, emphatically, "We can do this to each other, or we can decide not to. It is a choice."

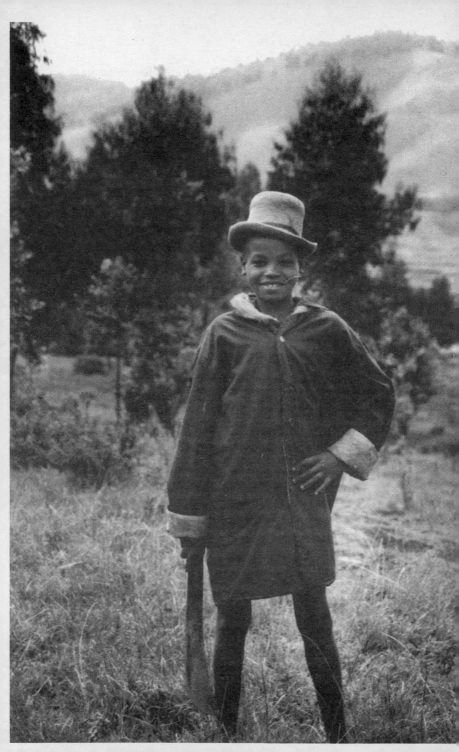

IN RWANDA, WE DANCED

Immunology drew me to HIV/AIDS, in the mid-1980s a new disease, the science of which was virtually unexplored, the politics of which would define how it would be explored. I was accepted for a year-long fellowship with the Canadian Medical Research Council, to do research on HIV/AIDS in children in Rwanda, and in 1987 I left for Africa. Before leaving, I had read almost everything I could find on HIV/AIDS in children, but I could find almost nothing about Rwanda and its history. The organizations that I contacted for information offered variants of the casual reply, "Relax. You'll find out all you need to know when you get there. Enjoy it." I went to Rwanda as a scientist who wanted to be a doctor. I came back wondering if either would be enough.

I arrived in Nairobi, Kenya, having had too much vodka at the Moscow airport with a relentlessly friendly man who wanted to hear "everything" about the West. I paid my first bribe, a "special fee in U.S. cash dollars only," at the Kenyatta airport because my immunization papers were not stapled properly into my passport. That first day, I fell in and out of sleep to the sounds of people speaking a different language outside my ground-floor hotel window. It was hot and dry. I woke intermittently to trace the slow walk of a gecko lizard that crawled across the ceiling and to see the silhouettes of blue-shirted security guards listlessly carrying long plastic billy clubs as they passed my window and peered in at me.

The next day I was supposed to go to a conference on rural health in east Africa, but the city was too interesting to ignore. I wandered out, feeling my difference in a sea of black faces. Car horns and gasoline and diesel fumes mixed with raw sewage in a miasma of smells and sound. People were friendly and offered broad smiles beneath constantly sweated brows. Boys repaired potholes on the roads with rocks and begged for payment from passing drivers. Girls sold newspapers, giant tomatoes and small bunches of bananas to drivers stopped at street lights. Some street lights worked, most didn't. There were street children everywhere in the city's core, and people maimed from disease or accident begged at nearly every corner. Store clerks moved them on, but the beggars were tolerated as long as they gave the illusion of passing by. Most beggars slept in the back alleys, covering themselves with cardboard boxes and plastic shopping bags. The smoke from cooking fires lit in large LIDO milk cans caught my eye as I looked down an alley. A man in a well-ironed short-sleeved shirt and pants that were too big had been watching me and sensed my newness. He gently stopped me, saying, "No, this is not good for you to do, bwana. It is very dangerous for you. Thank you, bwana." Why is he thanking me? I thought.

I had lunch at the street-level café of the Colonial Hotel, an old but freshly painted hangout for rich white residents, high-end foreign journalists and tourists, and a one-time curiosity stop for backpackers writing postcards home. More of the blue-shirted security guards I had seen throughout the city kept beggars and hawkers well away from the wrought-iron fence that separated the terrace from the sidewalk. I felt my privilege and the history of my white skin as an old sun-damaged woman with a British accent said, "I am horrified at the state of these eggs—they are completely over-poached. Do you understand? You do speak English, don't you?" The black waitress in her starched white cotton hat and apron was ordered to bring the manager to the table. He apologized repeatedly, obsequiously removing the offending eggs. "He, apparently, speaks English," the old woman said, as the manager spoke sternly to the waitress in Kikuyu, one of Kenya's tribal languages. Other patrons looked on in silent recognition of the gravity of the offence, while a different waitress brought a second plate of eggs.

I flew from Nairobi to Rwanda, where Dr. Jean-Marc Michel met me at the airport. He and his family were Seventh-Day Adventists, part of a large cadre of Christian missionaries in Rwanda. I had corresponded with him to arrange my research in Rwanda. He was a friend of Brian Lynne, a fellow medical student who had met Jean-Marc in Uganda some years before. "He is a great doctor," Brian told me. I moved into a spare bedroom in his family's home in the Kimihurura district of Kigali.

My first night in Rwanda, I ate a quick dinner and fell asleep to the sounds of house guards along the dirt road communicating with each other through an odd array of oral clicks and what sounded like strange bird calls. Early the next morning just below my open window, a rooster crowed repeatedly in a staccato chorus that never seemed to complete itself. I got up before everyone else and wandered beyond the gate to the street.

The morning air was cool. A clear blue sky promised a hot midday sun. It was the dry season, and the dirt road was as hard as rock. The top layer of the heavily packed ochre soil had turned to a fine sand that formed into dust clouds with each step I took. Small clusters of cows and goats were being herded along by barefoot boys. Other children walked balancing enormous pots on their heads, and the smoke from cooking fires could be seen rising from just inside the thatched fences of the less affluent compounds. Broken glass was cemented into the top of the solid walls of the more wealthy compounds, and the occasional vehicle emerged through heavy sheet-metal gates that were swung open and then quickly closed by zamus, the house watchmen. Servants walked to the nearby market to buy fresh supplies for the day, and girls in blue tunics and boys in beige school shirts and shorts walked together in small groups to school. They seemed surprised to see a muzungu—a white man—walking, rather than driving, on the dirt road. The children laughed and giggled together as one offered me a morning greeting—"Miriway, amakuru"—and stood staring and smiling shyly as I replied. Some men who walked by together holding hands—a custom in Rwanda—chided the children and smiled politely at me.

I walked the road to the top of a hill and could see the city coming alive, billows of blue smoke from cooking fires resting like a blanket over the valleys of the hilled city. Kimihurura was not the wealthiest district of Kigali but one that mixed resident muzungus—doctors, businessmen, missionaries and mid-level embassy officials—with relatively wealthy Rwandans who were usually low- to mid-level government and military officials or businessmen on the rise.

I began my research that week after meeting Drs. Philippe Van de Perre and Philippe Lepage, both Belgians, the former a pediatrician, the latter an immunologist at Kigali's main hospital, the Centre Hospitalier de Kigali, known around the country as le CHK. Most foreign doctors in Rwanda were either French or Belgian, and most were there for two years in lieu of military service. Lepage and Van de Perre were different: they had been in Rwanda for many years and were likely to stay for more. I was to study clinical case definitions of pediatric AIDS, most specifically an unconfirmed set of abnormal characteristics of the head and face among children who had been infected with the virus during their mother's pregnancy. Craniofacial dysmorphy had been identified in New York City in the early 1980s among Hispanic, African-American, white and racially mixed infants of HIV-infected IV drug users and crack addicts. Racial mixing in New York and the presence of other conditions such as fetal alcohol syndrome, which is often accompanied by craniofacial dysmorphy, made it difficult to determine whether HIV infection during pregnancy could cause such an appearance. It was an important question because even without a cure for AIDS, early identification of HIV in infants could result in early specialized treatment and care.

Rwanda was apparently a perfect place to study whether or not an HIV-related craniofacial dysmorphy existed. The country was free of drug abuse; alcohol abuse among young women was rare. Rwandans were separated into two main ethnic groups: a Hutu majority and a Tutsi minority. Intermarriage between Hutus and Tutsis had been common for generations, and there was no discernible racial difference between the two. The "forest people"—or pygmy Twa—were a smaller minority (1 percent) that, speaking a different language and being animists, were generally looked down upon as an anomalous underclass.

The Rwandan King Rwabugiri, who ruled during the late nineteenth century, created an ethnic class system that distinguished the Hutu agriculturalist from the Tutsi cattle pastoralist and established the Tutsi as the dominant ruling class of the kingdom. Both shared the same language—Kinyarwanda—and culture, and though rare, a Hutu could accumulate enough wealth to amass cattle, thus becoming a pastoralist and a Tutsi. German colonial masters exploited the division between the groups, using the Tutsis as their chosen native overlords in an often brutally enforced system of colonial control. Relying on the "Hamitic hypothesis," German doctors and anthropologists claimed that Tutsis could be distinguished from Hutus on the basis of scientifically measured differences in the shape and form of their heads and faces, and on other physical characteristics like height. These external markers were said to indicate the difference between the intelligent Tutsi and the more docile Hutu. The Hamitic hypothesis held that the Tutsi had come from a Nile Valley Caucasoid race that likely had Christian origins, thus making the Tutsi that much closer to the apparently civilized race of Europeans, and ostensibly that much further from the barbaric African. The interplay of culture, politics and economics that had characterized the Hutu and Tutsi boundaries, now had the imprimatur of science—the same specious science that inspired the eugenics movement in the West in the late nineteenth and early twentieth centuries. When Belgium took control of Rwanda after the First World War, it centralized power in a single chief and gave the Tutsis control of the judicial system. The Belgians would further reinforce "objective" ethnic differences, counting Hutus and Tutsis in a 1933 census, and indelibly marking Rwandans as one or the other with state-issued identity cards.

For a year I carried out my study, drawing HIV-positive children from the pediatrics ward and clinic. Each day I assessed the facial characteristics of the children, looking for differences between them and children who had not been infected with HIV. I measured carefully, unaware of what had been done in a similar way but for different purposes by white men before me. The ethnic differences between Rwandans were rarely, if ever, discussed openly, especially with muzungus. And yet, muzungus had had a culpable if not fatal hand in their construction. Rwandans had been measured then as I was doing now.

AIDS—or Slims disease, as it was referred to then in Africa—was rampant in Rwanda and throughout the sub-Saharan region of the continent more generally. The virus was spread silently for many years. Illness came later. In adults it began with a persistent cough or infection of the mouth, then unremitting diarrhea, and then a litany of other infections and cancers accompanied by a slow wasting (hence the name Slims) over a year or two as the immune system gradually failed. There were rumours of entire villages in neighbouring Uganda having been wiped out by the disease, and as hospital wards full of people wasting away in Kigali and elsewhere in central Africa attested, such rumours had to be taken seriously.

HIV was spread by men using prostitutes along transnational urban and rural trucking routes. Soldiers constantly on the move also spread the disease. It migrated into the officers' corps, and then on to the urban elites—teachers, nurses, doctors, civil servants and others. As the disease gained a foothold, it began to be passed on to newborns during pregnancy. By 1987, in some regions of Rwanda upwards of 20 percent of the population was estimated to be infected. Among those tested in Kigali, 14 percent of all adults carried the virus, and 4 percent of all children were known to be infected.

On the surface, Rwanda, with its rolling hills and polite people, was an idyllic place, referred to as the "Switzerland of Africa" in travel brochures. I was struck by the quiet whispers in which people spoke. Rwandans often held hands as they talked: careful, nearly breathless "nnn"s or "ehhh"s indicated agreement, while silence seemed to invite more discussion. "Yego"—yes—meant the conversation was coming to a close. And yet, beneath this agreeable calm, and beyond the few districts like Kimihurura, there was a grinding poverty that left most struggling with daily life and hoping for something better through the many aid and development projects that dotted the country. By the mid-1980s, even before the onslaught of AIDS, average life expectancy in Rwanda was forty-four years—a far cry from the seventy-two years that one could then expect to live in the West—and nearly three out of five children died before the age of five. Poverty left many sick, broken and hoping for relief or treatment at the clinics and hospitals largely supported by the foreign aid of "development assistance." Beyond the rare private practitioner, health care was delivered by myriad non-governmental organizations and Christian charities like those supported by the Catholic church and the Adventists, though the system remained nominally under state control.

With seven million people in a territory the size of Maryland, Rwanda was the most densely populated country in the world, even in the rural areas where 80 percent of people lived. One day as Jean-Marc and I were driving to a remote health centre in the north of the country, we stopped by the roadside so that I could urinate. I walked well into what I thought was secluded bush. While I peed, I became aware that I was being watched. Many children had gathered, unobtrusively, apparently from nowhere. They stared and smiled at the white man peeing in the bushes. Coming from the vastness of Canada, it was a strange feeling for me, that even in the bush I could not be alone.

I bought an old white pedal moped to get around Kigali. Every morning as I made my way from the Kimihurura district to the CHK, men at a roadside drink-stand cheered and waved as the engine failed and I pedalled the moped the final forty metres to the crest of the hill just beyond the St. Famille Cathedral. "Umva, muzungu!" they screamed. "Umva!" (Go, whiteman! Go!) It had become a daily ritual, and we expected to see each other. As I reached the top of the hill, I would give a victory wave and they would toast me with their raised bottles of Fanta.

I would arrive at the CHK just before seven every morning. Like any hospital it was a place where the sick and the maimed collected. The hospital gates were crowded with beggars. Then, as it was elsewhere in Africa and much of the developing world, polio was rampant. Every street corner in every village, town and city was literally crawling with beggars who had limbs paralyzed from polio, usually contracted in childhood. The lucky had families who could afford "bicycle chairs," bicycles modified so that they could be pedalled by hand rather than by foot and that allowed for limp, useless legs to be strapped to the frame in some manner. Others could get crutches or braces, usually from a charity or NGO program, but too many could get nothing and survived by begging.

The very rich and the very sick might arrive at the CHK in one of the country's few ambulances, but most patients were carried by neighbours on improvised stretchers. There were usually about eight men per stretcher. Four or five men would carry it on their shoulders, and the others would walk alongside until it was their turn to carry. With each stretcher there were usually two or three women, also neighbours, who carried food, sheeting for the hospital bed and pots for cooking. The women would feed and stay with whoever was sick.

Others outside the hospital, like those with elephantiasis— relatively rare even in Rwanda—would inch along, dragging gigantically swollen legs or feet behind them. A short old man who had elephantiasis and lived in the bushes across the street from the hospital soon became an unofficial guard of my moped. His foot was the size of a bucket, a festering weight that grew bigger over the years. It had toes stuck somewhere on its front, like barnacles stuck to a beached boat. Every morning he dragged his wrapped foot behind him, moving forward on his good leg using a walking stick that was at least two feet taller than him. He left a trail a foot wide and about half an inch deep etched in the red soil. I asked him one day why his walking stick was taller than him. "It's good for keeping the thieves away," he said. He would get his foot "fixed"—amputated—someday soon, he told me more than once. "But not now," he said. "I can still walk."

From the hospital gates, I would make my way to the pediatrics ward. Hawkers sold eggs, bananas and sorghum to

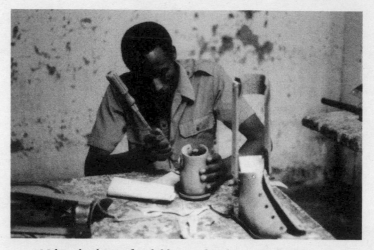

Making leg braces for children with polio in Kigali

the waiting mothers, and curt officials from the Ministry of
Health arrived in air-conditioned vehicles for their important
business. The cool morning air smelled of the Dettol used to
disinfect the communal latrines behind the hospital gates. The
smoke from small cooking fires that dotted the road to the hospital smelled of charcoal and left a slight but noticeable grey
cloud in the cold, breezeless morning air. Clutches of children
huddled with their mothers around the fires for warmth. Most
had arrived hours earlier; many had arrived the night before,
having travelled, in some cases, a hundred kilometres or more
from the countryside. They were hoping for what would be a
more definitive diagnosis and treatment from the European
hospital doctors. Some of the doctors were white, and at least
some of the Rwandan doctors had been trained in Europe or
the United States. The mothers waited obediently outside the
clinic. The children brought to the CHK were most often very
sick, having already passed through their village health centre,
or regional hospital. Often they had pneumonias or worsening
diarrhea unresponsive to initial treatment, or other chronic

diseases like polio or tuberculosis. Some children had the new wasting disease, AIDS.

We started each day with rounds on the children's ward. The yellow of the freshly painted walls was meant to brighten the dimly lit ward, but instead gave it a sallow look and a depressing feel. Children lay on cots or on beds manufactured in the 1940s or on cheap foam mattresses purchased from importers in the small Muslim quarter of Kigali. The mattresses reeked of old urine and Dettol. Unlike the children's wards at McMaster University Hospital back in Canada, there were no cartoon characters painted on the walls and no toys.

It was an unhappy place, governed by rules that were impossible to keep. Mothers stayed with their sick children. Healthy siblings who had been forced to make the trip as well slept with the patient, under the bed, or somewhere outside the hospital grounds. Sometimes it was difficult to tell who was the patient and who was a sibling. Doctors and nurses often scolded mothers for the presence of their unsick children, sitting on or under the bed of their sick brother or sister. Nurses moved slowly but efficiently to get lab results and charts as we made our way around the ward from one bed to another. Lab reports were often missing or lost, and parents held on to X-rays so they wouldn't be mislaid. Sometimes these X-rays had been taken years before. These could be useful for comparison, but more often they were as useful as an old lottery ticket.

From ward rounds, we would go to the children's outpatient clinic, where we would also draw patients for our research. Outside were hundreds of mothers, dutifully lined up around the downtown hospital block with their children. I saw one young girl, about five years old, with a meningitis-like illness. She had been brought from the countryside by her mother the night before and had waited through the night to see the white doctors. She had a stiff neck and a headache, was vastly underweight and had a cough and a fever. Her father had died a few months before of Slims, and now her mother was getting regular fevers. The girl needed a lumbar puncture to confirm her diagnosis. Crouched over the examining table, I sweated against her terrified screams and held her still as Dr. Lepage carefully put the needle between two vertebrae in her lower back. The girl tried to bite me, and the nurse grabbed her flailing arms and screamed at her, "Ummera!" After Dr. Lepage had drawn out a pus-coloured fluid, the girl, now cradled in her mother's arms, still resisted me as I started an IV line for an antibiotic.

"Ummera, what does it mean?" I asked the nurse.

"It means courage," she replied. "Sometimes you just have to find your courage. There is nothing else you can do."

My research was going well, and soon I became friends with Susan Allen, a professor from the University of San Francisco who was running a research project on AIDS in Rwanda. Her living quarters and office were in a house behind the CHK, and I was often there for meetings or for dinner. Susan loved parties, and nearly every weekend her office-house was the gathering place for hospital staff, embassy expatriates and employees, as well as Susan's extensive team of Rwandans. We danced, we drank and we laughed long into the night.

I made some friends, among them Thérèse Bizimanna, a Hutu nurse and social worker whose husband was Tutsi. Thérèse was a thoughtful, friendly woman who took her work seriously. I once sat down to join her as she was talking with some other nurses. A few of them resented one of the Tutsi nurses at the hospital whose husband was a white Belgian doctor. After the others had left to get drinks, Thérèse remarked, "People who want to will always find a way to be jealous. These are just petty politics, like anywhere. They mean nothing." I asked her what it was like for her and her husband as an inter-ethnic couple. Her pause told me I had asked the wrong question. She said that in Rwanda, Hutus and Tutsis were free to live as they liked, to marry as they liked. "There are some problems of course, but no big problems, not really," she said. Her husband was nearby and overheard our conversation. Smiling, he pulled me up from my chair to join the men dancing a traditional warrior dance. "See, James, in Rwanda we dance together— Hutu and Tutsi and muzungus! Umva!"

Halfway through the year, Jean-Marc got a faculty position at the newly finished Adventist University in Mundende, in the north of the country. He and his family would leave Kigali, but my research at the CHK meant that I would stay. Accommodation was expensive and not easy to find in the city, so Jean-Marc made arrangements for me to share the guesthouse at the Kigali Adventist compound. I wasn't happy at the thought of living among church officials and visiting pastors. Jean-Marc and his family did not push or preach their religion to me, but by then I had seen enough of their community to know that I did not want to be immersed in it.

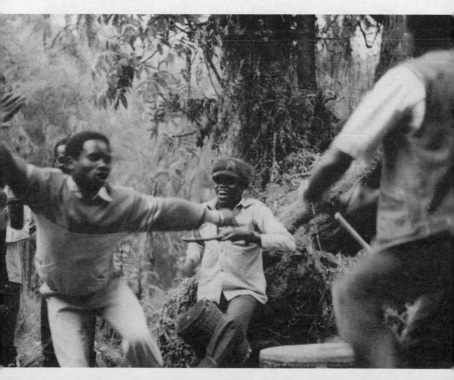

On my second night at the guesthouse, the chairman of Adventist publishing in sub-Saharan Africa stayed with me. He was from Kenya and asked me what I did. I told him, and he replied with an air of quiet forgiveness: "Yes, AIDS is a terrible blight. It is God's scourge for people who indulge in sex sin." For the next hour, building in a righteous intensity, he delivered a monologue replete with biblical quotes to support his conclusion. His rhetoric wasn't just religious. "AIDS is a white man's disease. You people are trying to blame Africa for your sexual immorality. More children die of diarrhea and measles than die of AIDS, so why should we worry about AIDS? The Russians have known about AIDS since before 1970—how can you say it is a new disease? Your homosexuals gave it to us." And on he went. He had no godly argument to justify children infected with AIDS, wives infected by husbands, or the thousands of people who contracted the disease through blood transfusions and unsterile hypodermic needles. In answer to my questions, he concluded in a heightened pitch, "God works—and punishes—in mysterious ways!"

The next morning I told Susan Allen about the sermon, and she offered me the guest room at the Project San Francisco office-house. It was perfect, right behind the hospital, and as long as I didn't mind sharing the room with the occasional guest, I could have it. Emile Fundira, Susan's project manager, was living there too. I jumped at the chance and moved in that night.

Emile was a Tutsi, and we had already become friends. Sharing a house, we became even better friends, having a beer together at night and visiting his family and friends on weekends. Emile told me how lucky he was to be working for Susan. By law, Tutsis, identified as such in all official identity papers, could constitute only 3 percent of any local employer's or government ministry's workforce, posing problems to the 14 percent of Tutsis who lived in the country. Many Tutsis tried to find work with NGOs, as embassy staff or with foreign

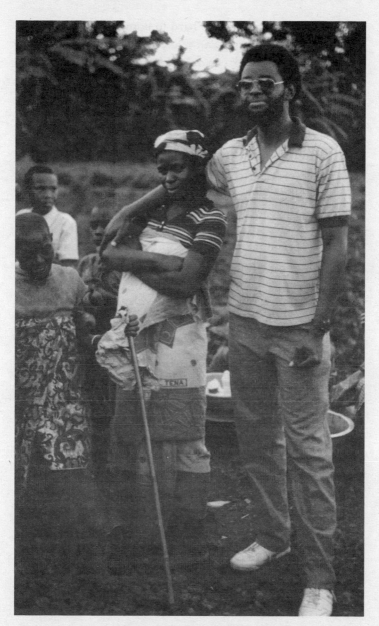

Emile with Hutu and Twa vendors at a market

researchers. These jobs were hard to come by, so most Tutsis had their own businesses and many traded beyond the country's borders. Whenever I enquired further, Emile, like others, was reluctant to say more, especially to an outsider. He would try to reassure me: "We're doing okay, so there is no reason to worry about these things now."

On Christmas Eve, Emile and I went with Susan and some other friends to the Nyanza Cathedral, perched on a hill in Butare province, the first and largest Christian mission to Rwanda, built by the Catholic White Fathers who had come in 1900. Ninety percent of Rwandans were Christian, and of these 60 percent were Catholic; the country was the most Christian in Africa. That night we walked up the steep hill, joining a steady stream of thousands coming from the countryside. Cathedral bells blended with the traditional drums being played outside the church's doors and in the villages in the surrounding hills. Drums had once been used to communicate between villages, bringing news of village life or warning of danger. Now, they were used in celebration. People had put on their finest clothes and carried fire torches in honour of Christmas. They were surprised to see a small group of muzungus led by Emile going to the cathedral, but most welcomed us and offered warm Christmas greetings of "Noeli Niza."

My body vibrated with the sound and power of the rhythms coming from the hundred boy and men drummers gathered around the church entrance. As women sang, drummers chorused back and forth to each other, weaving a chain song from hillside to cathedral. We managed to get inside, and people made room for us among the back pews. People prayed quietly as the drums roared outside. Soldiers stood throughout the church, in anticipation of the president's arrival. A model of national piety, the president and his family were supposed to come to the cathedral by helicopter. Their front-row pew sat waiting. The priests arrived late, the drumming stopped and the service started. It was a short, reverent service, and again the drums chorused. For whatever reason, the president never came. We joined the crowds walking down the hill, and went to a local bar for a calabash of gwa-gwa, the local banana beer.

Two days a week I worked at a clinic outside Mundende, a remote town a few kilometres from the border with Zaire, the former Belgian Congo. For most of the children, I was the first white man who had ever touched them. Some screamed in terror, for they had heard old—but true—stories of Belgians who would cut off children's hands if their parents did not produce enough rubber or other commodities for their colonial masters. Belgian King Leopold had taken the Congo under a "humanitarian mission" whose "humane and benevolent purposes" promised civilization and prosperity. Leopold had been "granted" the Congo colony at the Berlin Conference of 1884–85, where much of Africa was divided up among the Portuguese, French, British, Italian, German and Belgian empires. From 1895 to 1930, much rubber and teak was exported from the Congo, and more than 10 million people—half of the population—were killed or died under Leopold's "humanitarian" reign.

The village surroundings were beautiful—lush, green, fertile. And yet in this region one of the most common afflictions among children was kwashiorkor, a protein deficiency that led to malnutrition. It was not that children were not eating enough, but that they were not getting enough of the right foods. The village clinic had a "model home garden" set up by an NGO funded by the French government. The garden grew tubers, grains, soy, corn and other vegetables that, eaten in the right combination, would provide a balanced diet. The assumption was that people didn't know how to grow or prepare a balanced crop; with education they would learn, and the problem of kwashiorkor would be solved. A group of young, earnest and slightly arrogant expatriate aid workers tended the garden and offered training sessions to mothers and fathers who brought their children to the clinic. Almost all these aid workers wore Sony Walkmans, sometimes turned off but usually turned on, and I came to think of them as the "Walkman Crew." It was expected that parents would attend the teaching sessions before their children would be seen for regular health checks, but the Walkman Crew often lamented the poor attendance at the garden.

I was there trying to design a simpler way of monitoring growth on the children's medical charts. The clinic had a Therapeutic Feeding Centre, where children who were malnourished received specialized feeding. On one particular day, there were about thirty children in the feeding centre. All had skin sores, especially around their mouths, eyes and ears. The nurse would generously paint these with a gentian violet disinfectant, making the children look like small, unhappy clowns. Most had chronic coughs, and it was not clear if some also had TB. Most were from the poorest families in the outlying villages. Five of them, all toddlers or infants, had severely swollen bellies, feet and hands. They also had fine, slightly reddish hair, which indicated that their bodies lacked sufficient protein to make their hair grow normally. These children had severe protein energy malnutrition. Their joints were so swollen that it hurt them to move, and you have to move to eat. They cried only when they were moved, and most sat swollen and listless.

As well as the medicine they needed, every few hours they were fed a small syringe of carefully balanced liquefied food through a tube placed in their noses, down their throats and into their stomachs. About a week of this treatment would be enough to give them the strength to eat on their own. I had put tubes in four infants and was placing a tube in the last child when one of the girls pulled the tube from her nose, gagging and vomiting as she did. I hadn't taped the tube properly to the side of her face, and it would have to be inserted again. She

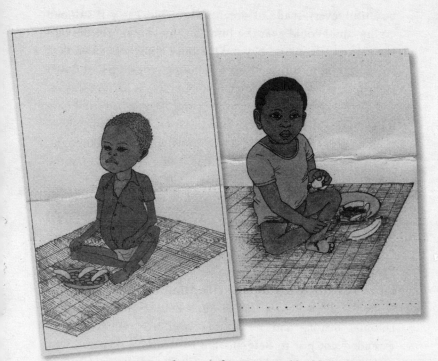

1987 teaching aids for parents and health workers
showing a malnourished and a well-nourished child

looked at me as I approached. She didn't cry but made the hollow, nasal begging sounds that I now knew were typical of those who are starving.

I sat down beside her and stroked her fine red hair. She started crying for her mother, "Mama-we, Mama-we!" (Mother, where are you?) I tried to touch one of her swollen hands. She pulled away from me, now screaming, "Mama-we!" I thought, I can't make her trust me and then hurt her again. I moved away and, sitting across the room from her, looked out the only window in the room. It was dark inside and cool. It was better that way for the children who had to sit or sleep for long hours while they tried not to move. The land beyond the window was beautiful, every shade of green imaginable. The girl stopped crying, and I could hear the birds outside. Except for the odd banana tree, the world beyond the busy clinic was an endless sea of carefully cultivated tea and coffee crops, up and down every hill, valley and terraced mountain. It was harvest season, and there were few mothers at the clinic. People had lived here for centuries, the most fertile land in Africa. And now they were planting cash crops. Of course they know what to eat, I thought. I walked back to the little girl and, ignoring her cries, I put the tube in. This time I taped it properly.

Every few weeks I worked at the Seventh-day Adventist hospital complex at Mugonero, just outside Kikuyu. I would help with the medical care of psychiatric patients or assist the Portuguese gynecologist, an Adventist missionary, with surgery. Zablon was the hospital manager. An Adventist himself, his salary was jointly paid by both the Ministry of Health and his church. Zablon held a not-so-quiet contempt for Rwanda's colonial history and its former overlords. His contempt extended not just to Belgians but to whites in general. One night over dinner at Zablon's house, the Portuguese doctor said that he had just arranged for parts for a broken ultrasound machine to be sent from Portugal. The machine had been idle for months since its arrival, waiting for parts from the Ministry of Health. In a few weeks it would be fixed. It would be of great use, he said, especially for difficult obstetrics cases. Zablon lamented that the hospital had to depend on "charity from the whites" in order to function. The Portuguese doctor took offence and said that the parts were coming not from whites, but from an Adventist friend in Portugal. "Whites are all the same," Zablon retorted with a laugh. "They will never change. Adventist or not, a leopard cannot change its spots. Only God can change what is, and He will show us how. We must have faith in God." The Portuguese doctor, looking for a way out of the argument without losing too much ground, agreed that "for all things, even those we do not understand, we must have faith in God." Zablon smiled as he ate his goat meat and looked around at his white guests. "Yes," he said. "And God loves even the leopards."

One day I was in a small village near Mugonero to help with a polio vaccination campaign. The clinic was in the middle of the village, and because our jeep had broken down on the way we were an hour late. Babies were crying. The air was humid and heavy with the heat. Still, mothers had come from all the neighbouring villages and lined up in the hundreds with their infants to get the vaccine. We'd been working for about an hour when one mother gently pushed her baby boy into my chest. He was beautiful, and so was she. She held his leg out to me. It was limp. I took the boy, and he smiled at me. He was a fat and happy baby who smelled of soap. His mother started to speak, and the nurse translated, telling me that his mother wanted me to fix his leg. She said he couldn't crawl like the other children and had been dragging the leg behind him for the last few weeks. I looked at the boy's health card as he played with my stethoscope. He had already had two doses of the vaccine. This was to be his final booster. Twice his mother had bathed him in the morning and walked miles to stand all day to get him the vaccine, and twice the vaccine failed. The problem had to be the cold chain—the vaccine had to be kept cold right up until it was used, otherwise it deteriorated. The boy started to cry, wanting to go back to his mother. "She has three daughters. He's her only son," the nurse said. I explained as gently as I could that the leg was never going to work properly. The mother stepped back from me as I spoke, holding her now happy baby to her chest. Rwandans rarely cry in public. For a brief moment, tears came down her cheeks. I reached out to touch her arm. I noticed the calluses on her hands as her son wriggled to turn to face me. I felt my own soft white palms with my fingers. Through the translating nurse I suggested that when the boy was older the mother could bring him to the Mugonero Hospital to see about a brace. She listened carefully, saying, "Nnn, ehhh," and finally "yego" as the nurse spoke.

The nurse told me that the mother had cried because she knew her son would be a bicycle-chair boy. "But he can go to school too," I said. "No," said the nurse, "they don't have the money for both." By now the mother's few tears had dried, leaving faint white salt marks on her black face. She bowed her head to me, turned and walked away to some waiting friends. I left the line to buy a Fanta, and it started to rain. The drink had been kept cold in the cooler at the roadside stand. I sat down on a big rock. The children laughed at the muzungu sitting in the rain while Michael Jackson's "Thriller" played on a battery-powered ghetto blaster. The clinic can't keep the fucking vaccine cold, I thought, and I hoped that the rain would mask my tears.

For NGOs and the governments that supported them, Rwanda was an administrative dream, divided as it was into ten prefectures and 145 communes and then into collines—or hills—of about a thousand people each. President Habyarimana had seized power in a military coup in 1973, overthrowing the Kayibanda government, which itself had survived by fomenting anti-Tutsi feeling and torment, an all-too-frequent strategy of elites clinging to power against the reality of a crumbling economy. In 1959, three years before Rwanda was granted independence from Belgium, the Hutu majority overthrew the ruling Tutsi king. Between 1959 and 1967, at least 20,000 Tutsis were massacred in Rwanda, and more than 300,000 Tutsis fled to neighbouring Zaire and Uganda. As refugees there, they learned English, but did not unlearn their allegiance to Rwanda. By 1987, at the height of the Cold War, wealthy Western nations had all but lined up to give to the tiny republic. The country was seen as a darling of the post-colonial international "development project"—a near perfect example of what could be achieved, with development aid properly applied. The United States, through its USAID program, the French and Belgians through their "cooperation" efforts, the Canadians through the Canadian International Development Agency, and even the Chinese and the Aga Khan supported the Rwandan government, tolerating a "benevolent" dictatorship as a necessary short-term cure for Africa's post-colonial instability. The problems of the past were, well, past—and everyone chose to offer a collective absolution. There was little talk of democracy. "They are not ready for it. Democracy is learned, never imposed," a senior USAID official reminded me.

I often went on weekends to Goma, Zaire, with Emile, Susan and other friends from Kigali. It was not far, and there was always music and dancing to be had at the Calabash Night Club. Emile's aunt lived in Goma. Like Emile, she was Tutsi, and I would learn over many visits that she had escaped from Rwanda in 1972, one of the victims of the pogroms. She had set

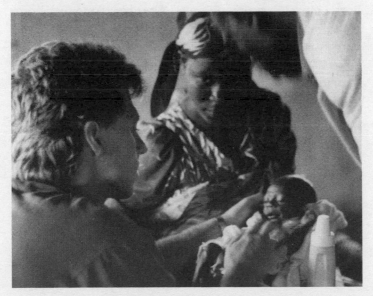

Examining a sick child at the Mundende clinic

up a small business in Goma and had managed to provide for her children. In the last year, though, she had gone bankrupt. Her brother, Suki, who had also fled in 1972, now helped her financially. I met Suki's son, Jimmy Carter. Suki worked for the Zaire government as a commissioner of public works and had travelled to the U.S. in search of foreign aid and investment. He had visited during Jimmy Carter's presidency and was so impressed with the country that he named his first son after its president. Suki was obsessed with his son's schooling. "Education," Suki said to Jimmy Carter, "is a treasure you can take anywhere, and no one can take it from you."

Since the 1973 coup, the political atmosphere inside Rwanda had calmed to a surface tranquility, and President Habyarimana had continued his rule over the central African paradise. But not without the help of the World Bank and the International Monetary Fund, whose structural-adjustment programs of the late 1980s resulted in drastic changes for Rwanda, now a model "developing state." Already anemic social programs were cut further. Under the new policies, user fees were introduced to health clinics and feeding centres, in an effort to make them "self-sufficient and efficient" and economically "sustainable." In 1988, two weeks after I had again taped the nasogastric tube to the nose of the little girl in Mundende, the government of Rwanda announced that feeding centres could no longer give out free food. Most mothers, and especially the most poor, stopped bringing their starving children. My research study on growth monitoring collapsed.

Late for my last trip from Mundende to Kigali, I managed to board the bus by climbing through a window. There was still room for one more on the bus, and a boy of about twelve was passed up through the window after me. He sat between me and three mothers with their infants. Once all the people were in, for the next half hour, chickens, goats, sacks of grain, shopping bags and bicycles were packed into every remaining space in the bus. Outside, goods were roped onto the roof and sides of the bus. The vehicle groaned, and soon we were on our way.

The boy spoke little French, but I learned his name was Uwimana. We talked off and on for the next few hours. He was going to live with his uncle in Kigali who could afford to feed him and pay his school fees. In return, Uwimana would clean his uncle's shop after school. At a rest stop three hours into the eight-hour journey, I bought myself and Uwimana each a boiled egg and a Fanta. He drank his Fanta and kept his egg for later. We continued, and talked a little more. He smiled innocently when he did not understand and grimaced when others around him drew attention to the fact that a muzungu was talking with him.

An hour later, at the edge of a small town, the bus rumbled to a stop on a potholed dirt road. I gave my backpack to Uwimana and got out with some other men to help change the flat tire. This was entertainment for those who remained on the bus, as muzungus didn't do such things. Two hours later, I climbed back inside the bus to find Uwimana and my small backpack gone. Some passengers smiled, watching to see what I would do. One man pointed to the town behind me. I crawled out the window and ran down the road, looking for the twelve-year-old thief. I searched everywhere among the small clutch of huts, drawing laughter from the men who sat on porches drinking gwa-gwa.

And then I saw him, sitting with his back to the road, behind one of the huts. I ran up and grabbed him forcefully by the shirt. "Uwimana—you thief!" I yelled, turning him to face me. He was crying. By now a small crowd had gathered, and I told them what had happened. One man slapped him, and others moved in to do the same. An older man stepped forward to protect him. Everyone deferred to the old man, who asked the boy what happened. Someone else had stolen the backpack, he said. Uwimana went after him, but the man ran too fast. Uwimana didn't want to go back on the bus empty-handed. I was ashamed. I put my hand on his shoulder. He pulled away and reached in his pocket for the egg. It was broken. I wouldn't take it, so he left it on a rock. Uwimana wouldn't come back to the bus with me. He stayed with the old man, to whom I gave some money to make sure Uwimana caught the next bus. I wanted to say sorry to him in Kinyarwanda, but I had never learned how. I climbed through the bus window and watched him staring at me as we drove away.

In May 1988, a week before my year in Rwanda was up, I had dinner with Paul, a Rwandan doctor at CHK. We had moved beyond a subordinate student-doctor relationship, and I considered him a friend. This was our chance for a final few beers together. We met at the Bar de Progress Moderne, a popular hangout off the expatriate strip of hotel bars and restaurants where officials mingled with muzungus, and where muzungus mingled freely with high-end prostitutes. We were each well into our third pint of Primus as I began to tell Paul about a meeting I had had earlier that day with an official at the minister of health's office. Throughout the year I had met regularly with the official, trying to get government approval for my research, approval that never seemed to come, though I had been allowed to continue without it. During our meetings the official would make frequent references to my visa, an unstated but real reminder that the length of my stay in Rwanda was in his hands. I laughed with Paul at the fact that approval had come on the day I had finished my research.

Paul knew the official by reputation. "Every Tutsi knows him," he said before pausing. "And every Tutsi hates him. It's the usual tactic," he said. "They always have a way to control, politely, without incident—or otherwise."

I asked what he meant by "otherwise." He took a mouthful

of beer, then looked into the bottom of his glass. He put his glass down and studied a giant red ant as it made its way across our table. "How does it feel to sit across the desk from a man who organized the murder of thousands of Tutsis in 1973?" he asked quietly. I shifted in my seat. Now the red ant had my full attention as well. I had never heard even casual references to this official. I asked him what he meant. He paused again. I watched him watch the ant crawl under our tabletop. The way Paul's hand moved quickly from his empty glass told me that he had said too much.

"So, back to Canada in a week. I can't believe it has been a year," he said. "What's on the agenda for next year? Muzungus always have agendas."

"Paul," I said, trying to formulate the question.

"Make sure you give me your address in Canada before you go," he cut in. "You never know when a friend might show up on your doorstep."

After a full year in the country—working, making friends—it was the first time that the reality of Rwanda's history had been acknowledged to me with any kind of intimacy. Here was reference to a massacre organized not by faceless people in history books but by people I knew, by people who had had some control over my life. With Paul's accidental comment, Rwanda's history was suddenly present, and I had felt Paul's anger at his vulnerability. I switched to scotch and drank heavily as I sat alone for the rest of the night in the bar. I left the country a week later to finish my medical training in Hamilton.

I wrote to Paul several times over the next two years. He never answered.

I returned to McMaster University with some research questions about AIDS and other diseases that needed answers. But what I had seen in Rwanda had raised questions not simply about failed vaccination strategies and inadequate clinical case definitions. My new questions were at first moral and then political ones about who gets what when, about why some get more than others, and most importantly, who decides.

I submitted reports on the research projects I had been involved in over the year to the Medical Research Council, which was delighted with my productivity. My research on craniofacial dysmorphy had gone very well. But there was something about it that bothered me. I presented my work at a few medical conferences, but despite strong encouragement from Drs. Lepage and Van de Perre and my faculty, I never did publish it.

In addition to the required reports, I also submitted a series of scattered reflections that I hoped someone would read. I told a story about an old woman I met on a bus. She was angry at white people and she had taken the opportunity to lecture me, through a translator, on the importance of respect and reverence for nature and for elders. This is important, she said, because they are together our past and our future. I recalled two hours I had spent in a remote village explaining to a mother how to treat diarrhea: "In the end, I knew she understood and that her child would get the right treatment rather than one that would make the diarrhea worse." I asked rhetorically, "Why does one child die of diarrhea in Africa while another in Canada survives this apparently innocuous illness?" I dismissed the phrase "Third World development" with all of "its inegalitarian and paternalistic overtones. It implies that we have reached some sort of Utopian ideal . . . where we are 'first' and the rest of the world is struggling to reach the same place . . . Are we so egocentric that we are unable to consider the possibility that other people's tomorrows are not necessarily ours for the taking today? The work of development is not apolitical. Failing to recognize this, one hazards the risk of a dangerous indifference to the effects of one's presence and work both overseas and at home as well as one's responsibilities as a doctor."

I finished with an account of how I had changed in my time in Rwanda. "It may seem naively idealistic, but I know that as long as we can imagine a better tomorrow, we can work towards a better tomorrow. Such idealism has seeded the world with some of its greatest accomplishments and social institutions. I can change my own life and practices to make these ideals live in what I do in my life today."

No one ever commented on my unsolicited ramble. I don't know if anyone ever read it.

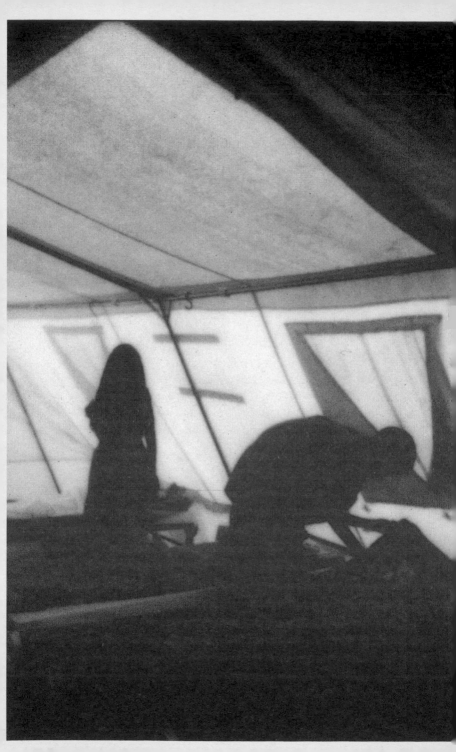

SEARCHING FOR HUMANITARIAN SPACE: MSF IN SOMALIA

What I had seen in Rwanda convinced me that I wanted to work in the developing world. I believed at the time that to be a doctor, to respond to the suffering of others, was to be apolitical. On November 9, 1989, I was watching TV in the surgeons' lounge at the McMaster hospital. A young East German man was swinging a sledgehammer against the Berlin Wall. The world had changed.

I had heard about MSF during medical school. Richard Heinzl, a medical student a year ahead of me, had gathered together a group of people to work with the Dutch section of MSF to establish a chapter in Canada. I didn't know much about MSF, but I knew that it had come out of the radical tide that swept through Europe and North America in the late sixties. Founded in Paris in 1971, by 1990 MSF had national chapters in Belgium, Holland, Spain, Luxembourg and Switzerland. It was now expanding farther, into northern Europe, North America, the Arab Emirates, Japan and China.

The history of MSF was one I would piece together from

official accounts, personal stories and the inevitable hagiography of tales told over too many drinks. I would learn that MSF had been formed by two groups of French doctors, one led by Raymond Borel and the other by Bernard Kouchner. Borel had worked with Secours Médical Française in eastern Pakistan (now Bangladesh) in the aftermath of the 1970 Bhola cyclone that had killed half a million people. Stuck in a morass of international politics, Borel and his team had to wait for permission to enter the country and became frustrated with relief agencies that they thought were too respectful of notions of non-interference and sovereignty. "When we saw people dying on the other side of the frontiers, we asked ourselves, 'What is this border? It doesn't mean anything to us,'" said Borel.

Kouchner had been working with the French Red Cross, which had been invited by the Nigerian government to work in Biafra in 1968. In keeping with the Red Cross's tradition of neutrality and discretion, Kouchner took an oath of silence. After a coup in newly independent Nigeria, across the country the Ibo people were slaughtered. The Ibo then declared the independence of their Biafran region. A brutal civil war ensued. Nigerian forces encircled the renegade region, imposed a blockade and left eight and a half million Biafrans to starve. One day, wounded villagers fleeing Nigerian soldiers overran the medical clinic where Kouchner and other French doctors were working. The doctors notified Red Cross headquarters and were ordered to abandon their posts. They refused, and in staying witnessed Nigerian troops slaughter unarmed men, women and children. The doctors were outraged by what they had seen and disgusted that the Red Cross's strict adherence to neutrality prevented them from speaking publicly about it. They quit the Red Cross, and when they returned to France they broke their oath of silence and told the world what they had witnessed. One of the earlier unofficial incarnations of the new group of French doctors was the Committee Against Genocide in Biafra.

Theirs was a reaction against the same view of humanitarian neutrality that had led the Red Cross to remain silent in its knowledge of the Nazi exterminations and labour camps during World War II. At that time, the Red Cross feared that if it spoke out, the Nazis would not let them assist prisoners of war. For millions, it would be a fatal choice.

On December 10, 1971, MSF was officially formed, a convergence of both the Borel and the Kouchner groups. From its conception, MSF refused to recognize borders as sacrosanct or as an impediment to action. While rejecting the silence of the Red Cross, MSF adhered to the principles of humanitarian action established in 1864 when the Red Cross was founded: the principle of universality, which asserts that all victims are worthy of assistance and protection wherever they may be; the principle of impartiality, which claims that assistance and protection must be given to all victims in a conflict, no matter which side they are on, regardless of race, religion, political or other affiliation, and given strictly and proportionately according to need, and need alone; and the principle of independence, which demands that humanitarian actors remain independent of political, economic, religious or other objectives. MSF would remain neutral to the political causes of conflict, but would not remain silent about the plight of its victims, nor would it remain silent in the face of war crimes, genocide and massive violations of human rights. MSF was born out of an understanding of the role humanitarians could play in shaping public opinion. It insisted on the responsibility not just to act but to speak out in solidarity against violations of human rights and international humanitarian law—violations that governments often worked hard to hide.

In 1979, MSF alerted the world to the plight of thousands of Vietnamese fleeing their country in small fishing boats. Since 1975, at least 400,000 people had fled Communist Vietnam by boat. Half had died at the hands of pirates who raped and looted, or in sea storms, or after running out of food and water while looking for refuge in neighbouring Thailand, Malaysia and Indonesia. In November 1978, Malaysia had closed its borders to the refugees. Bernard Kouchner, then leader of MSF, together with a group of French intellectuals that included Jean-Paul Sartre, wanted to send a cargo ship to the China Sea to rescue those who were stranded. Many inside MSF questioned whether it was feasible for a single ship to rescue all those on small fishing boats. They questioned the quality of medical care that was being proposed. And most important, they questioned whether the presence of the ship would encourage other people seeking a place in already overcrowded refugee camps to risk dying in the China Sea. For those that resisted Kouchner, the ship was seen as little more than a media stunt, and the difference of opinion forced Kouchner to split with MSF. He went ahead with the cargo ship, calling it *The Island of Light*. It soon abandoned its original mission and became a hospital ship that had little practical benefit, as it was too large to moor off the many small islands where the refugees had fled.

The more I learned about MSF, especially its willingness to question its own actions and its own myths, the more I wanted to join. The organization recognized—however quietly— that it had been founded on a mistaken judgment in Biafra. Like Oxfam and Christian missionaries working in Biafra, the Kouchner group of former Red Cross doctors believed they were siding with the victims when they took up the cause of the Biafran secessionists. And yet, General Ojukwu, the Biafran secessionist leader, had actually refused to allow a road route for food into Biafra, preferring to use the starving people as a media prop in his drive for Biafran independence. He only wanted telegenic airlifts of food that would build sympathy and support among Western publics. He worried that a road route might suggest the humanity of the Nigerian regime even in its military campaign to keep the country united.

Ojukwu's intransigence reinforced the Nigerian blockade and increased the starvation. MSF would later recognize its error in judgment, but the organization would not reject its commitment to speaking out. It was not afraid to confront dilemmas and it was not afraid to re-examine its own decisions in those contexts.

I volunteered as a founding member of MSF Canada along with a growing number of others across the country. (There were by now at least a hundred members across Canada, but the early people I most easily remember are Richard Heinzl—the official founder of MSF Canada—his brother John Heinzl, Jos Nolle from MSF Holland, Jim Lane, Ian Small, Ben Chapman, Vanessa Van Schoor, Marilyn McHarg, Chris Doll, Joni Guptill, Declan Hill and my brother Kevin Orbinski.) But I needed to pay off my medical school debt at the same time. I worked a number of locums, one of which unexpectedly turned into a more permanent position when I went to Orangeville, a town north of Toronto. I had taken over the practice and emergency shifts of Dr. John Turner, a doctor whose illness got worse over the months. I loved the medicine: assisting in surgeries at the hospital, and, in the emergency department, the immediacy of dealing with farm and car accidents, drownings, heart attacks, and drug overdoses. But mostly I loved getting to know people beyond their specific illnesses. One was a seventy-six-year-old woman who suffered from severe arthritic pain. She was dignified, a retired school principal who had never had so much as a parking ticket. She asked me to write her a character reference for court. She had been driving down the highway when she realized, "I'm seventy-six and heading for the grave and I have never broken the law. Screw it, I thought, and I put my foot to the floor. It was a damn good ride, and when I eventually stopped, the officer couldn't believe it was 'a little old lady' behind the wheel. I gave him my best smile and told him my shoe got stuck on the gas pedal. They're probably going to suspend my licence." We both laughed until we cried. I wrote her the reference letter.

Dr. Turner eventually died of his illness, and I took over his practice, but throughout I was drawn to what I had learned in Rwanda, to my questions, and to the idea of MSF. I wanted to be as useful as I could be as a doctor. I resolved to pass the practice on to someone else and, in the short term, hired a locum to cover when I was away.

My first mission with MSF was in Peru in 1991. I didn't see a single patient. But for the first time, I came to know something of the precariousness of war. I had gone to help in Carabamba and Caramarcos, two northern towns affected by an epidemic of cholera. It was the first time in the twentieth century that cholera had been seen anywhere in South America, and the disease was spreading rapidly. It had been brought to Peru by freighter ships from India emptying their contaminated ballast waters offshore. By the end of 1991, cholera had killed over two thousand people in coastal villages alone. Then fishermen sold their catch inland, and predictably, over a few short months, the epidemic had made its way along the trade routes up the mountains to the regions of Carabamba and Caramarcos. Death rates from cholera can approach 50 percent if not treated properly. Profuse diarrhea and vomiting can leave patients profoundly dehydrated and dead within hours. Treatment is relatively easy with oral and, if necessary, intravenous rehydration, and can decrease death rates to less than 1 to 2 percent. As a poor man's disease, cholera appears where there is a lack of clean drinking water and usually inadequate health care, inadequacies made worse by war.

President Fujimori was attempting to put down the Maoist Shining Path guerrilla movement. The guerrillas opposed the president's political and economic agenda. In turn Fujimora's efforts to stop the guerrillas from taking over a growing criminal trade in coca leaves (from which cocaine is extracted) were backed by the United States. The drug lords, the

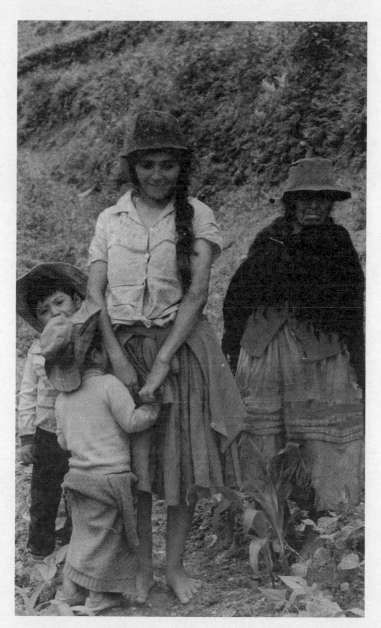

Carabamba, Peru

government forces and the guerrillas were all brutal in their methods, and it was the civilian population that suffered. Early in 1991, in the south of the country, guerrillas had killed two aid workers and several nuns. MSF could not get reassurances from the guerrillas that its humanitarian mission would be respected and had been forced to pull out of the region where it had been trying to help the Quechua Indians. The north, where I was going, was controlled by government forces.

It was mid-afternoon, and I settled in for my trip up the mountain by bus. It would be at least an eight-hour ride, and as I took my seat in the overcrowded vehicle, I was reminded of similar trips in Rwanda. People were dressed colourfully and proudly—some in traditional Peruvian garb—and they talked and laughed loudly and freely. I sat beside an old woman and her son who was in his mid-twenties. An hour or so outside of Lima, we shared sandwiches and drinks at a roadside café. We finished eating in the bus before the old woman and her son tried to get some sleep, despite the still lively but dimming chatter around us. About an hour later, the bus came to an unexpected military checkpoint. Everyone fell silent. A soldier in his early thirties boarded the bus, and after talking to the driver, walked directly to me. Wordlessly, he indicated with his rifle that I should get up. I looked to the old woman and her son, who both looked to the floor.

No one looked at me as I was followed off the bus by the soldier. My heart only started to race when I turned back to glance at the bus windows. No one was watching to see where I was going. I heard the bus engine turn off as the soldier directed me farther and farther away. I started to sweat as we went off the road into the bush. We walked for about thirty metres to a sandbagged wood-and-mud hut. I sat on a wooden chair before a wooden desk in a room with no windows, and I was questioned by a succession of more senior military officers. "Why are you here? Where are you going? Why is a Canadian interested in Peru? Have you been here before?" I felt my heart pounding again when I heard the engine start and the bus pull away. I realized that I was completely alone, and I felt a fear that I had never known before.

After about three hours I needed to urinate. The soldier kept staring at me, but wouldn't respond to me, and only shook his head, refusing to let me out. A half-hour later, another soldier replaced him, laughed sympathetically when I told him what I had to do, and took me out to the bushes. I was returned to the windowless hut. The other guard returned, and for another three hours I waited. I understood for the first time how easy it would be to simply disappear. Eventually they let me go, and I waited at the roadside for a bus back to Lima.

That night I drank heavily with the MSF team in Lima. They assured me that it was no big deal, that it probably meant the army was beginning a security sweep, and that for the next few days, we would wait it out in Lima. The experience had rattled me, but I became fascinated with how each of the two soldiers could see something so different when looking at a man—me—with a basic human need. I wrote in my diary: "If I had three mirrors I could look at each looking at me looking at them, and maybe I would see what each saw differently in me."

Days turned into weeks in Lima, and eventually I returned to Toronto. I couldn't go anywhere, as I had to pay off my student debt. MSF was recruiting for projects around the world, one of the most urgent of which was in northern Iraq. My friend Ian Small described the situation there in the aftermath of the 1991 Gulf War as "a God-damned hell for the Kurds. They were screwed by Bush and nailed by Saddam." Saddam Hussein had invaded Kuwait, and George H. W. Bush had organized a UN-mandated coalition to force out the Iraqi army. It was, in President Bush's words, the first united action in a "New World Order." Bush called on the three and a half million Kurds in northern Iraq and the Shiites in the south to revolt against

Saddam Hussein, but the war was relatively painless and easier than expected for the coalition forces.

Bush did not need to conquer Iraq, but feared that the country might descend into a civil war between the Shiites, Sunnis and Kurds, and that the entire Middle East region could be destabilized. Having responded to Bush's call to rise up, the Shiites and the Kurds were now effectively abandoned, and Saddam Hussein was free to crush their revolts. More than two million Iraqi Kurds began to flee over mountains to Turkey and to Iran to join the Kurdish communities there. They became trapped between an advancing Iraqi army and a border that Turkey was trying to close for fear that incoming refugees would inflame the long-held nationalist desires of Turkey's own Kurdish population. Living in the harsh mountain conditions, with no food and no shelter, men, women and children fell prey to the elements and to dysentery. In less than forty-eight hours, MSF flew in 2,500 tons of medical kits and other supplies as well as hundreds of medical personnel. Under pressure from the governments of the coalition forces, and Turkey and Iran, the UN declared northern Iraq a humanitarian zone. The UN Security Council called on Iraq to stop its suppression of the Kurds and the Shiites, and to allow humanitarian assistance in the north. It also authorized the United States and Britain to impose a no-fly zone over the area. Named Operation Provide Comfort by the Americans, the mission was ostensibly to protect the Kurds, but more than anything, it prevented their movement across borders and abetted the destabilization of the region. The MSF mission in northern Iraq saved thousands of lives, and I was bitterly disappointed that I could not be a part of it.

In the summer of 1992 I had found someone to replace me at my practice and had resigned myself to carrying debt a little longer. I went to Amsterdam to take MSF's course in health emergencies. I had just finished a medical course at the London

School of Hygiene and Tropical Medicine, and I was eager to put the technical certainties of what I had learned there in the context of health emergencies as MSF defined them. During the MSF course—in class, in the hallways and over beers—Somalia, Sudan and the former Yugoslavia were constant reference points, with our instructors returning to them again and again as though trying to make sense of something that didn't make sense any more.

While in Amsterdam, I met Jules Pieters, an imposing man who smoked cigarillos, and the head of the MSF emergency desk in Holland. He had a dry wit, and we got along well. Jules had emergency teams in Sudan, Afghanistan and the former Yugoslavia, and a small team still in northern Iraq. But it was in Somalia that he faced the most pressing crisis, and Jules's team of twenty in the town of Baidoa needed more doctors. He asked me to go. "It's not easy, but it's not impossible either," he said.

Civil war in Somalia had begun in 1990 with a popular uprising against Siad Barre, and MSF had been there ever since. Barre was ousted from power in January 1991, and rival clans were fighting each other for political control of the country. In the six months before my arrival in Somalia, 400,000 people had died in a war-induced famine. MSF was working throughout the country. And in what was now the largest relief operation in its history, the Red Cross was spending fully half of its budget for the entire world in Somalia. Looting of food aid was rampant, and threats to aid workers from warring clans were on the rise. The needs were overwhelming. Some of the old humanitarian rules of neutrality and independence seemed to be falling apart, and it wasn't clear what the new rules would be. For the first time ever, the Red Cross, MSF and other aid agencies were paying armed guards from various clans to protect aid workers and food supplies. By September 1992, four and a half million people of a population of nearly eight million were on the verge of starvation, and of these the Red Cross predicted that upwards of one and a half million could be dead within six months.

Jules explained to me that the MSF team had set up clinics where they saw several hundred patients every day. The team had sometimes difficult but good working relationships with clans and elders. The risks to our workers were mostly from random violence, but the UN, through the U.S. Air Force, would evacuate all NGOs if need be. We talked a few more times over several days. Each time I was drawn in more fully to the details of the situation in Baidoa, and was further impressed by Jules. I trusted him. Joni Guptill was already in Baidoa, and I spoke with her by satellite phone. "Yes," she said, "it's a little messed up here, but we're doing good work, and we need more doctors. I have to leave in two weeks, so we definitely need you." I asked her if she needed anything else. "Bring chocolate—I miss chocolate. And bring some good whisky." By the first week of October, I was on my way to Somalia. I arrived in Mombasa, Kenya, and hitched a ride on an American air force Hercules C-130 to Baidoa.

As the Red Cross had been doing for nearly a year before, the U.S. Air Force had been flying food into Somalia for the past six weeks. Approaching the runway from the air, I looked through my window to the sun-faded brown savannah soil. I could see the city of Baidoa in the distance, and a herd of camels grew bigger as we dropped in altitude. The pilot radioed over my headset that in five minutes we would touch down. I got up from the top of a 40-tonne shipment of grain—the most food the aircraft could carry given the fuel requirements for the four-hour return trip to Kenya. I had rearranged some of the 20-kilogram food bags into a cradle, but I hadn't been able to sleep because of Hank. Hank was a military techy, a farm boy from Illinois who had volunteered for a tour of duty with the U.S. Operation Lifeline in Somalia. He had just finished a tour in Iraq delivering aid for the Kurds, and spent the first hour of the two-hour flight telling me about his girlfriend back home. After that he told me stories of how some American soldiers had been shot at on runways unloading food in Somalia. His orders were to supervise the unloading of the shipment from inside the plane. He had put on his bulletproof vest and was getting nervous. "You've gotta wait till the Herc is emptied before you get out. Understand?" he said, his tone shifting from friendliness to command. I could see sweat beginning to collect in drops around his neck. *Either he knows what is really out there*, I thought, *or he has heard too many stories.*

As the rear cargo flap opened, about thirty Somali men clambered into the plane's belly even as it taxied to turn on the runway. When it came to a stop, Hank directed them to the strapped pallets of food. Within ten minutes, the plane was emptied, the food carried off to waiting Red Cross trucks. Hank screamed "Good luck!" as I climbed out the back of the Hercules and walked into a wall of heat. Armed men sat on top of the trucks. Around us were the bombed-out remnants of airport buildings and warehouses. A Land Cruiser drove at a recklessly high speed towards me on the shell-holed runway. There were two armed men on top, sitting behind a .50-calibre machine gun that had been welded to the vehicle's roof. Inside were a driver, two more armed men and a thirty-year-old blond woman in an MSF T-shirt. It was Joni. "I keep asking Hurzi to drive slower, but it's after lunch, and he's already had his khat. How are ya?" she said. Joni was a family doctor from Nova Scotia, beautiful and confident. Khat is a traditional herb chewed mainly by men in Somalia in the early afternoon or at night. It has amphetamines in it, so things tend to "get faster whether you want them to or not," Joni explained.

I smiled at Hurzi, a tall, thin man of about twenty-five. He was clearly in command of the other guards, three older than him, and one a sixteen-year-old boy named Abdul. Abdul tried to look tough, holding his AK-47 in one hand and a cigarette in the other. He didn't inhale, and the other men laughed at him as he coughed. Hurzi had fierce eyes and pulled at khat leaves with his teeth while he drove. He smiled at me, offering a few leaves. I declined, and he smiled again.

Joni told me, "I've got to get back to the Hawina feeding centre before dark, so we're going there right away. You can take a look around the city tomorrow." I was nervous with all the guns around, and especially with two AK-47s in the cab. "It's kinda like the Wild West here. You get used to it," Joni said. "The Hawina feeding centre is a mess—totally disorganized. The others aren't too bad, and we're setting up a few clinics in town as well, but I have to get some supplies out there before tonight. Get ready. This is like nothing you have seen before."

We drove too fast from the airstrip, through Baidoa, on our way to Hawina. Most of the main buildings in the city had been destroyed. Others were pockmarked by gunfire or had gaping holes from months of artillery and shellfire. Most houses had been looted or burned, and between them or in

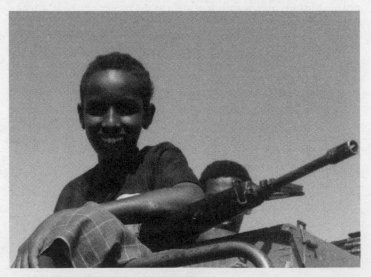

Abdul, my sixteen-year-old guard

them, people had set up shelters made of sticks with pieces of cloth or garbage bags draped over them.

The parched soil of the roads left a waist-high blanket of red-brown dust where people walked and where vehicles of armed clansmen and gangs passed. Skeletal figures in rags walked through the dust holding hands with their children; some carried empty cooking pots and other small belongings. The old walked with the aid of sticks. Young men walked with their arms held away from their sides to dispel the heat. Some women carried babies. Some people crawled along the road-side, too weak to walk. Others lay on the roadside, staring at us as we passed. Many were alive; some were dead. Over the past weeks, they had walked to Baidoa in the thousands from sur-rounding towns and villages. In what had been a city of 20,000 people, there were now an estimated 90,000. Many more had died in their villages or on their way to Baidoa. In the past eighteen months the countryside had been ravaged by com-peting clan militias and gangs that looted, raped, murdered and pillaged. Crops were stolen or destroyed and nothing had been planted. There were 300,000 more people starving in the towns and villages around the city. When MSF had arrived in Baidoa in early September, 350 people were dying every day. Now, they were dying at a rate of 1,700 a week, fifty times the normal death rate.

I could hear what I thought was machine-gun fire from somewhere in town. I asked Joni if that's what it was. "Yes. But they never fire at us." Why? I asked. "Because if we get shot, then the NGOs leave, and there's nobody left to pay protection money or salaries. They want us afraid and alive. So you should be afraid and happy, because it means you can work," she said. I stared at her, wondering if she was serious. Staring back at me, she said, "It's a little fucked up, isn't it?" As we approached Hawina, about thirty kilometres outside Baidoa, we could hear more gunfire. Travelling in groups of ten to thirty, people walked from the

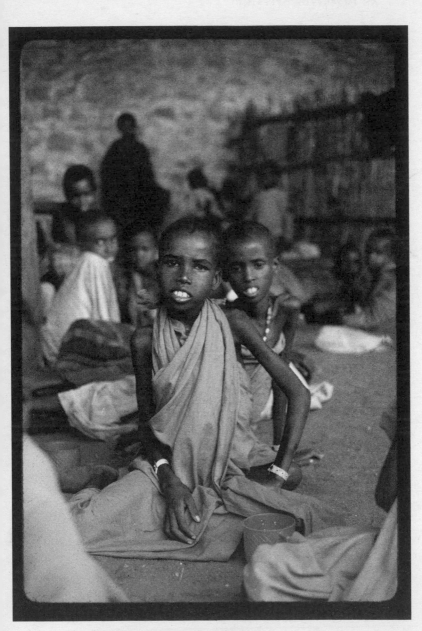

MSF Medical Feeding Centre, Baidoa

desert towards the small town, having abandoned the villages surrounding Hawina. Many crawled along the roadside beneath their last remnants of clothing, too weak to walk. Many had given up and simply lay still. As we drew nearer to the feeding centre, I watched people's faces. They were drawn, emaciated and covered in a fine dust blown into their skin from days of walking in the desert wind. Thousands sat inside the thistle barriers of the feeding centre, and thousands more waited outside. Bracing herself, Joni said, "Okay, let's go in."

She told me to start with the patients who could walk. In the next two hours, I examined a stream of thirty people—mothers with their children, fathers with their aged parents, and people from Hawina working at the feeding centre. The 32-degree heat was unrelenting, and many were dehydrated from the sun as well from dysentery. As I examined one, others stood silently waiting. There was shooting in the distance, and Hurzi was getting nervous, urging us to return to Baidoa. As we started to leave, the line-up of some seventy people simply vanished, disappearing into the thousands already sitting on the parched soil.

The chief of the Hawina village came running to our vehicle. He had organized his village to set up the feeding centre and to provide whatever food and water they could find. In the last weeks, in a massive airlift operation, the Red Cross and CARE had been able to supply some food and water pumps to Baidoa and its outlying villages. The flow of people from the villages had slowed, but still not enough food was getting through. The Red Cross and CARE were paying $10,000 a day to warlords for airport landing rights in Baidoa. Some food was being diverted to clans as a protection payment, and about another 20 percent was being stolen from warehouses or looted on the roads to the feeding centres. The chief had a small boy with him. Ali was the four-year-old son of the chief's friend from another village. Ten days before, near death, Ali's father had carried his son to Hawina. He died the day after arriving. Ali's entire family was dead. Now he was smiling, holding the chief's notebook in one hand and Joni's hand in the other. "Ali's lucky the chief is looking after him," Joni said. "Right now, if you have no family, you die." The chief knew Joni was leaving the next day and had brought some gifts from the village to thank her. As he gave her the gifts, he asked Joni to take Ali back to Canada with her. She paused, looked away, and then fought tears as she asked me to keep an eye on him.

The heat of the day was starting to lift, and we drove back to Baidoa. Hurzi and the guards were agitated. Night was falling, and it was the most likely time to be caught in a surprise attack by gangs or rival clan militias. Nearby gunfire was close enough to make Hurzi drive as fast as he could through the night to the MSF compound. The guards cocked their weapons and one man sat on the roof behind the welded machine gun, ready to fire. The vehicle was a classic Somali "Technical" or "Mad Max," as they had come to be called. In addition to military tanks, jeeps and mobile artillery, Technicals now crowded the country's roads. They were civilian vehicles, pickup trucks or Land Cruisers designed for rough terrain, transformed into versatile and formidable killing machines. The weapons welded to vehicles had been supplied to Siad Barre by the Soviets and then the Americans during the Cold War. Some larger Technicals had Soviet MiG air-to-air missile launchers welded to their flatbeds. In 1977 the Soviets shifted their support to neighbouring Marxist Ethiopia, which was at war with Somalia. The vacuum in support for Somalia was instantly filled by the Americans. Through the 1980s, Conoco and other American corporations explored Somalia extensively for oil, finding some significant deposits. These remained undeveloped, but the Untied States established a naval and military base in the country to oversee its interests in the Persian Gulf and the Red Sea. American weapons and aid buttressed the Barre regime. The last American arms shipment—$50 million worth—arrived in 1990 only months before the fall of Barre to the rebels and just before the Americans pulled out to their embassy in Nairobi.

Inside the MSF compound, a team of twenty were working well into the night preparing for the next day. Some lined up for a shower to cool down. I met Willem Oderwald, a Dutch nurse who was clearly the informal leader among the medical team. He welcomed me warmly and explained that Baidoa was the epicentre of the famine. Once known as the City of Heaven, it had been renamed the City of Death by the international media. In the Baidoa region, 40 percent of all children under five and 40 percent of people over sixty-five had died in the last few months. Of those children that were still alive, 95 percent were severely malnourished. Most adults were not much better. "There is a school bus that drives around town to pick up the dead from the streets," Willem explained, "but there is only one

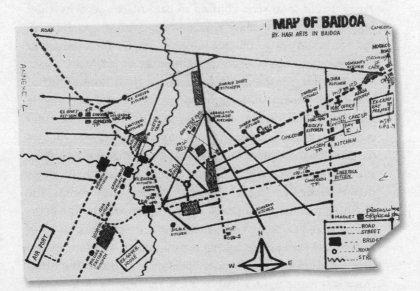

A hand-drawn map of Baidoa locating
feeding centres and NGO offices

bus, and there are too many dead. It's a small problem," he said wryly. "We need either another school bus or fewer dead. Since we don't have another school bus, we need fewer dead. We are glad you are here. It's nothing personal, just logical, really," he said, smiling.

Since arriving in Baidoa, MSF had set up five clinics and was trying to open others. MSF provided medical care at the thirty-two feeding centres in the city and surrounding villages as the Red Cross and CARE tried to get food to them. Somalis were being trained by MSF to work in a temporary field hospital that was under construction, but poor security was delaying progress. As we ate, Willem told me that the team was exhausted from the work, anxious and scared, and now drinking too much. There had been kidnappings of aid workers in Mogadishu, two hundred kilometres from us, the number of armed gangs was increasing there, and there were rumours that gangs would soon start coming to Baidoa. The security rules were strict. You had to have a walkie-talkie with you at all times, and you could not go outside the compound walls, even across the street to the MSF warehouse, without an armed guard.

The MSF compound was a former guest house built of stone and cement with eight rooms and two Eastern-style squatting toilets, one of which Wayne Ulrich, the MSF logistics coordinator, had converted to an improvised shower. One of the rooms was the office and radio room, another was a kitchen, another a combined dining and meeting room; expatriates slept three or four in each of the remaining guest rooms. The finishing touches on a new stone wall surrounding the compound were just being completed. Two armed guards sat in an improvised tower overlooking the main gate, and four others slept on mattresses in the inner open-air compound. The living space was made tighter still by a few thin and bony hens that clucked around the compound day and night. Across the street the MSF warehouse was filled with medical supplies, and its inner compound housed MSF's twelve rented vehicles and some eighty armed guards and drivers at night. We were paying $120 per vehicle per day. We also had to cover the cost of black-market fuel, repairs and the salaries for guards and drivers. And the prices were going up as the security situation worsened.

Dana van Alphen, the MSF head of mission, was a thirty-something Romanian neurologist who smoked constantly. "Two packs, never more than three a day. It's the only thing that keeps me calm," she said. "In this place, hurricanes can start anywhere. Someone has to stay calm." Dana never stopped talking—sometimes balancing three conversations at once—barking orders, easing anxieties and negotiating deals. Everyone trusted her. Her word was gold. The guards and clan elders deferred to her, which made the Somali women adore her. One elder later told me, "The only reason Dana doesn't carry a gun is because she is afraid she would use it."

"So you're James. Jesus Christ," she said to me, "it's about time you got here. Where the fuck have you been? Jules has been promising you to me for weeks. The medical coordination is a mess," she said.

"Medical coordination? I'm a doctor," I said. "I have no experience with coordination."

"Didn't Jules ask you? Well, now I'm telling you. You are the med-co," Dana said. "Don't worry, I'll help. Don't look so shocked. You haven't been here long enough, and there's already enough shock to go around."

That night, Dana's main concern was a rumour that General Morgan of neighbouring Bardera would attack the forces of Gen. Mohamed Aidid, which controlled Baidoa. I went with her to the CARE office to meet Merv, a retired special operations officer with the Australian army and now the coordinator of CARE in Baidoa. He reassured us. There was no evidence of troop movements, and, he reasoned, Morgan wasn't strong enough to hold Bardera and Baidoa if Aidid counterattacked, which he certainly would do. "Nothing's happening. Relax," said Merv. "Have a whisky before you go back."

When we got back to the compound Dana told me she was worried about the team. "They're scared and they are getting confused," she said. "They're shitting in the shower and showering in the shit. People are getting sick. We need some order here." Six of the team of twenty-one had diarrhea, malaria, dengue fever or something else. In the last week, two had been flown out to Nairobi with hepatitis. I identified the source of the disease when I saw the yellow eyes of the cook. He was immediately given a leave and replaced. By the end of the day, I felt like I had lived a lifetime in another world.

Early the next morning, Joni left from the airstrip for Kenya and then on to Canada. Hurzi and his crew became my driver and protectors. Hurzi pointed out that Abdul, my sixteen-year-old guard, was limping and asked me to look at his foot. Abdul had a tropical ulcer, which I promised to treat later. We drove to an MSF clinic beside the river in the centre of town. We passed through the central market. Fat women sat like immovable rocks, calling buyers to their stalls where they sold cloth, sacks of looted food, pots and other wares. Men squatted in small groups chewing khat while drawing attention to cheap mattresses, generators, fuel or khat for sale. I heard sporadic gunfire from nearby streets. The cash-rich and mobile had long since left. Only those without other choices remained.

I got out of the Land Cruiser and walked to the river, where at least five thousand people were living among bombed-out Italian-style villas along the bank. The bushes and trees surrounding the town were bare of leaves and bark. People had eaten anything they could find, and a green-brown froth stained the lips of many who camped by the river. I stopped near an old woman. Diarrhea had dried on the back of her legs. She saw me looking and tried to cover herself with her shawl.

Others sat or lay listless in the morning sun. Swarms of flies were everywhere, feeding on the green saliva, on purulent nasal and eye mucus, on skin sores and on the fetid pools of water that people had crawled to drink from by the riverbank.

A boy of about five walked towards me, his hands held open, asking for food. I felt nausea as he approached. "He is cursed," Hurzi cautioned. "There are more like him coming from the villages." At first I thought the boy had been shot in the face. He had a gaping hole eight inches in diameter just below his right cheekbone. The jawbone was exposed, and the flesh around the opening was rotting black. Through the hole I could see his tongue moving as he tried to talk to me. He was suffering from cancrum oris, a very rare effect of prolonged starvation, where immunity is all but nil and the normal bacteria of the mouth proliferate and begin feeding on proximate flesh. I had only seen old pictures of it in tropical-medicine textbooks. This was real, and for a moment I had to turn away. Disease follows hunger and will likely kill before the body expires from starvation. Like the old woman, the boy needed medicine, and they both needed food to allow the medicine to work.

Hundreds waited outside the clinic. Inside, Katrina, a Dutch MSF nurse, organized the staff for the day's work. Diarrhea was the most immediate killer, so we set up a series of rooms where oral rehydration salts and IV fluids could be administered. Clean water was delivered to the clinics by two donkey carts each pulling a 200-litre drum. Respiratory and bowel infections and malaria were the next most aggressive killers, so Somali staff were trained to diagnose the illnesses and to dispense the right treatments. We had a bandage room for the many who came with traumatic injuries and with the boils, skin sores and ulcers that are so common with starvation. Many had abscesses from untreated gunshot wounds. I treated a line of patients, showing the staff how to open and clean an abscess, and I cleaned and dressed the tropical ulcer on Abdul's foot. More serious cases were transported to the town's only hospital, where the International Medical Committee, an NGO, had one pediatrician and a physician's assistant to treat hundreds of wounded adults and children.

I went to each of our five clinics and to several feeding centres with Hurzi and my guards. By late afternoon, the heat was intense. I returned to talk with Dana in the radio room at the MSF compound. "The only treasures in Somalia are food, fuel, and now the U.S. dollars of the NGOs and the Red Cross," she explained. "There's no government and the clans are fighting each other for the treasures." Somalia was a Sunni Islamic country divided into clans and sub-clans. It had been colonized in the north by the British in 1886 and by the Italians in the south in 1889. After World War II, it had been an Italian UN protectorate until its independence in 1960. Now, Somalia was a country no more. Instead, in the jargon of the post–Cold War world, it was a "failed nation state." It got that way after being abandoned by the UN and the international community as it began a spiral into civil war in 1988. The dictator Siad Barre had responded to Ethiopian-funded rebels in the neglected northern region of Somalia by bombing the cities of Hargeisa and Burao into rubble, killing tens of thousands. There was little protest from the international community.

Late in 1990, as the rebellion spread, UN and foreign diplomats fled to neighbouring Kenya. In January 1991, Barre's forces in Mogadishu fell to the rebels, and he fled to exile. Over the course of his twenty-one-year dictatorship, Barre had fuelled tensions between the clans in order to hold on to power. The tensions now exploded into open clan warfare. Most urban centres were destroyed, and political institutions collapsed. Massacres, looting and systematic destruction across the country caused millions to flee their homes. Over half a million of the country's nearly eight million people took boats to

Yemen or walked to Kenya and Ethiopia for refuge and survival. The Red Cross and a handful of NGOs worked with hundreds of Somali health care professionals and volunteers who remained in the country. Together, what they were able to provide was little more than a drop of water in a desert of need.

Without counting those dead from a lack of food, by March of 1992 at least 41,000 people—almost all civilians— had been killed or wounded in the fighting in Mogadishu alone. While it sent troops to the former Yugoslavia, the United Nations Security Council voted in March 1992 to send only a humanitarian coordinator and a technical team to Somalia. In the previous months, the United States had gone to extraordinary lengths to defeat efforts at the Security Council to achieve a political end to the carnage. African members of the UN publicly accused the United States of having double standards on Africa and Yugoslavia. The March resolution had been watered down to a humanitarian mission because the United States would only be expected to donate 25 percent of the costs, whereas it would be obliged to pay 30 percent of the costs of a much more expensive political mission like the UN missions then under way in Cambodia, El Salvador, Yugoslavia, the African Sahara and elsewhere.

Since the start of the civil war, the International Red Cross had worked with the Somali Red Crescent Society to deliver up to 17,000 tons of food a month by air, land and sea. That was now a fraction of what was needed. Food was not only essential to life but had become, as Dana said, a treasure of civil war. The Red Cross and the NGOs found themselves caught in a protection racket with the warring clans. The armed clansmen demanded to be "hired" to "protect" workers against rival clans.

By April 1992, the crisis had worsened further. The UN Security Council created UNOSOM—United Nations Operation in Somalia—and authorized a special representative, Ambassador Mohammed Sahnoun, to facilitate compliance with a tenuous ceasefire agreement. The UN authorized fifty unarmed ceasefire monitors and five hundred peacekeepers. From the fall of 1990 to June 1992, UN humanitarian agencies had confined their efforts to minor evaluation sorties from their Nairobi offices. Now they returned to a capital city that was little more than rubble. It was divided by a contested "green line" that separated General Aidid's forces from those of Ali Mahdi, both of the same Hawiyee clan and rivals for power. At the same time, a growing number of breakaway gangs looted on either side of the green line.

The first UN aid coordination meeting in Mogadishu took place in the last week of June. United Nations humanitarian agencies, including the World Health Organization, the World Food Programme, UNICEF, the UN High Commissioner for Refugees, the UN Development Programme, and the newly formed Department of Humanitarian Affairs, competed with each other for control of coordination. In the end, each decided to be its own coordinator. By the beginning of July, only four of the promised fifty unarmed ceasefire monitors had arrived. By the end of July, the Red Cross declared that four and a half million people were on the verge of starvation in Somalia. The Security Council authorized an emergency airlift of food, as well as more peacekeepers to secure ports and to guard supplies. By August, it had authorized a total of five thousand peacekeepers, and yet those five hundred peacekeepers promised in April only began to arrive in mid-September. Now, by October, without consulting with the NGOs, the UN had come up with a " 100-Day Plan" for the Red Cross and NGOs to deliver food across the country. "It's a plan that's going nowhere," Dana told me. "Everyone is in charge, so no one is in charge except the one with the biggest gun. We are the good little humanitarians stuck in the middle, and it doesn't look like we're going to get unstuck any time soon."

I asked her how she had been able to get as far as she had with the clinics and feeding centres.

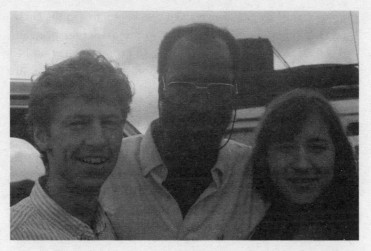

With Lesto and Dana

"You talk and you talk some more. And then you talk some more and you find a way," she said. "Right now, we're finding our way, but I'm not sure for how long or to where." Someone came into the radio room. "Ah, Lesto! Now here is a man who talks!" said Dana. Lesto was a clan elder and the vice-chairman of an alliance of clans in the Baidoa region, as well as the chief administrator for our project. Tall, dignified, impeccably dressed and a chain-smoker like Dana, he introduced himself warmly. Lesto and Dana immediately began discussing the need to hire more staff from a particular clan and to increase the guards' salaries.

As Dana and Lesto talked, I went with Hurzi and our guards to the Bay Camp, a kilometre down the road from the MSF compound. We had set up a clinic here a week before, and news had spread. About eight thousand people from outlying villages had collected in a field. From a distance, their shelters of sticks and garbage bags looked like birds' nests that had been flipped over to offer protection from the baking heat. I examined an old woman who told me through an interpreter that she was eighty-six. She had walked two kilometres to the clinic. It had taken her nearly seven hours in the 32-degree heat. She had collapsed on the side of the road, and someone had pushed her in a wheelbarrow for the last kilometre to the clinic. She had a bad fever and was short of breath from pneumonia. She had come to the clinic not for herself but to get medicine for her three-year-old grandchild, who had dysentery. She had left him at her shelter because she had heard there was an epidemic of measles at the camp. (There had been, and many children had died. In such circumstances, measles can kill up to half of infected children. Because of a lack of security, we had been unable to organize a vaccination campaign.) Each of her own three daughters and two sons, their husbands and wives and all of their children—except this three-year-old boy—had died over the preceding months. The Somali clinic staff was still new and needed more training. I showed the staff how to give the old woman an injection for her pneumonia. Hurzi and I drove the old woman back to her shelter. I treated the three-year-old boy. It made no rational sense to spend so much time away from the clinic treating one patient when there were so many. I don't know why I did, but I did.

When I returned that night to the MSF compound, Hurzi came to me with a group of eight guards, each with a medical problem. I held a small impromptu clinic in a corner of the compound. It would become a nightly ritual.

Over the next few weeks, we would organize and train staff to run eleven clinics, finish construction of the field hospital and try to give medical care at the feeding centres in and around Baidoa. I coordinated this, and with Rick Price—an excellent and much-respected British doctor, and the only other doctor on the team besides Dana and me—saw the more difficult patients in the clinics and feeding centres and trained staff for the field hospital.

The days were long for the team, and especially for Dana. She negotiated with clan elders, chiefs and a growing number of gang leaders. She talked with Lesto and others about local and national military movements, politics, salaries and security. She talked with MSF offices in Mogadishu, Nairobi and in Europe, with other MSF teams around the country and with other NGOs in Baidoa. She talked to the media by satellite phone and in person, trying to mobilize an international response. But mostly she talked about security issues, trying to keep track of which clan controlled what territory inside and outside Baidoa, and which posed a threat to us. Talking and smoking constantly, Dana had managed to achieve a delicate presence for MSF in Baidoa.

General Aidid controlled much of Mogadishu and all of Baidoa through armed clans or sub-clans loyal to him. In his territory, in his name, they were free to extort, or "protect" against looting from rival clans. Ali Mahdi had the allegiance of other clans or sub-clans in Mogadishu and around the country. In Baidoa, and around the country, clans and sub-clans constantly shifted from Mahdi to Aidid or the other way around. Freelance gangs were now coming to Baidoa, but MSF did not deal directly with food distribution, so we were not targeted in the way that the Red Cross and CARE were. Daily, they were forced to pay increasing amounts to "protect" their food aid.

Throughout the fall of 1992, there was a steady flow of media stars and personalities to Somalia. David Bowie's supermodel wife, Iman, Audrey Hepburn and Sophia Loren visited the country, bringing with them legions of journalists and with these, world attention. When Sophia Loren visited Baidoa, she went to the International Medical Committee, or IMC, hospital in the centre of the city. It was a media spectacle. An MSF logistician grabbed a photographer who was standing on the leg of a bedridden child and pushed the photographer against the wall in anger. The photographer had been trying to get the best shot of Sophia Loren holding a starving child. Others were more respectful. Mary Robinson, the president of Ireland, visited feeding centres run by the Irish aid groups GOAL and Concern. She spoke with many women and held their children. She went on to Mogadishu and to a refugee camp on the Kenyan border, and then she went to the UN headquarters in New York to press for immediate political and humanitarian action.

In Baidoa, by the end of October, we were treating a thousand people a day in the clinics and thousands more in feeding centres, but it was too dangerous to open the field hospital. The Red Cross, MSF and other NGOs continued to draw attention to the crisis in Somalia through the media, calling for full UN engagement and coordination of the relief effort. World Vision, CARE, the IMC and some other American NGOs were doing the same, while also lobbying the U.S. government to intervene militarily in the face of rising insecurity. Even without UN coordination, Red Cross, NGO and American military airlifts were getting more food into Baidoa, and delivery increased to the surrounding villages. This meant more food was being extorted or looted, but it also meant fewer new people were coming to Baidoa. Thousands had died in the city, and the population was now somewhere around eighty thousand. The death rate had dropped to twenty-five times the normal. There were fewer bodies on the street, but the school bus was still not able to collect all the dead. Security remained the main topic of conversation, but the team was drinking less at night, and the mood became less tense because, despite the difficulties, we were able to work. We held nightly medical coordination meetings, where we were even able to discuss special topics such as how to treat cancrum oris. Hurzi continued to organize my nightly clinic for the guards, some of whom now brought family members. Abdul's tropical ulcer was starting to improve with nightly dressing changes.

We were trying to help local aid committees by providing them with medical care, blankets, plastic sheeting for shelter, cooking pots and chlorine for water. One committee of elders, led by Abdulahi Hussein, had organized to assist war wounded and handicapped people who could not get to feeding centres. Another committee, led by Adan Hussein, set up an orphanage in a bombed-out library in the centre of town. Adan's committee went around to the feeding centres in the city gathering up orphaned children who had little chance of survival without adult help. I asked Adan to go to Hawina to get Ali and other orphans. Unlike us, Adan had no guards. Many committee members were shot, beaten or robbed by gangs and militias. Still, Adan's group collected as many orphans as it could. By the end of October, his group was caring for over 350 children. I asked Adan why he did what he did. After a long pause, he answered, "They are seeds for tomorrow's Somalia. Tomorrow's Somalia will be better—it must be. We want them to care for each other, so we must care for them today."

Jules—just back from the former Yugoslavia, where Bosnian Muslims were being slaughtered by President Milosevic's Serbs—came to see the situation in Baidoa for himself. He spent most of his time with Dana working on security and political issues, but he urged me to do more to support the informal local relief committees. A women's group took him to an orphanage that had been set up in an abandoned school. The group had some thirty infants, and most if not all of them would be dead in a week without medical care. The women wanted the infants moved to Adan's orphanage, where they could get at least some medical care from us. Jules was embarrassed as he cried twice while describing to me the condition that the children were in.

We were inundated with delegations of elders who came from outlying villages and towns like Hawina imploring us to bring aid. One came with a letter from the council of elders at Buurhakaba, about fifty kilometres from Baidoa on the road to Mogadishu. A French NGO, AICF, was already helping at the feeding centre, but medical care was lacking. Over the next two days,

Lesto and I checked and rechecked on safety and security in and around Buurhakaba and on the road to the city. I went with Hurzi and our guards on the hour-and-a-half drive along the shell-cratered road. Even though rival clans had agreed to let us pass, we drove at breakneck speeds of up to 150 km/h to avoid attracting gangs or thieves that could be hiding in the bush.

Thousands sat outside the feeding centre set up by the village elders in a former school. We entered the dark rooms of the centre, and as my eyes adjusted to the light, I could see that room after room was filled with mothers, fathers and children lying on the ground, too weak to stand or, in some cases, sit, with nothing between their skin and the cold cement floor. Flies swarmed over them and on them. I examined patient after patient. One man, Isaq, had arrived that morning after walking 120 kilometres over five days with his thirteen-year-old son on his back. They had been away from their house looking for food and returned to find that Isaq's wife had been raped, shot in the face and stuffed in a well with Isaq's four other children, who had been shot dead. Isaq and his son were both starving, and the boy's eyes bulged from deep in his face and stared into nowhere. His joints were covered in open sores. He was gasping for breath, and I listened to his heart pounding against his chest wall. It was too weak to stop fluid from backing up into his lungs. Three hours later Isaq's son died. He was the fifth to die since I had arrived. Hundreds of others had died that day in other feeding centres around Baidoa.

The smell and death and darkness were too much. I went out to sit in our Land Cruiser. Hurzi brought me a Coke and gave me a piece of cloth to wipe away my tears. I sat there for a long while and smoked a cigarette. Hurzi stood outside the Land Cruiser keeping the crowd away. Then he opened the door, waited a few moments and nodded to me that it was time to go back in. I nodded back and went inside. A few hours later, Isaq thanked me for trying to help his son. I asked what he would do now. He said that he would get strong again; that he would work at the feeding centre, and then he would go back to his farm with others from his village. The elders, AICF and I agreed on a medical program, and I left them some supplies until we could return.

We drove at the same breakneck speed on the way back. As we slowed to go around some potholes in the road, Hurzi slammed on the brakes and brought the Land Cruiser to a halt facing sideways on the road. "Ambush!" he screamed. I could see the nose of a pickup truck in the bushes a hundred metres ahead. Hurzi told me to lie under the Land Cruiser. Two guards went to the back of our vehicle and pulled out two rocket-propelled grenade launchers, or RPGs, that they had wrapped in blankets. Hurzi ordered three of the guards behind the bushes on either side of the road and one onto the roof of the Land Cruiser to cock and load the machine gun. No one talked. One of my guards winked at me as reassurance. My hands were shaking, and I thought I was going to urinate in my pants. "Don't worry," Hurzi said to me. "We have RPGs. I will die before you will die. And I will not die." He took long, confident strides up the road towards the pickup truck with his machine gun by his side. I could hear yelling and then silence. Hurzi

The Chief
OF Graves
Wants Book
to Write it
down People
those are
dieing !!?

Note from the graveyard keeper to me

returned and ordered us all back into the Land Cruiser. We drove on, the guards laughing. I asked Hurzi what he had said. "I told these animals they will die because I will not die," he said. I was puzzled for a moment and then understood.

That night, I felt a pain in my chest. At first I thought I had strained a muscle while moving a water pump at Buurhakaba earlier that day. But I had a fever. I asked Dana to examine me. "Don't tell me you've been showering in the shit too," she said. I had pneumonia. I can't remember what happened next. Dana told me later that I became short of breath and delirious with the fever. An American C-130 Hercules had taken some rifle fire earlier that day, and the American air force refused to fly in to Baidoa regardless of the circumstances. By satellite phone Merv called a friend who ran an air transport business in Nairobi. He agreed to fly in if Merv could get the clan militias to agree not to shoot at the plane. He did, and he and Dana arranged for CARE and MSF vehicles to provide light for the runway. I was flown to Nairobi and taken to the Aga Khan University Hospital.

After three days I was discharged, but the next day I was back in the Nairobi hospital for another three days with viral meningitis. I rested at the Nairobi MSF compound with Arjan Hehenkamp, the twenty-four-year-old administrator. After a few days, I was much lighter, but was feeling stronger. Jules had come again to advise on the Baidoa project. He told me that a ticket to Canada had been arranged for the end of the week. I couldn't sleep that night. There were three doctors in the entire Baidoa region, and thousands of people still dying. It was difficult but we were still able to work. I got up and went into the bathroom. I looked at my face in the mirror. Knowing what I knew, I had to try. I could not live with who I would be if I did not go back. The next day Jules and I agreed that I would fly to Baidoa.

I returned on November 7, 1992, with Hans Everts, who was to be the temporary head of mission while Dana was away on a much-needed break. The UN's Ambassador Sahnoun had resigned a few days before. For months he had painstakingly gained the respect of the various clans and had brokered several agreements that were holding. Perhaps he was forced to resign after he publicly criticized the UN agencies for breaking these agreements and for their lack of coordination. The UN in New York had ordered the immediate deployment of 2,500 peacekeepers, an announcement Sahnoun heard about over the BBC. There were rumours that the UN was mobilizing for something more than the already approved 5,000 peacekeepers. Within days of Sahnoun's departure, things got worse. Ships carrying food aid were shelled to prevent them from docking in ports controlled by rival clans; looting increased; clan and sub-clan alliances were splitting and reforming under different configurations.

On November 14, outside the MSF compound, the militia of a breakaway clan from Mogadishu tried to kidnap our British doctor, Rick Price. They fired into the ground by his feet and put a machine gun to his head. Our guards managed to get him inside. It was the first time a kidnapping had been attempted in Baidoa. That same day, CARE was looted, and an expatriate at Irish Concern and another from IMC were shot at by new gangs in the city. Hans and I spoke with Lesto. We knew that if the council of elders and chiefs couldn't deal with the escalating violence, we couldn't either.

The next day, we evacuated eighteen expatriates from our team, leaving me, Hans, Wayne Ulrich and our administrator, Dirk Matthysen, to oversee the program until the elders and chiefs could come up with an agreement for better security. Even with the increase in violence, not one of our 120 Somali staff stopped working. I tried to reassure them that we wanted to continue to work, but that we needed improved security to do so. Virtually all agreed with the decision to reduce the expatriate team until things got better. For the next few days, Dirk

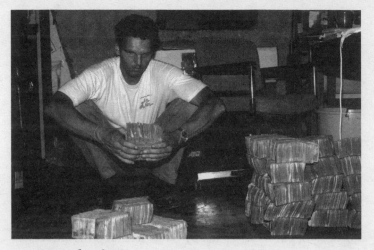

Money for salaries

paid salaries to the Somali staff from the office and organized another MSF water donkey for the clinics, Hans met with clan elders in the compound, Wayne ensured a steady stream of supplies from our warehouse to the clinics and hospital, and I supervised the clinics and some of the feeding centres. Lesto insisted on going with me everywhere.

A staff member at one of the clinics had been stealing large stocks of medicines and selling them on the black market. He had to be fired. When Lesto and I arrived, chiefs and elders from the villages that the clinic served were gathered outside the walled compound. Lesto spoke with them and then walked into the clinic with me. He went up to the man who was stealing medicines and spoke with him. The man answered Lesto with a dismissive gesture. Lesto grabbed his hair and pounded his face into the table where he was sitting. He pulled the man to the floor and kicked and beat him around the head and abdomen. The three clinic guards ran with me to restrain Lesto, who had taken a pistol out from under his shirt and was using it to beat the man, who lay curled in a fetal position covered in blood.

Lesto was covered in his own sweat and the man's blood, and his pistol shook as he forced it into the man's face. "We are not animals! We are not fucking animals!" Lesto screamed repeatedly in Somali, Italian and English, now pushing the nose of the gun into the back of the man's head. We were struggling to hold Lesto back, and then he stopped. The man crawled to the corner of the room. Lesto sat on the floor, spent, his Italian linen shirt torn. Sweating, he stared silently at the blood on the white compound wall.

"It's only pills. Why?" I asked. "Why this?"

The elders outside had told Lesto that the man had been raping women who came to the clinic. Standing up and adjusting his torn shirt, Lesto flicked his wrist towards the guards. "Give him to the chiefs," he commanded.

The next morning our safe was stolen from the MSF office. It was an inside job. Hans resigned, feeling himself too unfamiliar with the dynamics of the situation to be able to make confident decisions. Dirk, who had worked in Somalia for years, quit too. Willem, one of our best nurses, had been evacuated a few days before. He quit when he heard news of the safe being robbed. Jules and Dana returned from Nairobi that day, and the guards responsible for stealing the safe were fired. For the next week, Jules and Dana talked and talked some more with the elders, clan chiefs and other NGOs.

That week, I went to the Red Cross office to see about getting more food to some of the feeding centres. As Hurzi drove us down the alley, two Technicals came up tightly behind us, making it impossible to go anywhere but forward. At least sixty heavily armed men and several Technicals surrounded the Red Cross compound. They thought I was an International Red Cross delegate and ordered me to go inside the compound. I told them I was with MSF, but even though I had an MSF T-shirt on, they wanted confirmation from their leader inside. There was no way out but in. Hurzi agreed that I would talk, and that unless provoked he would stay in our vehicle with our guards until I came out.

Inside, I asked to speak to the Red Cross delegate in charge of food movements in town. "The fucking bitch is busy," a leader said. "That cunt-bitch will not see you now. Go. Go back to your MSF."

The Red Cross delegate sat surrounded by khat-chewing young men with sunglasses and AK-47s. "We are having a small discussion with our security men who can't seem to agree among themselves who is in charge," she said in French.

"No fucking French, fucking cunt-bitch!" the same leader screamed as he pounded the butt of his machine gun into the table.

"I think you had better leave us to it, while you still can," the delegate told me in English.

When I saw her again later that night, she told me that the dispute had been settled within an hour with a small increase in "salary."

That night I had tea with Hurzi. I wasn't sure if I could stay any longer. He told me that he would understand if I left, but that he did not want me to go. He swore by Allah that if I stayed he would die before I did. At ten o'clock that night I told Jules that I quit. Jules sat me down and explained in detail the measures he had taken to identify who had stolen the safe, and that the elders promised the fired men would not return. He convinced me too that our risk was not the same as that faced by the Red Cross or others handling food directly, and that if the local elders lost control, then we would go. I trusted Jules and I trusted Dana. And if Hurzi was going to go on, so was I. At 1:30 a.m., I unquit.

The following morning the chair of the council of clan chiefs and elders from Baidoa returned from Mogadishu. He had secured an agreement from Aidid to contain his faction of forces, which had been largely responsible for the increased violence in the city over the past weeks. The next couple of days were calm. The evacuated expat members of the team returned, and Jules went back to the former Yugoslavia and then on to Amsterdam.

Two days later I went back to Buurhakaba with more medical supplies and Katherine, an MSF nurse from Australia. We spent the day at the feeding centre. There were even more starving people, and, as in Baidoa, more gunshot injuries. Katherine selected people and started training them in how to give medical care. As we were leaving, several Technicals drove up to the feeding centre and demanded "taxes" for MSF to work there. As I talked with the armed men, a crowd gathered. We had agreed that MSF was not yet working there when shots rang out in the crowd. Hurzi immediately pushed Katherine into the Land Cruiser. A woman had been shot in the back. We lifted her into our vehicle and started an IV on her as we drove back through the crowd to the road to Baidoa. That day in Baidoa, shots had been fired at two MSF nurses, and two more nurses had briefly been held at gunpoint. CARE had been looted again, as had the Red Cross.

The UN's 100-Day Plan had all but broken down. Incredibly, the first of the five hundred peacekeepers in Mogadishu were seeking protection from armed clansmen. Ali Mahdi and Aidid intensified their fight for control of the city. Both Aidid and Mahdi were, as one elder told me, "choosing to create accidents and to make life more difficult for the NGOs." Each wanted to secure as much territory and as much food as possible before any new UN force arrived. On November 24, a UN World Food Program ship carrying 10,000 tons of food was struck by a shell off the coast of Mogadishu, and both Aidid and Mahdi attacked the UN peacekeeping troops already deployed in the city. Andrew Ignatios of USAID announced publicly that 80 percent of food was being diverted, stolen or looted. "That's bullshit," said Dana. "It's as high as 70 percent in some places, but it's probably closer to 20 or 30 percent overall. They are up to something with their big numbers."

The UN had begun talking about a massive military intervention as the only means of protecting the delivery of aid in Somalia. On November 25, 1992, George H. W. Bush declared that the United States was ready to deploy troops to Somalia to stop the diversion of aid. Overnight, fighting intensified in Mogadishu. Heavy artillery and Technicals were moved out of the city into the Baidoa region so they wouldn't be destroyed or seized by the Americans. Immediately clan fighting escalated in Baidoa and throughout the country. Dana had to leave for a family emergency. She was replaced by Wouter Van Empelen as coordinator. It was his first mission.

The elders and chiefs were urging us and other NGOs to continue our programs. Without them, thousands would die of starvation and disease. We reduced our teams, reasoning that fewer expatriates meant fewer risks, while the elders and chiefs sought a short-term political settlement until the Americans arrived. On November 29, the Americans announced that troops might be sent into Baidoa. Ali Mahdi in Mogadishu declared, "We will fight the Christian invaders." By late afternoon, his rival Aidid countered, "We will welcome the Americans."

That night I spoke with Jules in Amsterdam about the American plans to intervene. Given what I now knew about superpower politics in Somalia, I couldn't understand the American motivation. Was it oil? I asked Jules. "Nothing so basic," he laughed. "The American NGO lobbying effort has obviously had some effect but the Americans are the only superpower now, they don't have to worry about anything so trivial. Yugoslavia is not going well for them or the Europeans. It seems they have essentially decided to let the Serbs win. But the slaughter of Bosnian Muslims is continuing and public opinion is turning against the West." George Bush had just lost the presidential election to Bill Clinton, and neither wanted to get involved militarily in the former Yugoslavia. Western powers conveniently argued that they could not take military action because it would endanger the UN peacekeepers who were on the ground there. Jules explained that Colin Powell, the chair of the U.S. Joint Chiefs of Staff, was keen for a military intervention in Muslim Somalia as long as it meant that U.S. forces would not be engaged in Bosnia. "Sending troops to Somalia would take the sting out of the accusation that the West was indifferent to the plight of Muslims," said Jules.

"It's a whole other world out there," I said.

"Yes," said Jules, "And like it or not, Somalia and you are in it."

The following morning, as we prepared to reduce the team, clan militias loyal to either Aidid or Mahdi openly fought for political control of Baidoa. The Red Cross, CARE and World Vision were all looted. A two-hour gunfight broke out outside the CARE office, and one of our logisticians was pinned down in the crossfire. In the market, six bystanders and numerous gunmen were killed as rival militias clashed. Food trucks were looted as they approached feeding centres. Technicals drove through the walls of feeding centres to get at food stores. At one feeding centre, people were trapped under the wheels of a military vehicle as it drove through the compound wall. The men on top—clad in Mickey Mouse T-shirts and Vuarnet sunglasses and wearing Sony Walkmans—did not even turn their heads as women and children screamed beneath their tires. That afternoon we evacuated most of our team of twenty.

On December 3, the UN Security Council approved the U.S.-led United International Task Force for the purposes of humanitarian relief. The humanitarian intervention was to be not a UN mission but a U.S.-led mission sanctioned by the UN. Its relationship to the already established UNOSOM was never made clear. The Americans called it Operation Restore Hope. Again, clan fighting and looting escalated.

By December 5, only Wouter Van Empelen, our new project administrator, Arjan Hehenkamp, and I remained in Baidoa for MSF. All other NGOs in Baidoa had reduced their staffs to similar skeleton teams. Adan Hussein, leaders from women's groups and others came to the compound to check on our safety and to urge us to stay if we could. The chiefs and elders tried to reassure us, warning us of coming battles in the city and telling us where we should or should not go. Lesto in his own vehicle with its own guards, as well as an extra vehicle of guards, accompanied me with Hurzi and his crew from clinic to clinic, from feeding centre to feeding centre, as we supported our national staff, saw patients and delivered supplies. Our clinics were still caring for a thousand patients a day. We could get to only three or four clinics and the same number of feeding centres each day. It was enough to keep them supplied and to reassure our staff that we were still in Baidoa. Not one staff member quit.

Arjan kept paying salaries. He sent medical supplies to Buurhakaba, Hawina and some other villages with elders and

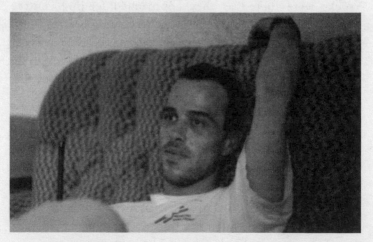

Arjan Hehenkamp

others brave enough to travel. Some supplies were looted, and some got through. Wouter—as Dana had done before—talked to MSF in Mogadishu and in Europe, other NGOs and the press, and kept an obsessive focus on politics and military movements. By now the winter rains had started, so Hurzi organized my regular evening clinic in one of the empty expatriate bedrooms. Abdul's tropical ulcer was worse, but he had quit smoking, so I gave him the wristwatch I had promised him if he did so. I was smoking more.

One morning, militias fought outside the stone wall of our compound. We took cover behind a heavy cement wall. After about ten minutes, the shooting stopped. Five men and a woman who had been shot were carried into the compound where I could care for them. A few minutes later, a single gunshot rang out, and a woman screamed outside the compound wall. She came running in, carrying a four-year-old girl who was bleeding from her chest. I lay the girl on a white plastic picnic table inside our compound. Her oversized dress slipped easily from her shoulder to her waist. She had a bullet hole in the upper right of her chest wall and needed a chest tube urgently, but I had none and could find nothing with which to improvise. Lesto and Hurzi drove me, the girl and the other wounded to the IMC team at the hospital. They were not there, but were trapped in their compound across the street by a gang threatening to loot. I found a chest tube and started to cut into the girl's chest while a Somali nurse held the gasping child. I could hear screaming outside. Two armed gunmen wearing sunglasses came into the hospital room carrying a wounded man. "Fix him!" they screamed at me. The nurse stepped back from the table and pressed her back against the wall. I watched a bloodstained piece of gauze fall from her hand to the floor. I began to sweat. "All these guns make me nervous," I told the gunmen. I put the tube into the girl and it made a popping sound as the pressure building inside her chest was relieved. The girl screamed, and I could feel the salt of sweat in my eyes. "Fix him now!" the gunman screamed at me again. Lesto calmed them down. The nurse attended to the girl as I put some sutures in the man's wound. The IMC team arrived, and we returned to the MSF compound.

Two remaining members of an MSF team in nearby Kandesere were being held hostage. Another MSF team in Kismayo had been evacuated completely. CARE had been looted again, as had two of our clinics. More people had been killed in the market and at new roadblocks set up throughout Baidoa. The NGOs all met at the Red Cross. We had been warned by clan elders to move out as many expatriates, especially women, as possible. We agreed to try to keep food coming in and our programs running for the 80,000 people still in Baidoa and, if possible, for the 300,000 people in surrounding villages. The Americans agreed that if they were asked they would airlift remaining NGO staff out by helicopter. Late that afternoon, the two MSF team members from Kandesere were released. They left on the last C-130 that delivered food to Baidoa that day.

I continued to go with Lesto and Hurzi in our convoy of vehicles and guards to our clinics. There were many orphaned children sleeping outside the clinics, and Lesto paid adults to take them to Adan's orphanage or to feed them whatever food could be bought on the black market. There were also many people with gunshot injuries. I examined one boy who had been shot through the hip. His mother had come from her village to Baidoa a month before with six children. Now, except for this twelve-year-old son, all were dead. I opened a massive abscess that had formed in his groin around the wound. Because we were so short of staff, Lesto was helping, but he had never done anything like this before. He was fumbling with gauze and getting blood on his clothes. Suddenly, he just stopped and walked out of the clinic.

I finished packing and dressing the wound and went outside. I found Lesto sitting in the Land Cruiser, smoking. His eyes were bloodshot and swollen. "I can't do this any more, James. I can't stand to see people suffering like this any more. It is too much. It is too much." We went to his house so that he could change his bloodied clothes. He took off his shirt and sat on his bed. "I must go to Mogadishu now," he said. "I must see my imam. I need Allah's protection in this madness."

"Take this for now," I said, and I gave him the St. Christopher medal that my friend Ian Small had given me in September in Amsterdam. Lesto cried again and put it in his wallet. He left immediately. He returned the next afternoon with a leather amulet around his neck. Pointing to the ground, he said, "I tell you before Allah, James, I am strong. This is my fuckin' land."

For the next week, amidst rumours that the Americans were coming, Aidid and Mahdi militias clashed in Mogadishu and Baidoa, and factions within each group began to fight with each other. The food stocks of the Red Cross and CARE continued to be the main targets of looting, but other NGOs and UNICEF were being hit too. In Baidoa, between ten and fifty militiamen were killed in gun battles every day, and many more civilians died or were wounded in the crossfire. We brought two Land Cruisers with .50-calibre machine guns welded to their roofs inside our compound at night for added protection. I hid a suitcase of medical supplies and a high-frequency radio on the roof behind the chimney. In addition to fifteen of our armed guards, Lesto stayed with us inside the compound. Wouter, Arjan and I slept in the room with the thickest cement walls. The other seventy guards protected the warehouse across the street.

On the morning of December 8, I went to the Baidoa airstrip to meet a C-130 coming in with medical supplies for our clinics. Shooting started not far from the runway, and the plane didn't even stop after it had touched down. The techy threw the boxes from the rear of the plane before it took off again. I collected the supplies and went back to the MSF compound.

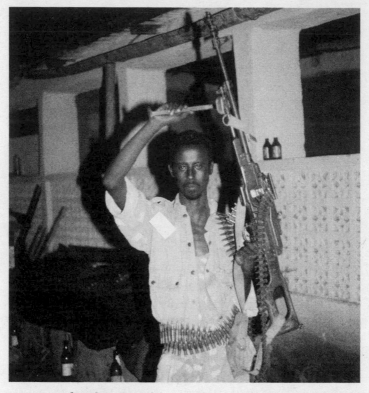

One of our house guards

As soon as I arrived, a clan chief who lived across the street was brought to me. Chief Hussein Mohamed Derir was feverish and delirious with pneumonia. I put him in one of our empty rooms and treated him with the newly arrived IV antibiotics. I was worried that he might die, and I feared the repercussions this might have for us. Together with his five armed guards, I slept in the room with him. I woke in the morning to find the chief and his guards gone. An hour later, Chief Derir walked into the compound with about twenty heavily armed clansmen. He dropped to his knees. He kissed my feet a hundred times. I tried to stop him, but he insisted.

"I swear before Allah all my clan will sleep in your bed to protect you!" he said.

I spent the day at the clinics with Lesto and Hurzi, avoiding parts of the city the elders had warned us to avoid. In the late afternoon, U.S. fighter jets flew over Baidoa as our guards and people in the neighbourhoods cheered. That night, Chief Derir and his clansmen stayed with our guards in the compound fighting off looters.

In the two weeks since George Bush Sr. had announced he was going to send troops to Somalia, the country had seen some of its most intense fighting and looting. That same night, December 9, more than 250 kilometres away, news of which was leaked a few hours in advance and timed for prime-time coverage in the United States, the Americans landed on the beaches of Mogadishu. Thousands of cheering Somalis waved green branches welcoming the U.S. Marines, Army Rangers, SEALs and Delta Force soldiers as dozens of helicopters and fighter jets flew overhead and hovercrafts delivered more of the U.S. intervention force that within weeks would number 37,000 troops. The American soldiers were met by a force of about six hundred cameramen and international journalists waiting to capture their arrival. News crews caught on tape a group of American marines arresting two armed Somali guards asleep in a warehouse of food. Bernard Kouchner, now the French minister for humanitarian affairs, was photographed on the morning of December 10 carrying a sack of grain on his shoulder through the American-held sand to Mogadishu. It was a media success. Operation Restore Hope had begun.

The following morning, I was at the river clinic in the centre of town with Lesto and Hurzi when Wouter called me on the walkie-talkie. He told me to return to the MSF compound, as casualties from artillery fire had been brought in. Fighting in Baidoa had escalated as hundreds of Technicals moved through the city, escaping from Mogadishu and on their way to Ethiopia. Fighting and looting erupted around us as Aidid announced over the radio from Mogadishu that Mahdi would control Baidoa. Aidid's governor in Baidoa refused to leave his compound a few hundred metres down the road from ours. Aidid had sent his undersecretary with heavy artillery to expel him. Our convoy arrived back at the compound to find it surrounded by our guards and all of our vehicles. All the Somali women staff were crying and praying inside. I treated five men, all with severe injuries, one with half his face blown off. Wouter and Arjan were shocked. They had never seen open wounds before.

In Kismayo, about three hundred kilometres from us, Somali staff working for MSF had been killed by looters. The militia of the warlord Colonel Omar Jesse, an ally of Aidid's, massacred between one and two hundred people thought to be loyal to General Morgan, the son-in-law of Siad Barre. The expatriate MSF team as well as all other NGOs had managed to evacuate to Mogadishu. All roads out of Baidoa were now too unsafe to travel. Chief Derir arrived from across the street with an anti-aircraft gun welded to the flatbed of a twelve-wheel truck. He parked it outside our gate and came in for tea. "You will never die, I swear before Allah," he said. He had also brought several sick members of his clan for treatment. That night, there was very heavy fighting outside our compound. Chief Derir's clan, with Hurzi in charge of our guards, fought off looters and rival militias with heavy machine guns, RPGs and anti-aircraft gunfire. Hurzi came to our room to reassure us every fifteen minutes. Wouter, Arjan and I sat on the floor eating cinnamon rolls that our cook Mohamed had made for us to help us "feel at home."

World Vision, IMC and CARE were in direct contact with the marines. They each gave information about when the Americans would arrive in Baidoa that conflicted with what Jules was hearing from American officials in Amsterdam and from MSF staff in

Mogadishu. We had not called for a military intervention, but many other NGOs had, and they now offered strategic information to facilitate the arrival of the American forces. Each changing rumour and BBC report brought a fresh outbreak of clan fighting. I kept working at the clinics with our Somali staff and at as many feeding centres as we could safely get to in our convoy. Hurzi continued to organize the evening compound clinic, where I was now seeing upwards of thirty guards and their family members each night. Looting continued, and Mohamed served gin and Cokes with our evening cinnamon rolls.

Tensions were high throughout the city. Some of our guards were angry that others had been fired after our safe was robbed. They knew that Lesto had been involved in deciding who would be fired. One night I was asleep in my room when I heard a commotion in the inner compound. Hurzi came to get me. I walked out to see Lesto seated in a white plastic chair. A guard was holding a machine gun to his head, and a group of other guards were screaming at him. The guards thought Lesto had charged MSF $260 each for some new mattresses Wouter had asked him to buy for the guards. They had confused the currency. Lesto had billed 260,000 Somali shillings—or $60—for all of the new mattresses. I explained the misunderstanding and said we would buy two mattresses for each guard's comfort. Lesto was released.

On December 11, I made the following diary entry at 11:30 p.m.: "860 patients seen by staff today in the clinics, thousands treated in feeding centres. Numbers down today because a woman was raped in Clinic Number 2 this afternoon. Also had to close Clinic Number 1 this morning because of clan shooting outside: reopened this afternoon. Staff working hard: all tired and scared about violence as gangs flee the Americans in Mogadishu. Still hundreds dying every day in and around Baidoa from starvation. American fighter jets now flying overhead almost hourly during the day. Not making much difference. The Red Cross was looted last night, and CARE International attacked—6 guards killed, as a Technical drove through a wall. CARE now digging foxholes around their compound. Irish GOAL vehicle shot up and looted in market. An Armoured Personnel Carrier drove into a crowd today as gangs clashed. Six militia killed, 50 bystanders shot dead. Another shoot-out outside our house this afternoon. Staff tell us to expect looting of our house tonight. Talked to media tonight in Amsterdam and Toronto by sat-phone. BBC Radio announces marines having problems in Mogadishu as they attempt to disarm clans. US embassy car looted. NGOs are now calling it 'Moga-Disney.' BBC says marines will not be in Baidoa for at least another five days. Immediate shooting outside our compound following BBC report."

The next day MSF publicly condemned the way the United States had handled its troop deployments. The situation outside Mogadishu had been made worse by the announcement that troops were coming though they had not yet arrived. That night we invited the elders and clan chiefs to our compound for a meeting with the NGOs to try to deal with the violence. There was heavy machine-gun fire outside as we met. After a long discussion, the elders and chiefs declared, "It is our duty to protect you," and decided to create a police force while we waited for the Americans to come. Some NGOs were skeptical, but in the absence of any alternatives, we all agreed to give it a try. Over the next few days, there were fewer Technicals coming in from Mogadishu, while the near hourly flights of American fighter jets continued. "What are they going to do? Bomb us?" said Lesto. "How many innocents will they kill? They are not so stupid, but they *are* useless to stop what is happening on the ground!" The police force reclaimed a stolen Red Cross vehicle: "a small stone of victory for the new house we are building," an elder said to me. The chair of the elders committee went to the CARE compound to talk down a heavily armed gunman described as "Rambo" who was shooting at people from the compound roof.

Still, major looting and fighting continued, especially at night as we ate our cinnamon rolls and drank our gin and Cokes behind our heavily guarded cement wall. I continued to travel with my convoy by day, but Lesto no longer came with Hurzi and me. Patients were still sitting in the hundreds at feeding centres, and dozens still lined up at the clinics. Many were starving to death. At one clinic, Laughi, one of our staff, asked me to see an old woman who lay in the corner of the examining room. Her daughter was adjusting the blanket that Laughi had given her to cover her mother. I listened to the last beat of the old woman's heart. Her eyes wide open, she gave several rapid gasps that sounded through my stethoscope like the flutter of a bird's wings. Her daughter covered her mother's face with the blanket and walked outside.

On the way back from the Bay Camp clinic, Hurzi stopped to give a soccer ball to some children playing with a dead bird at the graveyard where the school bus was still bringing its collected bodies. Tens of thousands were now buried there in shallow graves. The children laughed and I sweated in the hot sun. "Salaam Aleikum," Arjan said to them from the MSF compound as they played with my walkie-talkie. Adan Hussein from the orphanage stopped by during my nightly clinic with some sweets for us to make sure that "despite all the troubles in Baidoa," we would feel welcomed. An elder told me that marines had been spotted at an abandoned airstrip outside Buurhakaba. That night Voice of America reported a "military success in seizing control of an airstrip near Baidoa." American planes dropped millions of paper leaflets that descended like clouds of locusts from the sky. The leaflets had a cartoon of an American soldier shaking the hand of a Somali man. Inscribed in Somali were the words "We come in Peace." An elder told me the inscription was spelled wrong. Journalists were everywhere,

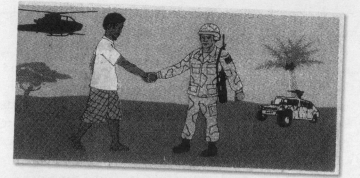

One of the millions of leaflets dropped by US forces
before they arrived in Baidoa

and with their arrival, the price of fuel and security skyrocketed.
Some of the media were staying at our compound, as it was
considered the safest in the city. I treated their fevers and illnesses as arguments broke out among them over who would file
first from our radio room.

An American envoy arrived in Baidoa on December 15 and
told us that the troops would be there soon. The elders were
told that the marines would disarm the clans and seize
Technicals. Chief Derir didn't want to lose his anti-aircraft truck
because he thought he might need it again when the Americans
left. He wanted to move it back into his walled compound, but
was worried that we would think he was breaking his promise
to protect us. We agreed that he would protect us with bazookas
and RPGs from the surrounding rooftops until the Americans
arrived. Arjan, Wouter and I were exhausted, and I wasn't sure
how much longer I could keep going.

On December 16, I woke at five in the morning because my bed
was shaking. My mosquito net was flapping above me like a curtain caught in a wild wind. Outside my room, a dust storm
whirled around the inner compound, and a black Cobra gunship

helicopter with no lights hovered overhead. I could only see its silhouette against the last of the night stars. I put on some pants and went outside. Children were smiling and dancing. Adults were clapping and hugging each other. Hundreds lined the streets as at least twenty F-14 fighter jets flew low over the city, weaving in and out in figure-eights. Below them Cobras and other helicopters flew in zigzag patterns and hovered over the Red Cross and NGO compounds. My body shook with the force of the rotors, and I could not hear people cheering though I could see that they were. Then, from down the road where Aidid's governor used to live, scores of American tanks, troop carriers, APCs and Humvees streamed into the city. Marines in Oakley sunglasses and tightly strapped helmets, body armour, flak jackets and with war-painted faces manoeuvred forward from building to building as people cheered. Some of the marines smiled and waved from their vehicles. It all felt like theatre. The last American vehicles to pass us were flanked by a few French Foreign Legion jeeps with machine guns mounted on their tops. The French soldiers wore light uniforms, bandanas, neckerchiefs and Vuarnet sunglasses. None of these soldiers smiled, and some had torn the sleeves off their uniforms. I turned to Lesto and said, "They're finally here. How do you think they'll do?"

"The Americans?" he replied. "We'll see. They don't like body bags. But the French Foreign Legion? Nobody fucks with the French Foreign Legion."

The Americans held a meeting with the NGOs at the IMC compound that morning. It was a media circus, with ABC, CNN, NBC and other American and European news carriers and print journalists all gathered. One aid worker observed to me that there was one journalist for every marine in Baidoa. His numbers were a little off, but not by much. Col. Werner Hellmer of the marines was in charge of the meeting. He was a short, solid man in his mid-forties with a firm jaw, rolled-up sleeves and huge biceps. He informed us that for now our guards would be allowed to carry guns but only inside our vehicles. Technicals, rooftop weapons, RPGs and other weapons were forbidden and would be seen as "hostiles." Whether this meant the Americans would confiscate weapons was not clear. Hellmer told us that his forces would secure Baidoa and then hand over to Australian troops who were part of a twenty-eight-country UN coalition of peacekeepers in Somalia. Once the aid was secure, the Americans planned to get out. "By mid-January at the latest," he said.

Hellmer asked us about our major security concerns. Some described certain areas of the city that were particularly danger-ous, and Wouter told him about the gangs on the road to Buurhakaba. Colonel Hellmer shuffled on his feet a moment before answering Wouter: "Well, don't you worry. We'll be taking the aid workers out there, and if any of them bad boys come out of the bushes, they'd better be ready for one hell of a significant emotional experience." After the meeting, the Americans in one of their trucks were filmed bringing food to an orphanage. They were accompanied by about a hundred heavily armed marines in a convoy of military vehicles.

At another meeting later that day, Hellmer laughed at what a "hassle" the media were and apologized when one of the orphanage staff pointed out that the marines had forgotten to unload the food once the media had got their shots. During that meeting, machine-gun fire broke out outside our ware-house. Arjan radioed Wouter, who then informed Hellmer. Within five minutes there was a Cobra helicopter overhead and three heavily armed American Humvees at our compound. The elders, our guards and neighbours were impressed. I went to all of our clinics with Hurzi. The gangs and Technicals had disap-peared into the desert and outlying villages. No one carried a gun openly. The staff and patients were jubilant. Laughi said, "Now we have a chance to build a new Somalia."

The next day I went to the temporary hospital we had built, which, though empty of patients and stocked with supplies, had

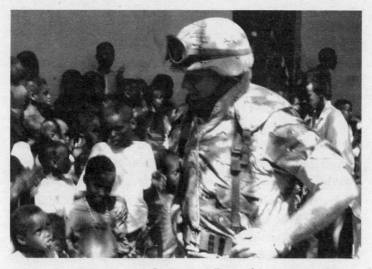

Col. Werner Hellmer of the U.S. Marines

never been looted. Not a single blanket or pill was missing. Our guards had done well. There was some sporadic machine-gun fire in the city, but the Americans were quick to show an intimidating response. They never fired a shot. Almost hourly, C-130s flew into the now heavily secured Baidoa airport delivering food and military hardware.

That night, while Cobras hovered over our compound, Hurzi and I cut the evening clinic short as our guards danced with Chief Derir's clan. Wouter, Arjan and I got very drunk. The next morning before breakfast a delegation of elders arrived from Buurhakaba with gifts to thank us for the supplies we had managed to get through to them over the past weeks. They wanted us to return as soon as possible, as there were still "many starving people." Outside our compound gate, two smiling five- or six-year-old girls had set up a stall selling single cigarettes, tea, candies, boiled eggs and red plastic cups from feeding centres. That morning many of our staff went to the airport on their own to greet our returning expatriate team. By the time our vehicles got to the airport, they were full of the clinic staff we had picked up along the way. Within hours all our clinics and feeding centres were operational. We opened the temporary hospital the next morning.

I attended a meeting that afternoon with the NGOs, several UN officials, Colonel Hellmer and Donald Teitelbaum, a cultural liaison officer from the State Department who was rumoured to also be with the CIA. Teitelbaum said that the United States wanted a system of proportional representation for the clans on a Baidoa political committee. A UNICEF representative who had worked in Somalia for many years said that the plan did not account for the clan structure and complex alliances that had existed across various regions of the country for centuries. The Americans seemed confused by the comment, and John Marks, an official with the UN's Somalia desk, UNOSOM, suggested that the discussion be reconvened later at the UNOSOM office. The meeting ended with the various officials agreeing that the situation was complicated and would require careful consideration. The clan elders and chiefs had not been invited to the meeting.

I left to go to the Bakiin Hotel on the outskirts of town where the legion of journalists covering the American deployment were staying. I checked in on an Italian journalist who had a bad case of malaria that I had treated the day before. The technicians from the NBC crew were packing up their satellite equipment to go to Kismayo, the next deployment site. Only the sick Italian remained. In Baidoa, the media circus was over.

Later that afternoon Lesto and the chiefs and elders had three camels and several goats killed and cooked to celebrate the "new peace." John Marks, the chair of the Somali National Association, Wouter and the heads of other NGOs all made speeches before the hundreds who had gathered to eat rice and meat. I was given fresh camel milk and the first piece of the best goat liver. It must have been a very old goat, but I ate it anyway. The milk was better. Meanwhile, across the street

American marines came for Chief Derir's anti-aircraft truck. It was taken without incident.

That night the chiefs and elders organized what they called their Liberty Party in the block surrounding our compound. It was a fantastic night. Hundreds of people were there for singing and traditional Somali warrior dancing, dramatic skits performed by women and children and, of course, more speeches. Poetry and song are honoured traditions in Somalia's oral culture, and singers and poets are revered as wise intellectuals and have a near rock-star status. The best poets came and to a rapt crowd recited old and new poems about the horrors of Siad Barre, about battles of the past three years, about MSF in Baidoa, about looters, about dignity and about courage, and they praised Allah and the "New Peace."

I left the next morning by C-130 for a hotel in Mombasa. I slept solidly for three days, ordering room service and leaving my room only twice, to get newspapers and cigarettes. The Americans and other troops were now in eight major centres across the country, and so intimidating were their forces that the Americans had opened fire only twice. Six other Technicals that militias had hidden in Baidoa had been seized. Red Cross and UNICEF workers were now urging the Americans to spread into the countryside where more Technicals had been moved by the warlords. UNICEF's Sean Devereux urged the troops to fan out from Kismayo, which the warlord Colonel Jess with his five thousand men had once controlled. Jess's militia was now in the countryside, looting and pillaging in the villages.

I returned to Baidoa on Christmas Eve and was in charge as Wouter and Arjan left for a week. The work continued, with a day off for Christmas as marines patrolled the city and Cobras hovered overhead. On New Year's Day, George Bush Sr. flew into Baidoa. I was among the aid workers who met him amidst heavy security at a school in the centre of town. He asked me if the situation was safer since the marines had arrived. I answered yes, and asked him why he had not brought his wife, Barbara. She wanted to stay at the White House, he said. "To pack?" I asked. He looked at me for a moment and then laughed. At a press conference later, Bush said, "I don't think there will be any leaving of the Somali people to suffer the fate they have been suffering. We will do our mission and there will be follow-up missions of peacekeeping. We are the peacemakers now. Hope Restores." The day after Bush left Baidoa, I attended a memorial service at the Irish Concern compound for UNICEF's Sean Devereux. He had been shot dead that morning outside his office in Kismayo by some of his own guards who were allegedly loyal to Colonel Jess's militia.

In September 1992, the mortality rate in Baidoa had been 1,700 a week. By the beginning of January 1993, it was down to fewer than 50. We were able to launch a measles vaccination campaign for the city. The clinics were all functional, and feeding centres in the surrounding villages were getting food from the Red Cross and CARE. Rick Price had organized an impromptu soccer league among NGOs and several local teams. The Australian peacekeepers had sent their first reconnaissance team to Baidoa to begin taking over from the Americans. In Mogadishu and the rest of the country, troops from twenty-four countries were arriving to take over from the Americans. UNOSOM was distributing seeds. It had opened schools in Mogadishu and was planning to build more across the country. It still was not clear who—the Americans or UNOSOM—was steering the political process and thus the political future of Somalia. It was clear, though, that in this "complicated situation," someone had to steer.

Wouter returned from his Christmas break. It was time for me to go back to my practice. Over the next few days I prepared to leave for Amsterdam and from there on to Toronto. I said goodbye to Adan Hussein, the chiefs and elders I had come to know, to the clinic staff, the guards and the expatriate team. I went to Buurhakaba one last time. Isaq was leaving for his village that day with a group of men. As we left the town, I saw

SOMALI REPUBLIC
Sabiye Village

To: M.S.F. HEAD OFFICE

BAIDOA

SUBJ:- Request to get helped homanitarianly/.

We are the elders of SAABIYE Village
Distreot of Baidoa. We ask kindly that M.S.F.
officers to consider our request which consist,
to have been supplied an emergence Medicine, Clo-
this, Blankets and tents.=

Our people are dying unbelivably 60
persons daily. We are buring people nedly an covering
them with sacks. They are mostly Children and Old
ones. The different kind of illness which are spreading now in this area are: Measles, Yellowfever, Malaria, diaharea, cough and etc..=

We should be very grateful if you would
provide us an immediate delivery of above mentioned
itms, before it would be very late. We need badly to be
helped in all possible aspect.=

Please visit us as eye-witness in order to
evaluate our prevaiting problems and solve then soon.=
Thank you in advance and with regards. Badly we hasten
to offer you our most sincere congratulation and hearty
good wishes:

MERRY CHRISTMAS AND HAPPY NEW YEAR 1993
°°°

WE ARE ELDERS SABIYE VILLAGE
1. Mahamed Addow Shoobey (Chairman).
2. Abdirashiid Sheik Mat Abaas(Vice
3. Sheik Mahamed Abaas   (Mulah).

Baidoa, 25/12/1992

"Request to get help"

125

a group of children laughing and swimming in a water hole. The sun dappled on the water and on their black skin. We stopped to take some pictures of camels. Farmers were singing in the fields. Hurzi said it was the first time in three years he had heard singing in the fields. I needed to say goodbye to Lesto and Hurzi. What can you say to the men who have saved your life? You can only say thank you and mean it. I gave them each a wallet. Inside of each I had put a piece of paper on which I had written, "Thank you. You are with me always, and I with you. James Orbinski." I left Baidoa on January 7.

I spent a week with Jules and the MSF medical department going over what had happened in Baidoa. Before leaving Amsterdam for Toronto, I met Michel Lotrowska, an MSF logistician who had just returned from Monrovia, Liberia. The civil war in Liberia was brutal, with thousands of civilians massacred and hundreds of thousands displaced and suffering from starvation and disease. Unlike Somalia there was little media attention, and there were no UN-sanctioned troops in the country. "Why did you stay?" I asked.

"Because it was possible to do something, even something small that helped," Michel answered immediately. He paused and then said, "Once you're there, there is no other choice."

"I know exactly what you mean," I replied.

I returned to my practice north of Toronto. One of my patients came to see me with her week-old newborn. I knew her and her two older children well. Her infant had cradle cap, a common problem among infants that usually goes away on its own, and was having trouble latching on to the breast. The public health nurse and a pediatrician had seen both the mother and her child several times in the last week. As I examined the baby, I couldn't help but think of the Somali children in the feeding centres I had been treating only weeks before. Sensing my distance, the mother cried and lifted her baby away from me and held the baby to her chest. She asked me to decide where I wanted to be: "Somalia or here?" She left the examining room, and with a waiting room full of patients and my nurse, Dianne, calling me on the phone, I sat there in silence with the door closed. Dianne called again, and then again.

I went to see Brother Benedict at the monastery in Oka that weekend. I was struggling with questions about humanitarianism and politics and the relationship between the two. I was unsure whether to continue working with MSF.

"Well, it seems to me that you must take the plunge," Benedict said. "Perhaps you already have. But be sure to come up for air if you can."

Somalia's three-year civil war had been put on hold by Operation Restore Hope, but it was by no means over. When the Americans arrived, it was never completely clear whether they were simply going to intimidate the warlords or actually disarm them. Initially, intimidation worked, and weapons were seized in Baidoa and a few other places. In late January 1993, the Americans thwarted an attack on American and Belgian forces in Kismayo. Belgian forces remained, and allowed the clan forces of Siad Barre's son-in-law to infiltrate and reoccupy the town. A month later, riots erupted in Mogadishu against the American-led forces and those NGOs like CARE that had called for the intervention. Over four days, several Somalis were killed and up to ninety injured as U.S. forces fought running battles with thousands of rioters. Now the Americans were claiming that they never said they would disarm the warlords without their consent. The Americans wanted out of Somalia.

Around the country, each of the UN's twenty-four nations involved on the ground had a different policy on disarmament, and the implementation was haphazard. In Kismayo, feeding centres were looted after their Somali guards were disarmed by Belgian UN troops. In Baidoa, the marines became the target of

Somali ambushes and hit-and-run shootings. A marine was killed in mid-January and another wounded in a separate incident. In retaliation, the marines assaulted several towns and villages around Baidoa. By the time they withdrew from Baidoa in mid-January, marines on patrol were being stoned by angry youths. A Concern aid worker was murdered in a robbery on the road to Baidoa from Mogadishu, and in Bardera, the Red Cross was robbed and a delegate assassinated.

Overall the Australian troops did a much better job of maintaining security in Baidoa. But even then, two MSF guards were shot in a robbery. An MSF clinic guard was shot dead by an Australian soldier, and another time, an Australian soldier was shot and killed. The safe at the MSF compound was robbed again by our own guards, the head of mission having been forced to open the safe with a machine gun to his head. By the beginning of March, Baidoa was so dangerous that ten Australian troops began sleeping in the MSF compound at night. A Somali MSF nurse was murdered. Death threats, kidnappings of expatriate aid workers and the robbery at the compound left MSF with no choice but to close its program in Baidoa. Confronting similar difficulties, the Red Cross withdrew completely from Baidoa.

By May, there had been some improvement across the country in the delivery of bulk food, but many of the most vulnerable were still without food. In Mogadishu half of the undernourished children were still not receiving food. Security was worse than it had ever been, and the credibility of UN forces was beyond repair. The rules of engagement—the rules under which troops can use force—were extremely liberal and open to interpretation. In many cases there were no rules. American soldiers often beat and humiliated people at military checkpoints and while searching their homes. One marine was demoted and fined a month's pay after firing his rocket launcher and injuring two boys, one of whom had allegedly stolen the soldier's sunglasses.

Among some soldiers racism fuelled brutal behaviour, which then flourished in a climate of almost total impunity. At a Belgian camp near Mogadishu, "trophy photos" were taken of two Belgian soldiers swinging and roasting a child over a fire. In Kismayo, Belgians shot and killed an armed Somali man, tied his body behind their tank and dragged him through the streets. A Belgian helicopter opened fire on farmers in a field. The helicopter then landed and soldiers took the farmers' watermelons. When a farmer later protested, he was beaten and told, "You and the field belong to us." Children caught stealing were frequently bound and held captive without food or water in stifling heat. One child held in a metal container cried for two days and was eventually found dead. Around the country, UN soldiers drove repeatedly and recklessly at high speeds through crowds, killing several children and adults and injuring many more. They most often did this with impunity, and without apology or compensation paid to their victims.

On March 4, in what soldiers had nicknamed Operation Nig-Nog, Canadian soldiers in the town of Belet Weyne shot two men who were running away from the base, allegedly after stealing. Both were shot in the back: one died, having been shot execution style in the back of the head. On March 16 a sixteen-year-old Somali boy, Shidane Omar Arone, was tortured and beaten to death by soldiers from the Canadian Airborne Regiment while dozens of other Canadian soldiers looked on. On May 19 two Canadians were charged with murder, and later the Canadian government disbanded the disgraced regiment. When the Italians took over from the Canadians, they cleared the area around their compound by beating the displaced people who had gathered there. UN member states were largely responsible for the conduct of their troops, and the UN had no mechanisms to send back the unfit or to discipline the offenders. It was no surprise that humiliation in the face of racism, torture and murder now fed a seething rage among Somalis towards the soldiers of the UN humanitarian intervention.

The media circus was over and the Americans were packing up to leave, but the difficult task of confronting Somalia's warlords and the country's politics remained. It was first intended that Operation Restore Hope would hand over its responsibilities to a reinforced UNOSOM by mid-January 1993. The transition didn't actually happen until the beginning of May. The 37,000-strong U.S.-led international task force, UNITAF, was replaced by a smaller force of 16,000 peacekeepers expected to cover 90 percent of the country, much of which had not yet been secured by UNITAF. With troops from twenty-four other countries in Somalia, the United States left a Rapid Reaction Force of 4,000 under its own command to support UNOSOM. As my MSF friend Jonathan Brock wrote to me from Somalia, "It seems that Clinton's policy is to pull out with as little press as possible. All the NGOs are rethinking their policy and doing some heavy duty cost-benefit analysis."

In the spring of 1993, The Economist wrote that the Americans had succeeded in the "relatively modest task of securing the delivery of aid"; they had then handed UNOSOM a "poisoned chalice." The declared intention of UNOSOM was to help Somalia rebuild its economic, political and social life from the ruins of civil war and to re-establish civil authority throughout the country. Reconciliation conferences among the warlords and elders were arranged by UNOSOM. Efforts were made to organize police forces and a functioning justice system and to coordinate the aid and development work necessary to prevent a return to war. The UN had agreed that Admiral Jonathan Howe, the former undersecretary of defense for George Bush, would lead UNOSOM. Howe then stepped up UNOSOM's efforts to disarm local militias. The plan did not sit well with Aidid in Mogadishu. The humanitarian intervention soured further as the process continued without him. Aidid stepped up aggressive military manoeuvres and radio broadcasts against the UN, and UNOSOM gave little ground. Though the U.S. special envoy to Somalia,

Robert Oakley, would say that "the problem of clan warfare is virtually gone," tensions in Mogadishu had long since spilled over to allied clans and sub-clans elsewhere in the country. As Oakley left Somalia, he concluded that "violence is a Somali trait." He admitted that "you can't travel around Mogadishu in a car without being in great danger of robbery" but argued that Operation Restore Hope had been a success because "at least you can walk around with food."

Admiral Howe moved to disarm Aidid, apparently in a previously agreed arms transfer. On June 5, twenty-four Pakistani UN peacekeepers were killed in three successive waves of a well-planned ambush led by Aidid's forces in Mogadishu. Within two days the UN Security Council had approved "all necessary means" to capture Aidid. Using gunship helicopters from the American Rapid Reaction Force and ground troops from other forces, UNOSOM launched attacks on Aidid's headquarters on June 12. They had the wrong address and raided the house next door. Tensions rose and demonstrations spread through the city as UNOSOM forces withdrew to their bases and limited themselves to helicopter patrols. In Mogadishu, over the next few days, twenty Somalis were killed as Pakistani troops fired into crowds of demonstrators. A few days later, on the morning of June 17, Moroccan soldiers were engaged in a battle with Aidid's forces whose snipers then took cover in a hospital and in the buildings around it. The Moroccan forces were initially reluctant to attack the hospital, but with no warnings given or evacuation of the staff or 380 patients permitted, artillery fire, missiles from American gunship helicopters and a full ground assault on the hospital by French soldiers followed. Four Moroccan soldiers and at least nine patients and other civilians died. On July 12, UNOSOM launched a helicopter attack on the house of a senior Aidid aide where a meeting, which UNOSOM alleged was political, was taking place. It was mid-morning and there were many people on the street. At least fifty-four Somalis were killed, among them religious and clan elders, women and children. No weapons were found in the house. An enraged crowd killed four international journalists.

By the end of July, Aidid was claiming to represent the Somali nation against the "colonialist aggressor." In turn, Aidid was portrayed on CNN as a "mad mullah" Somali insurgent. Clashes between Aidid and UNOSOM, and killings, continued throughout the summer. On October 3, 1993, eighteen American servicemen and about a thousand Somalis were killed after a U.S. Black Hawk helicopter was shot down during a botched daylight raid on an Aidid compound. The body of an American ranger was photographed being dragged through the streets of Mogadishu by an angry crowd. By mid-October, UNOSOM had lost seventy-four men, and between five and ten thousand Somalis had been killed "collaterally" by UN-sanctioned forces.

After the October 3 killings, UNOSOM and Aidid agreed to a ceasefire, and on November 16 the UN Security Council revoked the order for Aidid's arrest. In mid-December Aidid attended a Reconciliation Conference held in Ethiopia. The Clinton administration decided to withdraw all U.S. forces from the country by March 1994, and a number of the other countries began scaling back their presence in response. By the end of 1993, some positive signals had emerged, including the establishment of district councils in some areas as well as the re-establishment of judicial and police structures in Mogadishu (although the city remained divided by its green line into northern and southern halves).

Back in Canada I had decided to take the plunge. Throughout 1993 I worked with others to build MSF Canada. I was in Amsterdam so often that the desk clerk at the Hotel Smit knew me by name and knew that I liked a few beers at night. The office in Amsterdam drew together MSF workers from all over the world. The state of the organization's projects in such places as Angola, Colombia and, of course, Somalia was regular fodder for discussion over too many drinks. My friend Chris Cushing had been shot at in Sarajevo and openly wondered whether the work was worth the risk. Jos Nolle, who had worked in Mozambique amidst shifting rebel lines, was sure that as long as we could negotiate space to work and as long as what we were doing was respected, we had to at least try.

In Baidoa, we had saved nearly 100,000 people. That the situation in Somalia had changed so dramatically in the past few months did not alter this fact. It was definitely worth it, and I was working hard to pay off my medical-school debt so that I could continue to work with MSF.

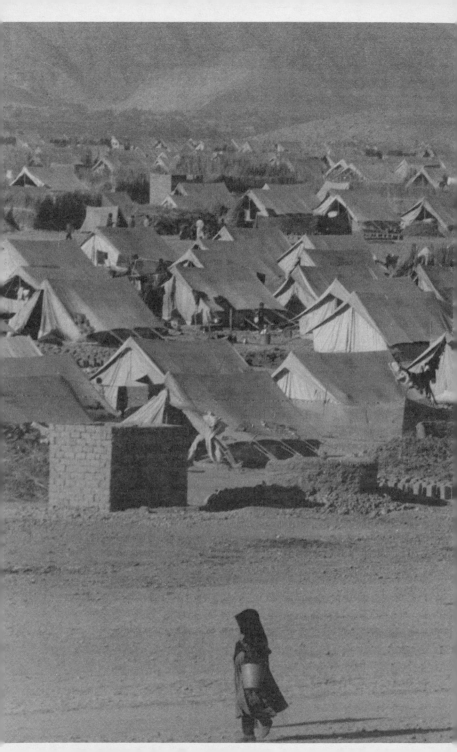

AFGHANISTAN:
NO SCARS, NO STORY, NO LIFE

There were MSF emergency relief projects in twenty countries at war, and there were MSF initiatives in forty other countries in the developing world. MSF was working with street kids in Brazil and in much of South America; it had expanded into medical social work in some parts of Asia, and was building and training for long-term medical laboratories in Cambodia. By 1993, the need to respond to a growing number of emergencies meant that MSF was stretched ever more thinly.

The UN was expanding its sphere of operations too. In the some forty-five years since it was founded in 1945, the UN had launched fourteen peacekeeping missions. In the less than four years since the end of the Cold War, it had launched thirteen more. Now the UN was doing everything from monitoring the ceasefire in Cyprus, to organizing elections in Cambodia and El Salvador, to protecting aid in Bosnia. It wasn't only the UN that was changing. As Western governments shifted their foreign-policy objectives away from development, they closed some embassies in developing countries and downgraded others to regional or consular offices. The NGOs that had grown or emerged during the Cold War to respond to the developing world's needs now found much of their government funding cut. The West began to rely on emergency humanitarian assistance as its response to a rising number of civil wars around the world, and funding to humanitarian relief organizations increased. Predictably, NGOs that had previously been engaged in long-term development work shifted their focus.

At a conference I was invited to towards the end of 1993, Barbara McDougall, then Canada's minister of foreign affairs, declared that it was "not a perfect world, but one of virulent nationalism, famine and abuse of human rights." André Legault, an academic at the same conference, noted that "the end of the Cold War has not meant peace, but war. There is no New World Order," he said, but "a juxtaposition of multiple disorders." I spoke about the military humanitarian intervention in Somalia, criticizing its failures and abuses, insisting on the need to keep military and humanitarian actions separate from one another, and on the responsibility of aid agencies to be witnesses to what was actually happening on the ground. A Romanian general pounded on the table as he shouted, "Your so-called witnessing is dangerous! You must be part of the international community, not critical of it!" Another academic took exception to my apparent naiveté, instructing, "There are always a few bad apples. We are talking about money. Countries act and allocate resources only in their own interests. When humanitarian principles are in their interests, then they will spend money."

By the end of the year, I had handed over my practice to another doctor. A week later, I was in Amsterdam, preparing to go to Tibet. I was to go for a year to set up a tuberculosis treatment program for nomads in a remote region of the Tibetan plateau. The Chinese government had delayed official approval and travel visas for the project, so I did some research for the MSF medical department as I waited. One night in mid-January, Jules met me at the Smit Hotel for a few beers. "Tibet is taking longer than expected. How do you feel about helping me out in Afghanistan?" he asked. "Wayne Ulrich arrived there two days ago and is coordinating logistics. He has a good handle on things. I need a medical coordinator on a plane tomorrow. Will you go?" I knew Kabul was being shelled and that 150,000 people had fled the capital. Jules said, "I am not asking you to go to Kabul, but to Jalalabad, where it seems most of the civilians are heading." Jalalabad was more than 200 kilometres from Kabul, and it was the middle of winter. "Let's see what we can do for them," said Jules.

I spent the next morning in Jules's office reading as much information as I could get. Afghanistan's was a forgotten war. The Soviets had invaded in 1979 and installed a communist prime minister. Jimmy Carter used the CIA to support the mujahideen rebels in a jihad that over the next ten years defeated the communists. China, neighbouring Arab states, Saudi Arabia and Pakistan also supported the mujahideen. The Soviets withdrew in February 1989, leaving one and a half million people dead and the country in ruins. The government of Prime Minister Najibullah still had the support of the Russians and held on to power by allying itself with factions from within the now divided mujahideen. The CIA continued its proxy war through the mujahideen until December 1991. April 1992 marked the beginning of fighting among the nine mujahideen factions. Najibullah took refuge in the UN compound in Kabul. Fighting flared along ethnic, linguistic and religious lines that formed the basis of an ever-shifting patchwork of alliances where parties could fight each other in one part of the country and be allies in another. Little else but money and weapons caused alliances to shift. And there were plenty of both.

With Russia and the United States out of Afghanistan, the fate of the country was left in the hands of those who did have interests there: Pakistan, India, Russia, Iran and China. Officially, each country called for a cessation of the civil war. Unofficially, each backed its horse with arms and political support. The civil war intensified in January 1994, after the warlord Dostum, an old communist, joined with his archrival Hekmatyar, a theocrat, to overthrow the warlords Rabbani and Masoud in Kabul. The city was shelled relentlessly, and even hospitals were bombed. MSF publicly condemned the indiscriminate bombing and continued to treat the hundreds of injured throughout the city.

Jules admitted to me that Afghanistan could be a deadly place for aid workers. More than 550 MSF nurses and doctors had worked in Afghanistan since 1980. It was one of the few NGOs, and often the only one, that provided medical aid during the Soviet occupation. Even with these solid humanitarian credentials, an MSF logistician had been assassinated in 1990, and MSF withdrew from the country until April 1992. The French and Belgian sections of MSF had been working in Kabul and Kunduz for years, but in early 1994, with the intensification of fighting, they had had to evacuate most of the team from Mazar-e-Sharif in the north. There were 12 million people in Afghanistan and an additional four million Afghan refugees in Pakistan. The no man's land between the two countries had become a haven for arms dealers and warlords who controlled the growing opium trade. Pakistan was now backing Hekmatyar and Dostum against Prime Minister Rabbani in Kabul. There was little chance that fighting would spread to Jalalabad, but, Jules said, "one never knows in Afghanistan. The security rules are strict and unbreakable. I am sure you will agree."

Only a year before, four people working with the UN refugee agency—the UNHCR—had been killed in Jalalabad, and it was still not clear by whom. Some suspected agents from Arab states who opposed any UN presence in the country, while others suspected communist allies of the former president.

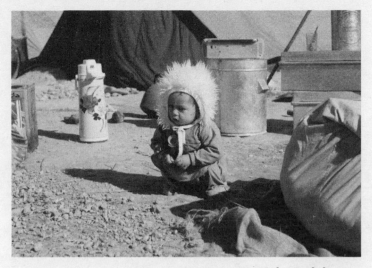

Girl at Sarshahi

Now, with fresh fighting in Kabul, the UN was understandably jittery and had arranged a thirty-six-hour ceasefire beginning on the morning of January 8, so they could evacuate from the city. One hundred and fifty thousand Afghanis took advantage of the break in fighting to also flee. Fifty thousand had gone north to Charikar, and the balance had started walking from Kabul to the Pakistan border. They walked the two hundred kilometres through the Khyber Pass of the Sulaiman Mountains towards Pakistan's Peshawar, but the Pakistani government—for the first time in the country's history—closed the border at Torkham to those seeking refuge from the war.

With the border closed, the crowd of 100,000 had walked back to Jalalabad: they had travelled three hundred kilometres on foot in ten days. Jalalabad's Shura, or governing elders' council, refused them entry into the city and insisted that they be absorbed into the three existing camps for displaced people. Located in a desert plain just inside the entrance to the Khyber Pass, these camps were twenty kilometres from the city. The

Russians had used the area as a tank base, and it was heavily laden with anti-tank mines laid by the mujahideen.

"So it's a refugee camp in a minefield?" I said.

"Not exactly," said Jules. "The camps themselves have been pretty much cleared, but no one is allowed outside the camp borders. They are clearly marked."

"So it's pretty much a refugee camp with a minefield keeping people in," I said.

"Yes, pretty much," said Jules.

That afternoon, Olivier Barthes, a French MSF doctor, called me by satellite phone to give me an idea of the medical needs at the camps. Olivier had been working in Kabul and had followed the group from the city. The situation was desperate. Many had died of exposure during the ten-day walk through the mountains and back again. The group had no fuel, vehicles or livestock and had run out of food. "They are just sitting in the desert outside Jalalabad, surrounded by mountains," Olivier said in broken English. They were the poorest people from Kabul, he explained. They were urbanites, not farmers. They had only what they could carry and were not much good in the mountains. "Right now we need tents, blankets, food and fuel. Wayne is working on these with the UN agencies," he told me. The UN was scrambling to get more funding for Jalalabad, and already MSF was trucking blankets and tents from warehouses in Pakistan. We agreed on the most likely medical priorities: clean water and clinics to treat diarrhea and common ailments. We would need to start a measles vaccination campaign and cholera prevention. Before leaving for the airport, I put in an order for emergency medical kits to be flown to Peshawar in Pakistan.

Late that afternoon, at Schiphol Airport, I met Dixon Chanda, a forty-five-year-old Zambian water engineer who had been working with MSF for the last two years. We travelled via Zurich to Karachi and then on to Peshawar. We made the twenty-two-hour trip without sleep. Wayne met us at the airport, and both Dixon and I slept on the drive to the MSF house. Annie, a forty-something logistician who had run the Peshawar office for two years, took us to a restaurant, but not before her two boys took me up into their tree house and showed me the "three ways you can get in and get out." Dr. Kalid, an Afghan refugee working at the MSF Peshawar office, joined us and explained something of Afghan culture and history. "You must clear everything with the shura in Jalalabad, the council of mujahideen commanders who control the Nangarhar province. Right now they are very nervous. This council has been stable for only a few months. As Western doctors you must understand that only women doctors and nurses can do gynecologic or obstetrical examinations."

Early the next morning we left by truck for Afghanistan. No one was flying in. The area was flooded with shoulder-mounted surface-to-air Stinger missiles. The CIA had supplied them nearly ten years earlier for use against Russian gunship helicopters and military transport planes, and they had turned the war in favour of the mujahideen. The CIA was now trying to buy them back at $150,000 apiece, but wasn't having much luck. In 1994, the U.S. government spent more trying to buy back the Stinger missiles than it did on funding humanitarian assistance in Afghanistan. In the same year, USAID shut down its humanitarian assistance program for Afghanistan.

We began our six-hour drive up through Pakistan's North-West Frontier Province to the border along a single-lane road that had to accommodate two-way mountain traffic. The road was in bad repair, except for the British-made gunner pillboxes and guardrails that had been built at the beginning of the twentieth century. A spotted grey fungus had grown into their thick cement; otherwise, they were in perfect condition. The brown mountains were rugged and as bare as a moonscape, except for their snowcaps. There were a few caves carved into their sides, and the rare family compound built on cliffs, usually three or four hundred metres from the roadside. Lone men wearing turbans and armed with rifles stood guard on top of the thick stone compound walls. These were the centuries-old tribal lands, known locally as No Man's Land, and, our driver told us, "ungovernable by any state: it is only sharia law and blood feuds here."

The people here were proud, independent and tough, and as in Somalia, organized by clan and tribe. The men were fierce fighters; a clan's honour was more important than an individual life; loyalty and hospitality as sacred as blood revenge, though still an uncertain guarantee of one's life. No one, not even the Pakistani police, would venture off the road that twisted up through the rocky mountains. No one slept as we dodged careening trucks laden with wares and with people sitting on the roofs, their musical horns blaring to announce their presence as they rounded a corner at full speed.

Still in No Man's Land, less than an hour from the Torkham border crossing, we stopped at a roadside market. Wayne wanted to get some of the supplies we needed, as most were not available in Afghanistan. Thousands of Afghan refugees, local boys and bearded men in gurtas and hats, and a few women in hijabs or head-to-ankle burkas, mingled with goats, shrouded tribal peoples, hawkers and traders with trucks and carts full of goods moving between tin-roofed stone stalls. The sun bore down on the brittle rock and on us. There was no plant life, and a cream-coloured dust covered everything. You could buy anything here: AK-47s, rocket launchers, opium, water pipes, pumps and household wares. Wayne scouted around for water cisterns for the clinics we would build, and pens, paper, shelving and canned food for us. One man offered me a kilo of hashish: "Afghan Gold—the best! I give you a good price!"

At Torkham, we crossed into the Nangarhar province of Afghanistan after anxious and officious Pakistani border guards searched our truck. Wayne was jovial and reassuring and stamped our passports himself while one of the guards went off to look for kerosene for the lamp. Once inside

Afghanistan, the road wound down the mountains like a creek finding the easiest way, and it was a surprisingly good road despite years of civil war. The Khyber Pass mountains were both strangely glorious and ominous. I had forgotten to bring sunglasses and I squinted at the bright sun reflecting off the cream-coloured terrain. I could see lone gunmen in turbans and full body shawls hunched over smoking fires in the mountains above the road. They were rumoured to be excellent marksmen, able to hit a moving target with a single shot from more than half a kilometre away.

It took just over two hours to drive the hundred kilometres from the border to the outskirts of Jalalabad, a barren plane just inside the meandering end of the mountain range. Some 35,000 people sat in the cold desert. Thousands of others had been absorbed into the three more-established camps. The UN was mapping out this new camp, already known as Sarshahi. It was late afternoon, and the cold night air was beginning to fall. Eighty perfectly straight rows of twenty-five tents each had been laid out, with about seven or eight people in each tent. There were thousands more people than tents, and men and boys dug holes and used heaps of rocky earth to make walls against the night wind. The night before, twenty old and young people had died of exposure. The women wore two or three winter coats and carried pots, bags and babies to their numbered plots marked with stakes in the soil. Bearded men carried bundles of heavier belongings that were wrapped in tablecloths, bedsheets and shawls. The children wore three or four layers of clothes and pushed wheelbarrows and bicycles loaded down with mattresses and other small household possessions. Some already had diarrhea from drinking contaminated water along their route; everyone was skinny, cold and miserable, and most, even the children, had hard eyes. Those with green-blue eyes were among the most beautiful people I have ever seen. One woman sat on a mound of earth. Her face showed her exhaustion, and she held her dead infant close to her chest.

Three crying children sat around her. One child had the watery eyes and the red rash on his face and arms of measles.

I met Olivier. A man of about thirty, he had a serious face behind wire-rimmed glasses and was worried about the prospect of measles and cholera spreading through the camp. In such a worn-out, exposed and stressed group, these two diseases alone could kill thousands within weeks. There were already several clusters of measles among the children. In the last year UNICEF had vaccinated against measles in Kabul, but in the midst of civil war had managed to reach only a quarter of the children, nowhere near the 90 percent necessary to prevent an outbreak. There was no way to be sure who and how many among the children in the camp had been vaccinated.

It took an hour to drive the remaining twenty kilometres into Jalalabad. We passed more people walking from Kabul, boys selling bread and fruit, the rusting carcasses of Russian tanks and armoured personnel carriers and the levelled remnants of an irrigation system that came from a river two kilometres away. The town of about forty thousand was teeming

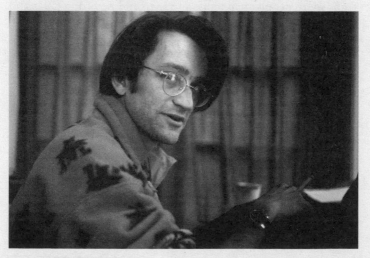

Dr. Olivier Barthes

with cars, donkey carts and pedestrians who moved slowly along treeless narrow roads and alleyways that separated mud-brick homes behind high stone compound walls. Women wearing shawls and head scarves—and some wearing burkas with coarse lattice grilles over the eyes that allowed them to see out but no one to see in—followed with children behind bearded men. Amputees and beggars walked among the crowds or sat along the roadsides looking for money and food. Small convoys of Land Cruisers and pickup trucks carrying armed men mixed with traders' trucks that passed slowly between the crowded market stalls lining the streets in the centre of town.

We went directly to the UN compound. The curt man in charge of the WHO was most concerned that I sign an agreement to cover the medical needs in the camps. I could see why the WHO had a reputation for being bureaucratic and ineffective in Afghanistan. I met Jeremy, the practical, friendly man in charge of the UNHCR in Jalalabad. "The shura won't let the people from Kabul into town. They are afraid of guerrilla attacks. We're scrambling," he said. "We are struggling to get the camp de-mined and to get in enough tents. We need you for water and sanitation and the medical bits at Sarshahi, and to support the overflow at the other camps." The UNHCR was not officially engaged here, Jeremy explained, as these were displaced persons within their own country and not refugees in another. He assured me with a wink that UNHCR tents and equipment would be "stored" in Jalalabad, and that he was "of course powerless to stop MSF from looting. But be careful of the shura," he warned. "They will loot everything."

Wayne thought he would have a house for us the next day. In the meantime, we went to the restaurant of the Pinnar Hotel, where a few heavily armed men looked at us, and especially at black-skinned Dixon, suspiciously. "Don't worry," Wayne said. "There's no way we could have got this far without permission from the shura commanders. These men know that as well as we do."

Wayne detailed the supplies coming in from MSF and the UNHCR. The UN World Food Program was having some trouble with its supply lines through Pakistan, but was confident it could get enough food in over the next few days. A Norwegian NGO was bringing in kerosene and stoves for the camps. Wayne and Dixon focused on water and sanitation, marking out sites for pit latrines on a photocopy of a hand-drawn map of Sarshahi. Olivier and I reviewed the medical priorities and the lists Olivier had already made of people in the camp and in Jalalabad who could be trained to work in the clinics we would set up.

We stayed at the hotel that night. It was so cold the next morning that my porcelain cup cracked as I poured hot water into it for tea. I tried to imagine walking three hundred kilo-metres with children. I couldn't.

By early morning word had spread that we had arrived, and about fifty people were outside the Pinnar Hotel looking for jobs. Some offered to work as translators, which we clearly needed. I interviewed about twenty young men. Some spoke English, poorly, but could not read or write it for translations. Of those that had better language skills, most were too young to be taken seriously at shura and other meetings, or too earnest to be taken seriously by me. We hired many of these younger men to work in the clinics that we would soon be opening, but I still needed a translator.

Abdul Aziz was a sixty-five-year-old chain-smoking Afghani who, before the Soviet occupation, had worked as a translator at the British embassy in Kabul. Abdul had a limp and carried a steel-tipped walking stick. "I have three wives and three heart attacks," he told me, "and I have nine daughters and two dead sons." He had a closely shaved white beard, bright green eyes and vertical lines wrinkled into his cheeks from far too much smoking. He came wrapped in a shawl and capped with a traditional Pakol hat. Jobs were scarce, but still Abdul enquired after the salary and whether it would be paid in

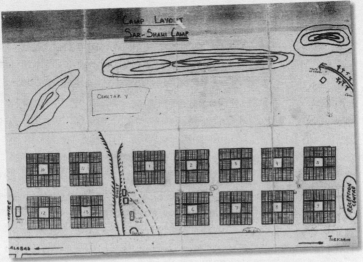

A hand-drawn map showing the layout for Sarshahi Camp

afghanis or dollars. "An afghani is not quite the same as a dollar. One buys a very dry fig, the other a very fat camel, if you see what I mean," he said with a smile. I said he would be paid in Pakistani rupees. "Thin camels and fat figs are not unwelcome," he replied. He seemed to never stop talking. He spoke French, Russian and Pashto, and his English was impeccable. The job was his when I asked him to write as I dictated a test letter. "I will write it one hundred times," he said. "I will even write it in my own blood, dear doctor. And then you will have something to fix." When I told him he was hired, he replied, "Ah, it just so happens I am available."

Abdul and I met with Dr. Wakali at his Ministry of Health office on the third floor of the nursing school building. The university campus had been badly shelled over the years of war, and the university itself had long since closed. Dr. Wakali readily committed some of his staff to work with us, knowing we could pay their salaries, which they were otherwise not getting. He pointed out that the Islamic Relief Agency was coming to help, and that the Jalalabad shura wanted them to work in the Sarshahi camp.

We then went to the Red Cross compound. The head of mission there was leery of depending on the UN for coordination, as "they may well leave." He too warned us about the shura and advised, "It is better to pay the shura something than to lose everything." The Red Cross was running a surgical hospital in Jalalabad, largely for land-mine victims. "There are about 10 million mostly Russian land mines, nearly one for every man, woman and child in the country," he said. "It is mostly the children and the goats that get hit, working or playing in the fields," he explained. "The anti-tank mines are buried deep, and need a heavy vehicle to detonate them, except in the sand, where anything can detonate them. The cluster bombs are coated in a green plastic, and look like butterflies to the children, so they pick them up, and, well, you know what happens." A British NGO and the UN ran a national mine-clearance program, but at their current pace, it would take them two hundred years to clear the country. Camp Sarshahi was being cleared now, and fifty anti-tank mines had been detonated in the last three days. He showed us their bomb shelter. "Every good home has one.

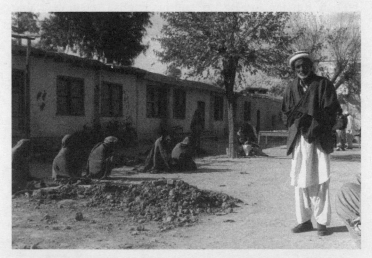

Abdul Aziz

Can't live here without it," he said. We were invited to use it, "if need be. Though try to get here before the shelling starts, and if you know when that is, let me know."

Providing water was a problem at Sarshahi Camp. Wayne had found two oil tankers and had had them cleaned out. On four daily runs to Sarshahi, they carried 7,000 litres of chlorinated river water. It was nowhere near enough, but it was a start. Unloading the water was the next problem. There was nothing to put it in. People filled cups, buckets and pots from the tankers, and chaos ensued as too many people struggled against each other for too long to get not enough water for drinking, cooking and bathing. Until boreholes could be drilled, we would have to store water in MSF bladder tanks that would arrive the next day from Pakistan. The runs would then at least be faster, while we looked for more trucks.

There were still not enough tents. Some of the fifty thousand people who had fled Kabul for Charikar were now heading to Jalalabad because of the extreme cold in the north. The Jalalabad shura would allow food distribution only to people with tents. Angry men in the camps shouted at the UN workers, who were unable to give them food. I met with the Sarshahi shura — a group of about twelve older men — that had formed in the camp. With Abdul translating, we sat in a circle on blankets covering the dirt ground inside the shura's tent. Every half hour or so a hollow boom halted our conversation, and the tent walls fluttered as anti-tank land mines were detonated nearby. We worked out a way to hire people from the camp, including the three doctors there. We agreed to procedures for monitoring disease outbreaks and counting the dead. We also established clear priorities: to dig latrines, to determine sites for water tanks and clinics and to keep the children and others from wandering into the minefield around the camp borders. We set up the first of three tent clinics with the supplies we had. Another ten people had died the night before, and another

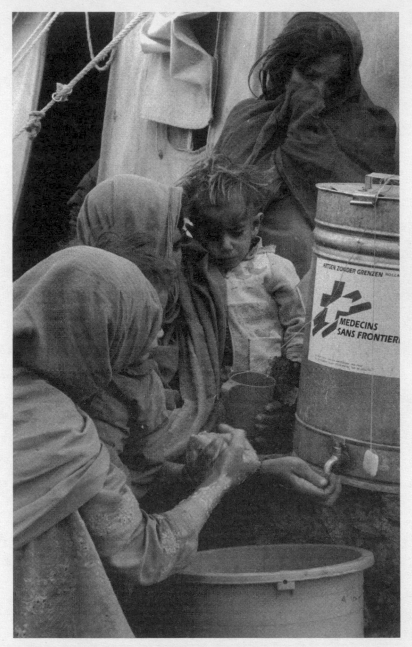

Refugee women and children gather water

six children had measles. Thousands more had arrived from Kabul. Men came looking for tents or temporary employment; women came for treatment for their children.

Wayne had found us a house not far from the centre of town with security and a cook provided by the owner, one of the shura commanders. The cook's first meal was peas fried in oil. I stuck with the Heinz baked beans and Mars bars we had bought in Peshawar. That night, Jules called me on the satellite phone looking for details he could use in a funding proposal he was preparing for the Canadian government. MSF had been drawing on its privately raised funds, but these were running short. Geoff Prescott, the MSF head of mission in Afghanistan, also came from Kabul to meet us. In his early thirties, Geoff was warm, direct and thorough. He impressed Abdul and the other Afghan men among us, and they were not easily impressed. Geoff explained that heavy shelling and fighting continued in the capital, and there were hundreds of casualties in the city. MSF was bringing in planeloads of medical supplies and surgical equipment to Peshawar and then overland through Jalalabad to our teams in Kabul, Kunduz and Mazar-e-Sharif. All available resources and workers were needed in Kabul and in Mazar-e-Sharif, and Geoff was reluctant to increase the size of the team in Jalalabad. What's more, security was uncertain in the area, and the Jalalabad shura was not yet stable. Geoff outlined the three most likely risks we would face: the fighting could spread to Jalalabad; disgruntled people from Kabul could turn violent if food distribution did not improve; and guerrillas from opposing factions could infiltrate Jalalabad or the camps and split or dishonour the shura. We were to travel with all vehicle lights on and with the armed escorts provided by the shura. We had to remain in our compound between 6 p.m. and 6 a.m. We could evacuate our compound only if it was under heavy attack. He emphasized "heavy" and then reminded us of the overland routes we could take to Pakistan. That night more people at the camp died of exposure.

By the following day we had two clinics up and running and started training a staff of twenty-four. With at least three more cases of measles, the prospect of an epidemic remained real. Cholera was a constant threat. Diarrhea, exhaustion, hunger, respiratory and skin infections and swollen, blistered feet were the most common problems. Massive blisters on some people's feet oozed fluid and blood, and the skin just above their ankles was nearly macerated from walking. Most people shivered in the cold and were silent as we cleaned and dressed their wounds. Only rarely did children cry out as their parents held them. Two women were in labour, but our female nurses hadn't yet arrived, and there were no female nurses or doctors in the camp. We arranged transport for them to the Afghan Obstetrics and Gynecology Hospital in Jalalabad.

More tents had arrived, but there still were not enough. Seven men from the camp had been killed and three injured at a military checkpoint the night before. They had tried to go into Jalalabad to protest to the shura about the lack of food for people without tents. Men now surrounded the UN tent, and a British UN employee screamed back at them, a red-faced outburst that lasted at least three minutes. His translator was a short, pear-shaped, happy man, who happened to be Abdul's brother. He held his smile as he looked to the ground and translated with fewer than five words. All stood silent, and Abdul whispered to me, "That man [the UN employee] has humiliated himself and does not know it. It doesn't help that he is British. My brother would like to bury himself under that rock." The situation was defused as truckloads of bladder tanks, tents, blankets and jerry cans arrived from Pakistan. We continued organizing and hiring for water points, pit latrines and more clinics.

As Abdul and I were getting into our vehicle, a father asked me to smuggle him and his nine-year-old daughter to Pakistan in one of the MSF trucks returning to Peshawar. His weather-beaten face gave him the look of a fifty-year-old, but he said he was thirty-five. His daughter had cancer, and his brother in Pakistan was trying to arrange treatment. Abdul suggested that they would both fit well under a few blankets in the rear. Because the truck was part of a returning convoy, it was not searched as it crossed the border.

Late that afternoon Abdul and I met with the shura in Jalalabad at the office of the governor, Haji Kadir. Scores of armed guards, pickup trucks and Land Cruisers surrounded the office. Abdul was searched, but I was not—"You are the guest," Abdul explained. Inside, about fifteen older men sat in thickly cushioned armchairs, sipping tea and whispering among themselves. An ornate hand-tiled peacock looked at us from a windowless wall. Kadir was allied with Hezb-e-Islami, and thus with Hekmatyar and Dostum. Of the other fifteen commanders, some were hard-line Islamic theocrats and were for the most part allied with Kadir. Others were tentatively allied with Kadir, but could easily shift allegiance to Rabbani in Kabul, if it proved to their advantage.

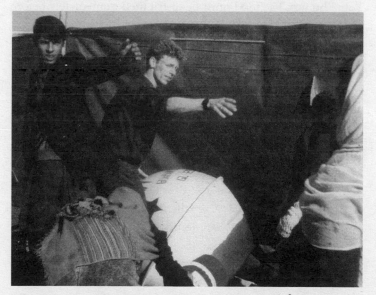

Trying to right a bladder tank that had tipped over

Kadir welcomed me and introduced me around and then sat silent for the rest of the time I was there. I thanked the shura for permission to work in Jalalabad, and then outlined what we were doing in the camp. I presented our worry about epidemics of measles and cholera, which could easily spread to Jalalabad. One of the commanders began to reply, and Abdul leaned over and whispered to me, "James, listen carefully. Smile at him now as I talk. Agree to nothing, except that we must come to an agreement. This man is the biggest killer and thief in all of Jalalabad. Do you see how fat he is?" I smiled and nodded at the commander. Stroking his beard, he smiled and nodded back. I raised the problem of those without tents going without food. Abdul immediately whispered in my ear, "You will get nowhere unless you offer them something." While our most immediate concern was food distribution, I said that we would need to rent secure warehouse space for standby cholera equipment. The fat man replied: "We cannot leave our brothers and sisters from Kabul hungry. The food must be distributed immediately before the tents arrive. We will be happy to provide warehouse space and security. Of course, there will be expenses." The governor nodded his agreement, and Abdul and I took our leave.

Over the next four weeks, shelling continued in Kabul, and Sarshahi swelled to fifty thousand people. Alliances and political support from outside states shifted around us as we worked. In mid-February, Pakistan closed its consulate in Jalalabad, though it was not clear why. A few days later, three Afghanis hijacked a school bus from Peshawar and drove to the Afghan embassy in Islamabad. The hijackers were killed in a commando raid by the Pakistani authorities. Afghan demonstrators then ransacked the Pakistani embassy in Kabul, and Pakistan withdrew its diplomats from the capital. The Jalalabad shura increased its visible security forces around the camps, and our vehicles were thoroughly searched by nervous men at new checkpoints along the road. Geoff kept our team to a minimum of seven expatriates, while our national staff swelled to nearly ninety and included drivers, as well as clinic, warehouse, logistical, water and sanitation staff. Hundreds more were now employed part time or under the UN food-for-work payment scheme to care for water tanks, dig latrines, count the dead and distribute food.

Several times a day I drove the one hour to and from the camps. I saw patients, trained staff and met with the shuras, UN agencies, other NGOs and a nervous Dr. Wakali at the Ministry of Health. Typical of UN initiatives, the World Food Program was inadequately funded by donor countries. The organization struggled to get enough food to the camps, delivering about 2,000 calories per person per day, well short of the 2,800 calories required in the cold weather. By now we had a full cholera-preparation program in place, with equipment on hand and staff trained in case of an outbreak. The Islamic Relief Agency had arrived, and together we had the necessary clinics in the camps for men and women. De-mining continued. We had enough bladder tanks, and five tanker trucks were doing forty runs a day as drilling rigs looked for water in the desert. With the UN we planned a measles vaccination campaign and trained an additional seventy temporary staff. We prepared for a nutritional survey to be conducted. Over the course of weeks, as these arrangements were made, Abdul accompanied me everywhere I went. He talked constantly, and his only request was to have time to pray four times a day, and then time to have a smoke. I joined him for the smokes.

Boredom was the biggest problem at the camps. Children made kites, played soccer with homemade rag balls and attended makeshift tent schools where they learned math and read the Koran. For hours at a time the older boys played rock toss: you toss a rock up in the air and try to pick as many rocks off the ground before having to catch the falling one. For me, night meant tallying statistics, writing training manuals, communicating with other MSF teams in the country, sending reports to Europe and trying to avoid peas fried in oil. There was little else to do except work.

Late one night, one of the guards came to wake me up. Even though it was extremely dangerous for anyone to be out at night, a young woman and her husband had arrived at the door. They had come from the Sarshahi camp and had walked through a minefield to bypass the military checkpoint. They had managed to get a lift the rest of the way to our compound. They had their only child, an infant less than a week old, with them. He was very sick, they said. I examined him, rewrapped his cold body and told them as gently as I could that their son was dead. Later that night I could hear the mother sobbing and the voice of her husband trying to console her from the spare room where they had been taken to sleep. The following morning there was silence in the truck as we drove them back to the camp. Not even Abdul spoke.

At the camp I walked with Abdul along the outer border, counting tents and the number of people in each to determine the sample size for the nutritional survey. Suddenly the earth shook and the air pounded against my face. Dust and small rocks fell from the air, and I heard children's screams coming from where, a few minutes before, I had passed a group of boys playing rock toss. I ran over. An anti-tank mine had exploded. The limbs, torsos and bloodstained clothes of three children were scattered around a crater in the sand as a beige dust cloud from the blast was carried off in the wind. Tripping over the clothes and flesh of their friends, other children ran away bleeding, screaming, crying and holding their ears.

A few days later, Lucie Blok, the MSF medical director, arrived to help with the measles vaccination campaign and the nutritional survey. She told me that a few weeks earlier in the former Yugoslavia, an MSF nurse had her ankle badly injured

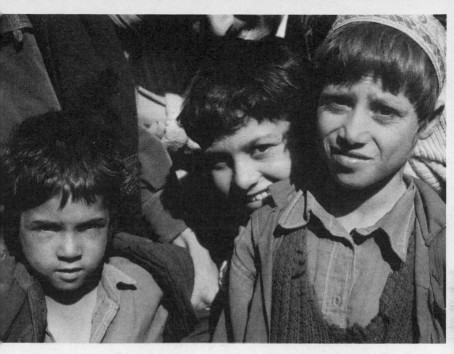

Boys at Camp Sarshahi

when Serb forces mortared her aid convoy as it travelled to a safe haven in Vukovar protected by UN peacekeepers. A few weeks before, sixty-eight people had died in a mortar attack on the Sarajevo marketplace. NATO had immediately declared that it would protect UN "safe havens" for Muslims. It hadn't.

Olivier and I had carefully mapped out the camp, and the night before our vaccination campaign was to start we marked fourteen temporary vaccination centres with green flags. Abdul and I went out early the next morning to make sure everything was ready. A truck with loudspeakers had driven through the camps the previous night telling parents to bring all children under five to one of the marked vaccination points. It was doing the same now. But all the flags were gone. I looked up into the surrounding mountains and could see a circle of green flags around a firepit billowing smoke. "Mujahideen," Abdul said. "Green is their colour." The campaign had been weeks in its preparation and coordination. We could not afford to fail. We drove towards the firepit, as far as the rugged terrain would let us, and walked the rest of the way, uphill for about three hundred metres. Abdul was slow, but we made it in about thirty minutes, and the commander walked down to meet us.

I explained anxiously that these were my flags and I wanted them back. Abdul spoke with the commander and then turned to me. "James, I am an old cat who still has three lives. One of them, I have just given to you. You are looking far too serious. I have told him that you are sorry for having taken his flags. He has agreed to lend them to you for the next three days. He is glad that they will be helping with the vaccination. He would like you to have some tea. Do you want two sugars or three? You may wish to offer him one of your cigarettes, otherwise he will claim those too."

First we had tea and a smoke, and then over the next three days, we vaccinated 95 percent of the children in the camp. The survey found that 18 percent of the children vaccinated were suffering from moderate to severe malnutrition. We now had a basis to demand more food from the World Food Program, and it had a basis to demand more money from donors.

The Tibet project was back on, and I was to return to Amsterdam within a week. Abdul invited me to dinner and to stay overnight with his family. As the guest, I was seated at the centre point along a wall on a bed of thick red carpets. Two young girls brought me cushions for my back. Another poured washing water over my hands and the hands of the other men as we sat. The young boys giggled and waited for the men to eat, while the women served the food. It was a slow, relaxed meal of goat meat and bread.

"The Russians were a sick army," said Abdul. "They would torture, and if a soldier liked your wife, they could rape at will. They had no honour, and some liked boys. Many young men killed themselves after this." An old man who lived across the street had joined us. He said in broken English that the Russians, like the British before them, learned that "no one conquers Afghanistan. We can't even conquer ourselves. Look at us now. It is shame on all of us." He had fought with the mujahideen and was missing the thumb and index finger of his left hand. They had been blown off when a bullet had exploded in the barrel of his rifle. He laughed. "American bullets in a Chinese rifle!" I asked him about the scars on his arms and face. The men spoke heatedly in Pashto and laughed as they recounted their battles against the Russians. Shaking a cigarette held between his ring and middle fingers, the old man turned to me and said, "No scars, no story, no life."

It was late as the women poured green or black tea for us. "Be careful," the old man said before leaving. "Trust Abdul. He is an old man who only laughs and sometimes cries now."

A few minutes later several bursts of machine-gun fire rang out from down the street.

"It is only a wedding," said Abdul.

"Who is getting married?" I asked.

"Who knows," said Abdul, pouring two generous glasses of Black Label, "but we'll celebrate anyway." We drank a few more glasses together. Half asking, half telling, Abdul said, "Afghanistan is a tough place, isn't it?"

"Yes, and sometimes a cruel place," I replied.

Abdul took a sup of his drink, and then said, "Yes, cruel is a better word."

A few days later, Abdul and I had a final smoke together. "I know we can be difficult, but don't let MSF forget us, James. And you, please do not forget me," he said. He gave me a small traditional Afghan carpet, a gift from his family. I gave him enough American money to buy several fat camels and a few dry figs.

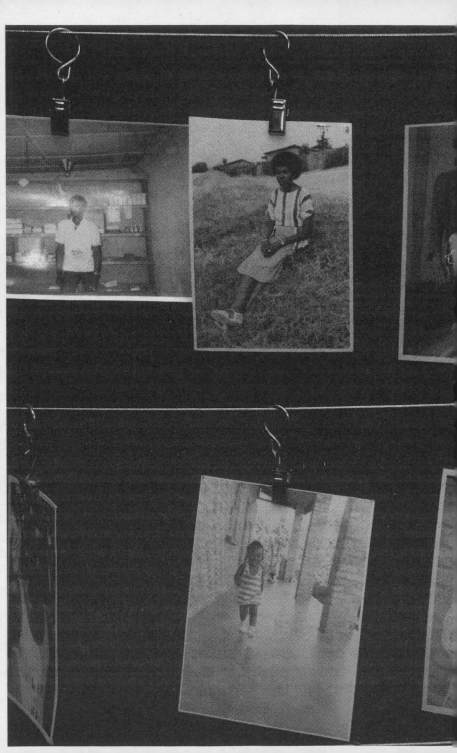

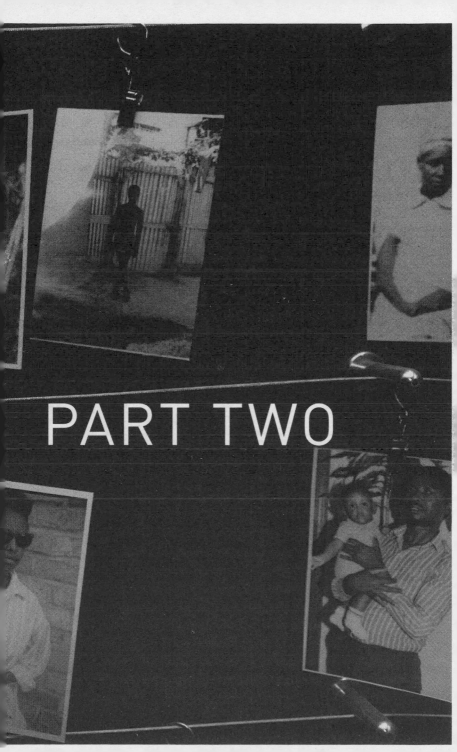

PART TWO

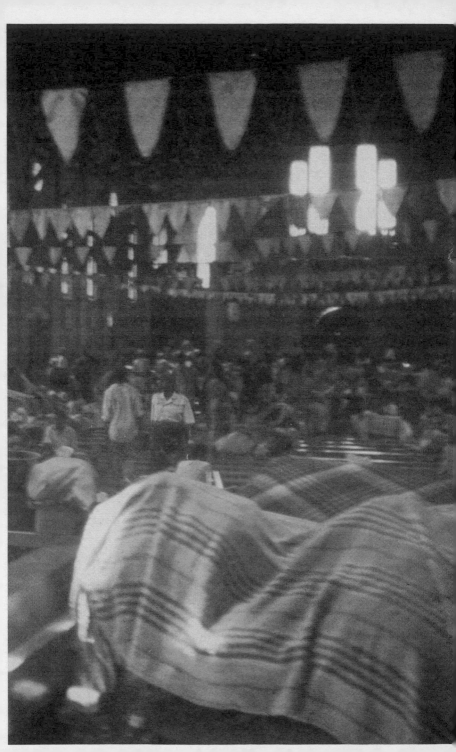

AN UNDOING

The genocide in Rwanda was my undoing. It was where I came to know intimately the fullness of what we are capable of as human beings. No illusions or fantasies were possible after this; no retreat into false hopes or comforting yearnings for a lost past.

I lost my questions, and for eighteen months afterwards existed in a kind of netherworld of confusion, trying to side-step memories that could impose themselves at any time. I struggled against what I knew and could not escape. I struggled to find a way to understand and regain my footing as a man, as a doctor and as a putative humanitarian. And I still struggle now when I confront memories of that time, memories that are no longer unspeakable, but still unbearable.

It is easy to imagine that war and genocide come from a place outside of ourselves. But genocide is not an accident of nature, nor an act of God. It is an act of man—a human choice. And genocide is not war, itself another human choice— ostensibly a choice with agreed-upon rules. In genocide there are no rules, save, of course, to be thorough, to finish the job. That's what genocide is: an effort to finish the job of completely erasing the other, his actuality and his possibility. And once started, it is usually efficient.

The genocide in Rwanda was the most efficient genocide of the twentieth century, more efficient than the Turks over the Armenians, the Khmer Rouge over its unwanted, the Nazis over the Jews and those others it defined as a threat to the Reich. Not bad, if you pride yourself on efficiency. In Rwanda the choice of those who controlled the government was to kill every member of the Tutsi enemy together with their Hutu sympathizers. This was to be a low-tech genocide, carried out with clubs and machetes placed in the hands of a discontented youth who were mobilized by radio.

From April to July 1994—just fourteen weeks—85 percent of all Tutsis in Rwanda, one million men, women and children, would be exterminated, four times the number that would die over the four years of war in the former Yugoslavia. Half a million people were injured, and more than half of Rwandans— four million people—became displaced in their own country or became refugees in another. The UN lost fourteen peacekeepers. MSF and the Red Cross lost no expatriates, but did lose hundreds of nurses, doctors and other national staff, most of them Tutsis, who were taken out of medical facilities and murdered— assassinated in cold blood by the roadside, in rivers, in wells and in farmers' fields.

Jules first called me on May 12, 1994. I had returned to Canada from Afghanistan a few weeks earlier. I was still waiting to go to Tibet to start MSF's tuberculosis treatment program and was working at a hospital just outside Toronto. It was a perfect way to wait—nights spent in a rural emergency room, days spent canoeing. Jules told me that the Tibet mission was still on hold as MSF continued to negotiate details with the Chinese government and Tibetan authorities. Instead, he asked me to go to Rwanda. He was aware that I knew something of the country, something of its culture, geography and language. And I knew it was a place of dark secrets that had now exploded.

A lot had happened in Rwanda since I had left in 1988. President Habyarimana and his family had achieved a stranglehold on government and thus on the state. They had a licence to print money, to control the exchange rate, to receive foreign aid and to run up debts on the national account. Most of the benefits went to a small circle of Hutu elites and to Habyarimana's home region of northwest Rwanda. The president's wife was increasingly powerful, as were her brothers. Together they would come to be known as the Akuza, or the Little House. Akuza had a controlling hand in all major commerce in the country and in all major trade with Europe.

From the late 1980s, France vigorously supported the Habyarimana/Akuza dictatorship. The Belgians also maintained strong business interests in Rwanda, and thus kept a healthy political presence there, but they were now very much the little sister to France. France considered Rwanda among its vital national interests, if only to maintain an imperial fantasy of itself as a superpower. In fact, France was effectively a has-been power, except in la Francophonie of Africa. Rwanda, a French-speaking country, was to be France's minion, a pole of political and economic influence in the region, its line in the African sand. In terms of African policy, little was more important to the French than maintaining a bulwark against the very real Anglo-American interests in the Great Lakes region of Africa.

The United States had Mobutu's Zaire, a mineral-rich kleptocracy created and supported by the CIA since the early 1960s. But Zaire was disintegrating under Mobutu's rule. Museveni's neighbouring Uganda, a former British colony, was now a model developing state implementing with full vigour the structural adjustment programs of the World Bank and International

Monetary Fund. Uganda's health system crumbled with a lack of funding. After user fees were imposed on public services such as health and education, Uganda's HIV rate rose from 8 percent in 1990 to 18 percent in just four years. In Rwanda, the same economic shock therapy had been imposed with disastrous outcomes. Prices rose, consumption fell, incomes plummeted, while the cost of school fees, water and health care rose.

Coffee was Rwanda's major export. In 1989, after American coffee traders had lobbied successfully to remove quotas, world coffee prices fell by 50 percent. As global markets opened in the wake of the Cold War, other Rwandan commodities like tea and tin were subject to price drops that left government coffers empty. Already anemic social programs were cut further, and women like those I had treated in 1988 in Mundende had even less to feed their starving children. Drought struck in the south in 1989. The informal barter system that existed precariously inside a formalized monetary economy became even more tenuous for those who depended on it. By 1993, with upwards of 90 percent of Rwanda's population living below the poverty line, the country was formally ranked by the UN as the poorest place on earth.

There was trouble in what had once been called paradise. No one could make money without the hand of Akuza somewhere deep in the pot. Resentment grew among Hutus outside the northwest region over the Akuza hold on power. The excluded demanded access to government, which beyond the church was the only real source of power and its benefits in Rwanda. There were growing calls for multiparty reform to this one-party state. In response Akuza actively alienated moderate Hutus and united extremists under "Hutu Power." They recruited, trained and armed their own militia wings; the most notorious among them was the Interahamwe.

It wasn't hard to build militias. In 1988 I had asked a teenager who sometimes looked after my moped at the CHK whether he did anything else for a living. "I am a thief," he said, looking straight at me, his eyes far older than his face. "I do what I have to, to survive." He explained that his father had land only for his brothers and so he had none. He had neither an education nor cows, and so he had no wife. There was no work for him, and so he had no food. "For one such as me, how is it different if I die by someone else's hand or by my own hunger?" He paused and then said, "I used to feel ashamed, but shame is for those who have choices." By the time the genocide began, the Interahamwe militia was a 30,000-strong, carefully organized, nationwide Hutu force.

In 1989 Habyarimana declared that the 500,000 Tutsi refugees inside Uganda could not return to Rwanda. And they were now unwelcome in Uganda, despite the fact that a good number, including Paul Kagame, had fought on Museveni's side during Uganda's own recent civil war. Kagame was a loyal lieutenant of Museveni, but his first loyalty was to his own Tutsi people, and to their justified claim of a right of return to Rwanda. When Habyarimana rejected that claim, the Rwanda Patriotic Front was officially formed. With the RPF getting arms from suppliers in the United States, Paul Kagame—who had trained at the home of the 82nd Airborne and Special Operations Forces at Fort Bragg, North Carolina—launched the first RPF guerrilla incursion into Rwanda from Uganda, in October 1990.

Between 1990 and 1993, an estimated two thousand Tutsis were murdered in a series of massacres and pogroms, all allegedly isolated incidents at the hands of the private militias. As attacks on Tutsis inside Rwanda continued, so did RPF guerrilla incursions across the border. By mid-1992, attacks by RPF in the north and insecurity elsewhere had displaced between 200,000 and 300,000 people inside Rwanda.

France helped repel the rebel RPF attacks in 1990, with French military advisers offering training, arms and military intelligence on RPF movements to the Rwandan army. Some among the senior French officer corps referred to the RPF as Rwanda's

Khmer Noire, a reference to Cambodia's genocidal Khmer Rouge. From 1990 on, France had between six hundred and eleven hundred soldiers in Rwanda that trained and armed the Rwandan army, which grew from ten thousand to thirty thousand. French soldiers assisted in combat, in interrogating military prisoners and in enforcing control measures on the civilian population.

Habyarimana had a close personal relationship with President Mitterrand, and if he were to lose the fight against the RPF, it would be the first time that a regime loyal to France had been removed without prior French approval, possibly undermining the loyalty of France's other African client states. In February 1993 the French sent more than five hundred troops to "indirectly command" and assist the Rwandan forces in halting an RPF advance. The French sent arms and ammunition, up to twenty tons a day, enough to cut into the standing stocks of the French army itself. However, by the early summer of 1993, France had come to realize that short of actually taking over the country, it could not achieve its goals in Rwanda. And so it offered its support to internationally led negotiations between the Rwandan government and the RPF as the best, cheapest and most politically feasible option for its own foreign policy in Rwanda.

In August 1993, after months of negotiation at Arusha in Tanzania, a peace accord was brokered between Habyarimana and the RPF. Under Chapter 6 of the UN Charter, the Security Council sent a classic peacekeeping force to Rwanda. The UN began deploying peacekeepers in November, and by mid-December about 1,300 troops were in place, including 400 of the soon-to-be 1,000-strong Belgian paratrooper unit, which was to become the strong arm of UNAMIR, the UN Assistance Mission in Rwanda peacekeeping force. By January 1994 it was obvious to Major-General Roméo Dallaire, the Canadian UNAMIR commander, that the Arusha peace accords would do little to stop unrest, as Hutu extremists felt threatened that the accords would reduce their power. UNAMIR was poorly armed, had only two working armoured personnel carriers, or APCs, and was underfunded, understaffed and under-equipped. (Its budget was approved only two days before the beginning of the genocide.) On April 5, 1994, the day before the genocide started, the UN Security Council extended by four months the mandate of the peacekeeping force that had started its piece-meal arrival only four months before.

Throughout February and March 1994, groups of Tutsis and moderate Hutus were killed, and there were targeted political assassinations in Kigali and in the south of Rwanda. Thousands of machetes were imported and distributed, and hate propaganda spilled venomously from the commercial radio station, RTLM. Arms were distributed to Interahamwe from secret caches around the country. The government clearly had no intention of honouring the Arusha Peace Agreement and instead was looking for ways to provoke an all-out military confrontation with the RPF.

None of this was known publicly at the time, but all of it was known secretly to the diplomatic and intelligence services of the United States, Belgium and France and through detailed reports by General Dallaire to the UN. The French were particularly duplicitous; according to a report of the Belgian Senate, even as they made contingency plans for the evacuation of their nationals, they secretly continued to supply arms through Zaire to the government in Rwanda. On several occasions, UNAMIR identified and seized these shipments.

Years after the genocide, it would become widely known that on January 10, 1994, an informant told Dallaire that Hutu extremists were planning the "extermination" of prominent Tutsis, were training Interahamwe militias for the extermination of up to a thousand Tutsis every twenty minutes and were planning to kill a number of Belgian peacekeepers in order to provoke the withdrawal of UN forces. Dallaire informed UN headquarters in New York in a now-famous fax dated January 11.

Dallaire wanted the UN to provide asylum for the informant. He also wanted to raid identified arms caches in order to
prevent killings of Tutsis by Hutu extremists. Because an attempt
to confiscate arms had sparked violence and subsequent failure
for the UN operation in Somalia, Kofi Annan, then head of UN
peacekeeping operations, bluntly ordered Dallaire not to intervene. Instead, Dallaire was to inform the president of Rwanda
of what he knew. Dallaire was incredulous—"dumbfounded,"
he would say to me years later. UNAMIR was all but powerless,
and its credibility quickly waned. Over the next twelve weeks,
Dallaire used the phrase "the situation is deteriorating rapidly"
eleven times, and asked six times for reinforcements and for
permission to use the full provisions of his mandate to seize
arms caches. He got neither. Instead he was told to keep talking
with the Rwandan government even while some among them
were preparing for slaughter.

The genocide started in earnest on April 6, 1994, with a missile
attack on President Habyarimana's plane as it approached the
Kigali airport. The president had been returning from a peace
conference with the Burundian president in Arusha. All aboard
the plane were killed. Roadblocks immediately went up around
the city. Within the hour, the organized massacre had begun.
Throughout Rwanda, Tutsis and moderate Hutus were systematically and meticulously butchered. According to plan, mayors
and civic officials provided Tutsi names and addresses to the
Interahamwe militia. People were killed in their homes; or
killed after being assembled in churches, schools and hospitals;
or bused or marched to pit latrines or mass graves where they
were not shot but had their hands and feet cut off and were left
to bleed to death, unable to climb out of the graves. People
often begged—and paid—to have their children shot rather
than suffer this particular terror. In the southwestern town of
Butare, the Interahamwe militia offered the Hutu mayor a

choice: he could save his Tutsi wife and children if he gave up his wife's family—both her parents and her sister—to be killed. He made the deal.

Two days after the genocide began, the RPF entered Rwanda from its stronghold in Uganda. The country was now in an all-out civil war fought while a genocide raged. Within a week, every aid agency, every embassy, all the development and cooperation missions and UN agencies had evacuated their offices. They left behind the vast majority of their Rwandan staff and abandoned the Rwandan people to their fate. After April 6, 1994, only the Red Cross, MSF, two members of the UN Advance Humanitarian Team, and the UNAMIR peacekeeping force remained in Kigali.

Three days into the killings, France, Belgium and Italy sent three thousand paratroopers into Rwanda to evacuate their citizens, while Americans left by land convoy to meet 250 U.S. Marines waiting across the border in Burundi. The French landed a C-160 transport aircraft in Kigali to extract their expatriates, together with Habyarimana's wife, sixty children from an orphanage she patronized, their thirty-four helpers and 299 other Hutus, all said to be extremists. The French didn't just remove people, they also brought supplies. The Hercules was full of munitions and arms that were moved to the Rwanda Government Forces (RGF) military base not far from the airport.

In all, 3,900 foreign citizens were evacuated. Rwandans who managed to board evacuation trucks were taken off at roadblocks and killed while French and Belgian paratroopers looked on. Within three days of the president's plane being shot down, Hervé Le Guillouzic, the Red Cross medical coordinator in Kigali, said, "Yesterday, we were talking about thousands of dead. Today we can start with tens of thousands."

By April 14, the Belgian government had pulled out their 1,000-strong paratrooper unit—the fighting capacity of the UNAMIR peacekeeping force—after ten Belgian peacekeepers were beaten, mutilated and then killed by RGF Presidential Guard soldiers and militia forces. The ten had been protecting the moderate Hutu prime minister, who was later assassinated by RGF soldiers. She was shot in the face. As a parting gesture, a beer bottle was shoved into her vagina. On the tarmac of Kigali airport, disgusted by the death of their ten comrades, the Belgian soldiers stomped on their blue UN berets. It would be learned years later that the Belgian government not only withdrew its forces but, fearing international embarrassment, lobbied the United States and the UN to shut down the entire UNAMIR mission. It turned out that the assassinations of the ten Belgian peacekeepers had been orchestrated to provoke the very response that came.

Without arms and equipment and without the paratroopers themselves, UNAMIR was effectively emasculated. After the Somali debacle only a few months before, the United States and the UN would have little appetite to intervene. On the day that the president of Rwanda's plane had been shot down, the last U.S. warships moved out of the port of Mogadishu. The Hutu extremists determined that there wasn't a political hope in hell that the ships would be turned around. The calculations were prescient and accurate. The genocide could continue unimpeded.

MSF had been working in Rwanda since 1990, giving medical aid to people displaced from their homes by a simmering civil war there and in neighbouring Burundi. By the time the genocide started, MSF had 126 expatriates and hundreds of national staff working in the country. In the previous months, with increasingly violent demonstrations, political assassinations and massacres of Tutsis, MSF had established an emergency plan with the Red Cross to deal with the escalating numbers of wounded.

The week the genocide started, the situation across the country appeared chaotic. Like other agencies, MSF was responding materially to events as best it could. In retrospect, the response of MSF was technically near perfect, but politically uninformed. Although three of MSF's five operational centres had been working in the country since 1990, there had been no systematic effort to develop a coherent political analysis. Now a reactive response to the chaos on the ground was the best MSF could do, and this meant that no one knew or was able to infer just what was happening.

When Jules called me, both MSF and the Red Cross were having trouble finding doctors willing to go to Rwanda. And with good reason. In Kigali, Red Cross ambulances were being stopped and their patients dragged out and shot. The CHK had been shelled, and when thirteen Red Cross workers and twenty-one Tutsi orphans were killed, the Red Cross denounced the killings and temporarily suspended its operations. Because of its aid to victims of violence in those early months of 1994, MSF was seen by the Rwandan government army and the Interahamwe as pro-Tutsi. By the end of the first week of the genocide, Belgian nationals, MSF clinics and MSF living quarters were being attacked. Government soldiers and militia went door to door checking identity cards against prepared lists, looking for Tutsis. MSF harboured many Tutsi national staff and their families, and they were murdered either in MSF compounds or outside their doors. MSF evacuated all but fourteen of its expatriate staff. The CHK where I had worked in 1988 was no longer a hospital but a slaughterhouse, and the hospital was abandoned altogether after the killers thanked MSF for providing "a collection point for Tutsis." An MSF team returned on April 14, to find at least one thousand dead in the morgue and the hospital grounds littered with bodies hacked by machetes.

On April 20, 1994, at the University Hospital in the southern region of Butare, Dr. Rony Zachariah of MSF saw government soldiers round up 179 men, women and children, taking them out of the hospital in groups. They were beaten and then hacked to death. "I tried to intervene with the soldiers," Dr. Zachariah

said, "but they told me that these people were on their list."
Hutus among MSF staff were given machetes and ordered to kill
their Tutsi colleagues. Those that refused were labelled Tutsi sympathizers and killed. Dr. Zachariah heard one soldier say: "This
hospital stinks of Tutsi. We must clean up." Sabine, an MSF
nurse who was pregnant at the time, was a Hutu, but her name
appeared on the typed list of the commanding government
army officer. "Her husband is a Tutsi," he said. "And his baby is
going to be a Tutsi." She was killed by machete. At the National
University, Tutsi students were rounded up and shot. The killings
were relentless and accelerating exponentially.

By the end of April, in the Butare region alone, some
100,000 Tutsis had been massacred. The Red Cross reported
that across the country hundreds of thousands had been killed.
It being impossible to work at the CHK, MSF helped the Red
Cross to set up a makeshift hospital in the abandoned Kigali
Salesian Sisters School. Together, what remained of the MSF and
the Red Cross teams managed to keep the hospital running. But
the carnage around it was horrific. Within five hundred metres
of the hospital, René Caravielle, an MSF logistician, found a
young girl, "Marie Ange, aged nine [who] was propped up
against a tree trunk . . . her legs apart, and she was covered in
excrement, sperm and blood . . . in her mouth was a penis, cut
with a machete, that of her father . . . [Nearby] in a ditch with
stinking water were four bodies cut up, piled up, [her] parents
and older brothers."

Wouter Van Empelen had escaped from Butare into
Burundi with his MSF teammates and scores of patients and
national staff by throwing handfuls of money at the
Interahamwe killing squads while leading his convoy of vehicles at full speed to the border. Once there, a priest travelling
with them threatened the border guards with eternal damna-
tion if they didn't let the convoy pass. The convoy—and the
border guards—were saved. I would learn later that an MSF

France expatriate team had passed into Tanzania but were forced to abandon their national staff at the border. At least seventeen were massacred. The fate of the remaining twenty-three was likely the same; they were never heard from again.

Between emergency shifts, even before I received Jules's first call, I had been scanning the papers for news of what was happening in Rwanda. Media coverage was superficial at best. The media was preoccupied with the election of Nelson Mandela in post-apartheid South Africa, with the Bosnian crisis in Yugoslavia, and in North America with the O.J. Simpson trial. Events in Rwanda were reported in the back pages of every major newspaper in the world, but with little practical effect. I remember reading in April 1994 about the Holocaust film *Schindler's List*, which was opening in North American theatres. Moments after the evacuation of American nationals from Rwanda had been discussed in the White House press room, the U.S. State Department spokesman Michael McCurry urged that the film be shown worldwide. As McCurry said from the White House podium, "The most effective way to avoid the recurrence of genocidal tragedy is to ensure that past acts of genocide are not forgotten."

Rather than as genocide, the killings in Rwanda were portrayed as tribal infighting, a kind of Hobbesian violence inevitable in places like Africa. A few days into the genocide, an editorial in the *Wall Street Journal* noted that in Rwanda "the nation state hasn't taken root . . . and any attempt by outsiders to provide order would be deemed 'imperialism'. . . . Where there is no state to exercise a monopoly on violence and thereby curb private violence, something like a war of all against all is the default mode. For young men living lives of idleness and insecurity with no opportunities, being part of an armed band offers an escape from tedium, the pleasures of comradeship and opportunities for enrichment. Most of all it offers a modicum of security in a world without law." And yet, the Rwandan state was alive and well, its full apparatus trained and now harnessed to carry out genocide. No one wanted to admit that Rwanda was a highly competent, highly organized dictatorial state that had become that way through years of backing by the West.

The *New York Times* was not much better in its portrayal of the killings. On April 14, it reported "tens of thousands of deaths" but labelled the killings "tribal and political violence." And yet it was no secret that what was happening in Rwanda was genocide. On April 11, 1994, Jean-Philippe Ceppi, a journalist with the French newspaper *Libération*, had described Kigali as a city filled with the sounds of screams and gunfire. He saw the massacred and their killers. "Everyone was using the word genocide," Ceppi wrote. "Everybody knew."

Once the genocide started, the UN was indeed "seized of the matter" transpiring in Rwanda. But the Security Council— with the exception of New Zealand, Argentina, the Czech Republic and Spain—refused to recognize what was happening as genocide. Even with the private political lobbying and public statements by MSF and others, the UN became little more than a cowering paper lion, offering earnest resolutions and fine humanitarian rhetoric while the superpowers pursued their national interests.

Two weeks into the massacres, on April 21—only two days after it had voted to increase the UN force in Bosnia—the Security Council voted to withdraw what remained of the UN force in Rwanda, leaving a rump of 270 soldiers to act as an "intermediary" in bringing "the two parties" to a "cease-fire" and to "assist in the resumption of humanitarian relief operations." The Red Cross denounced the UN's "effective departure" from Rwanda. And though the order came from the Security Council, Dallaire refused, stating firmly, "I will not withdraw." He and a force of 470 volunteer peacekeepers stayed, protecting thousands of civilians in Kigali who had fled to the Amahoro Stadium, the King Faisal Hospital and other sites around the city. Dallaire persistently used the small number of journalists in the country to draw attention to the genocide and to the need to reinforce UNAMIR. For Dallaire, the media was "worth two battalions on the ground." But all this was to no avail. In the wake of the neutering April 21 resolution, mass killings inside Rwanda skyrocketed.

MSF and others scrambled to somehow change the climate of apparent indifference and feigned political powerlessness in the face of obvious genocide. Dr. Rony Zachariah and his MSF team managed to escape from the Butare region into Burundi, and told the world what they had seen. At a press conference in Brussels on April 28, the president of MSF Belgium, Reginald Moreels, labelled events in Rwanda as genocide. The day before, MSF had sent its general director, Jean-Pierre Luxen, to lobby the UN for the establishment of humanitarian corridors and civilian protection zones inside Rwanda. Luxen met with representatives of the American government and the president of the Security Council, New Zealand ambassador Colin Keating. The Belgian UN ambassador described Luxen's reports as "a knock out" that stunned the Security Council into silence, before it asked for an explanation from the Rwandan ambassador.

Keating pushed hard for the council to recognize genocide. The permanent five members—the great powers—would have none of it. Only after Keating threatened to publicly expose the council's debate did it agree that it would issue a statement. It would not, however, agree to use the word *genocide*. The April 30 statement condemned the breaches of humanitarian law in Rwanda, "recalling" that "the killing of members of an ethnic group with the intention of destroying such a group" was a "crime punishable under international law."

By recalling wording from the 1948 UN Convention on the Prevention and Punishment of Genocide while not naming the convention itself, nor naming the events in Rwanda as a genocide, the Security Council freed itself from the obligation to enforce the law against genocide.

By early May, with more than a million people displaced throughout the country, and with only eleven MSF expatriates able to work inside Rwanda, the organization expanded its teams in Tanzania, Burundi and Zaire to give assistance to Rwandan refugees fleeing the genocide. The fifteen journalists in Rwanda competed with the hundreds of journalists flocking from South Africa—its first multiparty elections now over—to Tanzania. The refugees, not the genocide, became the prominent story.

Throughout May, MSF, Oxfam, Human Rights Watch and Amnesty International publicly and repeatedly called for both firm political pressure on the genocidal government and immediate UN action in Rwanda to protect civilians. It was not an easy sell. Nothing could happen without the permanent five of the Security Council on board, and most especially the United States. With the image of a dead naked ranger being dragged through the streets of Mogadishu still fresh in American minds, the United States wanted to minimize its involvement in UN peacekeeping crises that were not in its immediate interests. Rwanda was not on the Clinton administration's list of major issues. The president's national security adviser, Anthony Lake, was consumed by the crises in Bosnia and Haiti. James Woods in the Defense Department's Bureau of African Affairs was told by his superiors that "if something happens in Rwanda-Burundi, we don't care. Take it off the list. U.S. national interest is not involved and we can't put all these silly humanitarian issues on lists . . . just make it go away."

On May 3, 1994, Clinton signed Presidential Decision Directive 25. It had been informal policy since October 1993, and in the wake of Somalia was designed to severely limit U.S. military involvement in international peacekeeping operations: "It is not U.S. policy to seek to expand either the number of UN peace operations or U.S. involvement in such operations." With PDD 25, for the Clinton administration Rwanda and its genocide went away and would stay away—at least until it was over.

But with growing international public and political pressure from MSF and others, the UN could no longer be seen to be passive. On May 17, still refusing to use the word *genocide,* the Security Council passed a resolution that would in theory expand UNAMIR, giving it a more explicit mandate to use force to protect civilians and the firepower and equipment to do so. The vote had been delayed three full days by the United States, which said it didn't have instructions from Washington on how to proceed. Among the last-minute changes to the resolution that the Americans had insisted upon was the stipulation that UNAMIR's new mandate would not be implemented until the Security Council had had the chance to review the situation further. Thus, even though the resolution authorized supplies, trucks, fifty armoured personnel carriers and 5,500 troops, in practice it was a farce. In the words of Security Council president Colin Keating, the United States had "essentially gutted the resolution . . . in reality the expansion [is] a fiction."

Not only did the great powers oppose the drive to stop the genocide, they actively obstructed, if not outright sabotaged, efforts to strengthen UNAMIR. While the May 17 resolution had imposed an arms embargo against the Rwandan government, secretly the French continued to send arms. As President Mitterrand declared on French television, "Our soldiers cannot be expected to become arbiters of the passions that are tearing apart so many countries." Meanwhile, the United States refused to jam the hate propaganda broadcasts on RTLM radio that incited people to kill Tutsis, saying such action would be a violation of international law. And both the U.S. and the U.K. used bureaucratic stall tactics to delay the delivery to UNAMIR of arms and equipment.

By now MSF had a concerted international campaign calling on governments and the UN to stop the genocide. On May 16, Dr. Jean-Hervé Bradol, then operations director at MSF Paris, returned from Kigali and declared on French television, "It is genocide . . . France knows the murderers very well, it arms them and equips them—we consider this to be a veritable policy of incitement . . . We have not heard the French state calling on the butchers of Kigali and Butare to restrain themselves and we have to stress that we are extremely shocked by this aspect of things." The next day MSF France published an open letter to President Mitterrand in the French daily Le Monde saying that "France—that bastion of human rights—has a serious responsibility . . . in Rwanda" and insisting that Mitterrand intervene against the "systematic, pro-grammed extermination of opponents by a faction supported and armed by France." On May 23, the New York Times published a letter to the editor from the MSF international secretary protesting the inadequacy of the UN Security Council's response to genocide and calling for urgent measures to stop it. On May 24, MSF made a formal submission to the UN Human Rights Commission on Rwanda. After hearing Dr. Zachariah's descriptions of events in Rwanda, the Canadian government called for an emergency ses-sion and special rapporteur to determine whether a genocide was in fact taking place in Rwanda.

Jules wanted me on standby, to be available to go as soon as it was possible to work and to assume the role of head of mission in Kigali. He wanted me to lead a surgical team and open the as yet never used King Faisal Hospital, where the UN was now pro-tecting six thousand civilians. I was to get medical care to as many people inside the city as possible. By mid-May, 500,000 had been massacred. I would leave for Rwanda a few days later. By early June I would be in Kigali.

Why did I go? I knew people in Rwanda—nurses, doctors and others at the Centre Hospitalier de Kigali, many of them Tutsis—people like my friend Paul, the doctor I had had a farewell dinner with a week before leaving Rwanda in 1988, and Thérèse, the nurse who had worked for Susan Allen. I trusted Jules implicitly. I had seen him in operation in Somalia and Afghanistan. He cared. He was smart and prudent, and he would never ask anyone to take a risk he himself was not prepared to take. If it proved impossible to work, then so be it. I was thirty-three, single and free. If I didn't at least try, I knew I could not live with myself. In theory I knew where I was going, but in retrospect, I had no idea.

I travelled to Europe with another Canadian, Jonathan Brock. A twenty-nine-year-old logistician, he had worked with MSF before and was studying medicine. He had prepared hastily for the trip and hadn't had his immunization shots, but brought the vaccines with him. I administered them to him in a bathroom at the airport moments before we boarded our plane. We were both nervous. I reassured him that I had every intention of returning home to Canada, and that we would stay only as long as it was possible to work.

Ten hours later we were in the MSF Amsterdam office. We met with team members Efke Bakke, a Dutch nurse who had worked in Liberia, and Eric Vreede, a Dutch anesthesiologist and former surgical resident with an unusually jovial disposition. We had coffee with Jules while he briefed me and then the others on the latest developments. The situation was changing rapidly. The Kigali airport, because of heavy shelling, was closed. "It's not clear that we can get in," said Jules. "Or that you'd want to," said someone from the emergency team who was passing through the office.

"Let's see what's possible, but only what's possible," I said.

"Of course. It's the only thing we can do," said Jules.

We left for Nairobi the next day. The team was anxious, but most managed to sleep on the plane. I didn't. Instead I pored over whatever documents Jules had been able to give me.

UN flights from Nairobi to Kigali were still suspended, so we stayed in a Nairobi hotel that night. We met some of the MSF Nairobi team for drinks and went over communication and logistics details with Juliana, the coordinator. The next morning, we flew from Nairobi to Uganda's Entebbe airport and then took a UN helicopter to Kabale, still in Uganda, where we stayed overnight at the Highland Hotel. I spent most of the early night trying to find a working phone to call MSF headquarters in Amsterdam. Later I checked the emergency supplies I had brought from Toronto, a personal supply for use on teammates or myself if needed. I had learned in Somalia not to depend on anyone other than myself. Most of what I had— broad-spectrum antibiotics, IV lines, ventilation tubes, plasma expander, a homemade mini surgical kit—had been given to me by the nurses at the emergency room where I had been working. I showed the kit to Eric so that he would know what we had in case he needed it.

The following morning we had a quick breakfast and made our way to the UN helicopter pad at Kabale to be picked up by a UNAMIR vehicle. We were nervous, even more so when we met some of the UN soldiers stationed at Kabale. The two Ghanaians were serious and sombre and had none of the bravado that I had seen so often among UN soldiers in Somalia. Though they were outside Rwanda, they knew only too well what was happening inside. The border, marked only by a knotted wooden pole over a dirt road, was a faint barrier between Rwanda and the rest of the world.

We drove with UN personnel over the border into the Akagara region of Rwanda, now controlled by the rebel Tutsi RPF army. We were in a Volkswagen minibus, driven by a Swiss UN security officer. His sweat showed through his shirt and his green safari vest. He smoked constantly. He and the minibus stank of Gitanes. As we drove through the region—a game park in northeast Rwanda—we saw bloated bodies in the river.

Swarms of flies hung in black tornadoes over corpses that had been snagged in branches along the shoreline. A feeling of stillness was everywhere, and the Volkswagen engine squealed along in a high-pitched diesel rev. The wind carried the semisweet rancid smell of rotting flesh. The driver lit another cigarette. The vehicle slowed as we approached a major pothole, and the sunlight glistened in a pool of blood on the road. Flies swarmed around the human meat that had been dragged to the roadside by a pack of wild dogs. Fat and calm, the dogs tore at chunks of flesh. As we entered a long stretch of road free of bodies, somebody spotted a herd of zebras. He wanted to take a photo. We stopped. We could see small cooking fires in the distance, and people ran away when they saw us. Vultures were sitting on tree branches, or hovering overhead. Surreal, fucking surreal, I thought. For the rest of the journey we were mute, not because we could not speak but because speaking would never be enough.

We passed through fourteen military checkpoints in the two-hour journey along the road to Kigali. This was a seriously guarded road. As we entered Kigali, formerly a city of 350,000 people, the only people we saw were the corpses on the street and in the gutters. The stench of death was everywhere. I lit a cigarette. We passed a pickup truck with about ten RPF soldiers in the back. "Some of this is RPF territory," our driver said. "Here, we are now their sometimes unwelcome guests." As we neared the UNAMIR headquarters, I could see the damage that had been done to the hilltop parliament building by heavy shelling. I looked out the open window, taking shorter breaths to somehow stop the smell from entering me. I held each breath a little longer. The breeze helped, but not much.

The Red Cross had organized the removal of most of the bodies from the early weeks of the genocide, about 100,000 in the city of Kigali alone. What we were seeing and smelling now were relatively fresh kills. I looked at the corpse of a woman on the side of the road. Her face had been torn off by wild dogs; her clothing was soaked with the leaking body fluid of the dead. I tried to remember why I was here.

We approached the UNAMIR headquarters, and I had to get focused. I lit another cigarette. MSF had five people staying with UNAMIR on the RPF side of the front line and four on the RGF side, working at the Red Cross hospital. My first task was to talk to all of them to figure out what was actually happening. We pulled into the heavily sandbagged headquarters. The walls of the main four-storey building—a hotel in its former life—had been shelled and were patched with scrap wood. Most of its windows were blown out and sealed with sandbags, the remaining ones striped with duct tape to stop glass from exploding into rooms. Rows of slightly used white UN jeeps and pickup trucks sat in the parking lot. Two soldiers sat atop a white APC with the black UN logo painted on its sides. One smoked, the other glared at us as we pulled in. I noticed the MSF logo on the doors of two of the vehicles. One of them, a Toyota Hilux pickup, had a flat tire. Two well-groomed Bangladeshi UN officers with clipboards were checking the engines and recording the licence plate numbers: "I'm checking for broken or missing bits," one told me in a thick Bangladeshi accent. "But I am guessing, you see. We can't start the engines. We don't have enough fuel."

Don MacNeil, a tanned, slightly dishevelled middle-aged Canadian, was second-in-command for UNAMIR's humanitarian operations. Cigarette in hand, MacNeil was listening to me talk to the Bangladeshis. He introduced himself to us. "Welcome to hell with no fuel," he said, reaching to shake my hand. The mood was matter of fact, as MacNeil turned to our Swiss driver, now more relaxed inside the compound. "How was the drive?"

"Not too bad," the driver said. "Not too many more bodies this time." Christ, I thought, how bad had it been?

Pepijn Boot, a logistician and one of the five MSF people on the RPF side of the front line, wanted to take me immediately to the Amahoro Stadium. Dirt was worn into the creases of his hands and up his forearms, his hair was greasy and unwashed, and his MSF T-shirt was stained with sweat and ochre-red soil. He made only a cursory effort to greet us, and his blue eyes looked through me as he insisted we go immediately to the stadium. We could travel only when a vehicle was free and a UN soldier available to drive. Boot had been in Rwanda only a week, but he seemed disoriented, desperate and confused.

The thirty-thousand-seat stadium, about a kilometre from the UNAMIR headquarters, had been turned into a logistics base for UNAMIR. Scores of damaged UN trucks, a few APCs and other white UN vehicles lined the playing field and, with no repair parts available, sat useless. "There's no fuel for these either," Pepijn said. The stadium also housed Tutsis who had fled the Interahamwe death squads and the Rwandan government army, and Hutus afraid of the advancing RPF, which was now in control of the territory around the stadium. Anyone who left would be killed outside. "There are about twelve thousand people here," Boot said. "We're trying to dig latrines, but we don't have enough shovels."

The stadium stank of shit, of old blood and of death. In the stands, people sat listlessly staring at us from under blue plastic tarps propped up with sticks. A few tarps fluttered in the light breeze as men tried to re-tie them with strips of torn cloth. People had ferreted out and defended their territory—the more powerful under the open-air stands, the weaker on them. Pepijn was alone, doing what he could for the people in the stadium. It wasn't for lack of trying, but it wasn't much.

What was called a clinic was set up in a changing room beneath the stands. Some two hundred people were crowded into a room designed for no more than thirty. The air was thick with the smell of too many people in too small a space for too long. The room was dark. Only occasionally did sunlight glisten through the door onto the olive-green walls. There were no beds, and only a few blankets wet with shit. A woman passed by me with a bucket of urine and feces as she walked out to the freshly dug latrines that Pepijn was organizing to the side of the playing field. A man writhed in pain; a woman sat with her screaming child. Another man, drenched in sweat, his legs covered in diarrhea, cried deliriously for water. "Agwa, agwa, agwa." I wanted to vomit.

"This woman is a nurse," Pepijn said quietly. She looked at me. Her eyes were empty. In one hand she had a half-full bucket of water with a UN seal on it, in the other a red plastic cup. She stepped over bodies, some sleeping, some moving, some dead, and walked towards the man screaming for water. "They bring only the sickest here, usually just before they die," Pepijn told me. "Moving the dead is a problem. Sometimes it takes days. We need everything: medicines, blankets, plastic sheeting, lumber for latrines, shovels." He paused, again his blue eyes looking through me. "We have nothing."

When I returned to the UNAMIR compound, Steven Kyler, a water and sanitation specialist on the MSF emergency team, approached me. He had been here two weeks. His fingernails were uncut, with almost half an inch of overgrowth, and his eyes darted about relentlessly. His words wandered in a kind of free association that would stop suddenly as he encountered a thought he could not express, and his eyes would look somewhere else.

Among other things, Steven was responsible for emergency preparations for the team's safety. He had made none. There was no water, no fuel, no food, no maps and no emergency medical supplies. There was no evacuation plan, other than the plan to make a plan. We had two vehicles, and as I now knew, one had a flat tire and neither had fuel.

We went upstairs to an office that had been hastily set up

on the third floor for MSF. The five-member team was living there. Some UN troops were housed above us, with more living quarters and offices—including Major-General Dallaire's—below. The office was a mess, and UNAMIR's was not in much better shape, even though it had been cleaned up after being shelled several times since the beginning of the genocide. There was no running water for drinking or sewage. The smell from the toilets that some still used, combined with the smell of hastily established latrines, left the place reeking of shit and not enough chlorine.

I met Giovanni Gabrini, an Italian surgeon, his wife, Dana Turati, a surgical nurse, and Jacques Ramsey, a doctor and the last of the five MSF expatriates on the RPF side of the front line. They had arrived a few days before us and were staying at the UNAMIR HQ. Jacques smiled warmly and appeared organized and determined. He was keen to get the King Faisal Hospital up and running. Neither of the UN's two functioning APCs was available, so after ensuring that everyone's flak jacket was the right fit, we made the three-kilometre drive to the hospital in a UN Land Cruiser driven by a soldier. We passed through several roundabouts and along a heavily shelled road, the actual front line between the RPF and the RGF.

As part of the Arusha Accords, the RPF had a battalion stationed inside Kigali to protect their political delegates. They had moved in a few days before the genocide began. In the early weeks of the genocide, Paul Kagame had broken a path to them from Uganda, creating a forward thrust for his advancing forces, who pushed to isolate the RGF forces inside the capital from those outside it. By late May the RGF's best troops—its Presidential Guard and four battalions of gendarmerie—had combined with the Interahamwe to launch a counteroffensive. Beyond Kigali the RPF were pushing the RGF to the west. The Interahamwe continued to massacre Tutsis as the RGF moved in behind it, and reports were coming into UNAMIR that as the RPF advanced, it was killing former Hutu government employees, agents and their families. Around the country the RPF put restrictions on where UNAMIR military inspectors could go, allegedly in an effort to conceal their activities, especially massacres.

In Kigali, most of the soldier-to-soldier combat took place at night. The fight between the two forces was in full swing, with the RPF making significant gains. In some areas the RGF was in retreat. Looting, mutiny and desertion were not uncommon. By day, snipers from both sides were holed up in abandoned houses and in trenches along the sides of the road. They could—and often did—fire at anyone or any vehicle that moved. We drove at full speed, slowing only as we approached the hospital gates.

The Faisal Hospital was a brand-new 150-bed facility that had never been used. It had been slated to open in June. It was well designed, and the beds and much of the equipment needed for a hospital were in the basement storage. Now the building was home to six thousand people seeking refuge from the killing squads and the civil war that raged beyond its grounds. Most had come from the district around the hospital in the early days of the genocide. A group of eleven Tunisian UN soldiers offered a veneer of protection from what was happening outside. Every room of the hospital's four floors was packed with people. Some still managed to get into the grounds, mostly at night, but as the city emptied and the fighting intensified, fewer and fewer did.

There were no beds on the wards. Blankets, pots, pans and whatever people could take with them as they fled covered every inch of floor space. The balconies, hallways, broom closets, stairwells and washrooms were packed with people who, lacking running water, had been unable to bathe for nearly two months. UNAMIR and the Red Cross had supplied a few small generators to power too few water pumps. Tents had been set up inside the perimeter of the six-foot wire-mesh fence that surrounded the hospital grounds. Cooking fires dotted the periphery of the building and the grounds of the open atrium at the centre of the building. The smell of burning wood was a welcome reprieve.

Inside, untreated sick and wounded were everywhere. Many people lay dying among those who just needed a place on the floor for their blankets and cooking pots. Ten minutes after arriving, I looked into one of the packed rooms and saw a woman with a club wound to her head lying on the floor convulsing in a seizure. One medical assistant and a few nurses lived among the people in the hospital grounds. They had done what they could and were overwhelmed.

As I was leaving to go back to UNAMIR HQ, I saw a young boy being chased by a group of older boys. They threw rocks at him as he ran to the UN guardhouse by the hospital gate, and he sat on the curb crying while the older boys jeered at him. I went over to him, and he told me his name was Lulu. He was

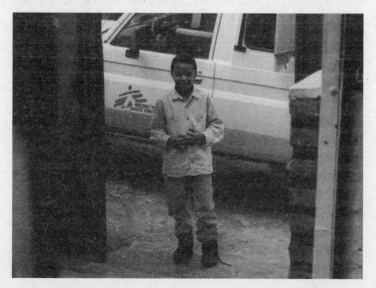

Lulu

nearly five years old and a Métis—half white and half Rwandan. Métis were given a rough ride in Rwanda in the best of times. I would learn later that his father was Belgian—so, whether his mother was Tutsi or Hutu, Lulu's was a deadly paternity. I sat with him for a moment, and he played with my pen. I asked him to hold on to it until I returned.

We drove at full speed back to the UNAMIR HQ, where I met with Don MacNeil. I already knew that it was too danger-ous to stay at the hospital overnight. "No way," MacNeil said, lighting a cigarette. "You'd be stupid. There's too much shelling and mortar fire at night, and if the shit hits the fan we don't have the firepower to send in a team to get your people out. And you can't come out on your own—there's heavy fighting all along that road at night. You don't want to be meeting any Interahamwe at the midnight hour. And if the front line shifts and some of the road falls to the RGF, you'd be fucked for sure. But it's up to you." MacNeil explained the radio system, which we synchronized with the MSF radios and walkie-talkies. His call sign was "Momma Poppa One," Dallaire's "Momma Poppa Zero" and MSF's "Momma Poppa Nine."

MacNeil described who held what territory in the city and where things were changing. The Faisal Hospital was now right at the margin of the front line, and the Red Cross hospi-tal was well within RGF territory. "The Faisal has taken a few hits, but no one has shelled the Red Cross hospital since early May," he said. "But the RGF is not too happy with MSF for call-ing them génocidaires and calling for UN intervention. The RPF is on an offensive. They are gradually taking the city, but that might change."

"What do you mean?" I asked.

"The French are playing games," MacNeil said. "They have spooks everywhere and are still getting arms through the embargo to the RGF. The RPF isn't too happy with MSF either. You know, the whole French thing. We'll see what happens."

The RGF and the Interahamwe were faltering militarily, but were relentless in their killing of Tutsi civilians. On the wall map of the city, MacNeil pointed to orphanages, churches, diplomatic compounds, an embassy house and the CHK hospital, places where people had gathered and that were sometimes within UNAMIR's reach. People were also hiding in houses throughout the city, many in the Kimihurura district where I had lived in 1988.

From the beginning of the genocide, more than ten thousand people had been rescued by UNAMIR soldiers who had nothing more than sidearms. Now, though UNAMIR knew there were people at each of these sites, the killing squads prevented their transfer to safe areas. Occasionally they were still able to get a few people out, but not many. "We don't even have enough fucking helmets. Hold on to that flak jacket—it's a hot item and there are no replacements," MacNeil said as he finished his third cigarette.

For anyone trapped in the city, to venture out meant certain death, but to stay was to wait for death. The RGF and Interahamwe surrounded the sites by day, or they weren't far off, showing up within minutes if anyone tried to escape. They would kill Tutsis and moderate Hutus between dusk and dawn. At this point, MacNeil explained, UNAMIR was down to fewer than 470 peacekeepers and was waiting for its newly promised fuel, weapons, supplies and reinforcements. Until these arrived, UNAMIR would at best be in a holding pattern, and if things got much worse, MacNeil said, "who knows?" It was not an inspiring meeting.

It was too dangerous for the MSF team to move around freely outside of the small area that UNAMIR occupied in RPF territory, and no one was allowed to go anywhere without my permission. For the most part, we travelled in UNAMIR vehicles with peacekeepers as our drivers. If we were crossing the front line, we travelled in an APC if one was available. There were only

two that worked, and these were for the entire UNAMIR operation across the country. Occasionally, we had no choice but to
move in "found" vehicles or those we "borrowed" from the UN
or the Red Cross.

MacNeil organized an APC to take me across the front line
to the Red Cross hospital. I wanted to meet the MSF team working there, and Philippe Gaillard, the head of mission for the
Red Cross. From inside the APC I couldn't see what was going
on outside, except through a small slit of bulletproof glass in
the armoured door. This didn't help me see much as snipers'
bullets ricocheted off our thick metal box as we rumbled up
and down hills, over potholed and shelled roads. After the third
bullet, I wanted to smoke, but the driver reminded me it was
against the rules.

We rattled up the final hill to the Red Cross hospital and
turned through the main gates in the surrounding brick wall.
Formerly a school, the makeshift hospital was made up of a
number of classroom buildings on a hillside, with administration offices just off the road near the bottom of the hill. It was
heavily sandbagged and clearly marked with twenty-square-foot
Red Cross flags on the roofs, walls and in the trees surrounding
the school compound. Like the Faisal, the hospital was densely
crowed, with about 2,500 people living in tents or in shelters
between the classrooms that served as hospital wards. MSF and
the Red Cross had been doing surgery here since the first week
of the genocide. Hutus and Tutsis had fled here as they had to
the Faisal, but many more injured had been brought here
because it was a functioning hospital. People were treated for
wounds inflicted by machetes, for injuries to their limbs caused
by the blasts of grenades and land mines, for bullet and shrapnel injuries and for crushed-chest injuries caused by being
buried alive. After surgery, the wounded had nowhere to go and
joined the others seeking refuge.

I met Philippe Gaillard. He had been in Rwanda for more

than seven months. He was a thin, bearded, dark-haired man with nicotine-stained hands and kind, intelligent eyes. No matter what the circumstance, he wore a tie and a brown blazer with the Red Cross pocket insignia. He looked nearly skeletal even under his blazer. He smoked constantly. We shook hands warmly, and I liked him immediately. He noted that the shelling around the city was getting closer to the hospital. "There is no getting through this, James. There is only being in it. If necessary we will get your people out," he assured me. "UNAMIR has promised us this. All we need do is ask."

Having seen the condition of UNAMIR, I wasn't satisfied. I wanted to better understand the situation for the MSF surgical team of four French expatriates: Patrick Henaux, an anesthetist; Madeline Boyer and Isabelle Lemasson, two surgical nurses; and Gilbert Hascoet, a logistician. I spoke at length with Gilbert, the team co-coordinator. He had worked in Mozambique with MSF during its civil war. He was very practical.

There were large numbers of Tutsis in the hospital who couldn't leave. The majority of the hospital patients were Hutus who had been wounded in the RPF offensive. Given MSF's repeated calls for UN intervention to stop the genocide and for the French president to intervene personally with the Rwandan regime to stop the killings, MSF was de facto seen by RGF and its militias as pro-Tutsi. The MSF team had gathered up all stickers, T-shirts and anything else with MSF insignia in the hospital, and they were now wearing the Red Cross insignia, but everyone knew MSF was working in the hospital. Gilbert felt that for now, while the Interahamwe and RGF were still respecting the Red Cross hospital, it was possible to work. We talked about contingency plans for the MSF team's evacuation. He agreed that they would be packed and ready to go at any time.

I returned in the APC to the Faisal to collect my team. Lulu was waiting for me at the main gate. He smiled as he gave me back my pen. I walked with him to the hospital building. His mother had been frantic for the last few hours. She was angry with her son but obviously relieved to find him. She cried as she picked him up and disappeared into the crowd.

We returned to UNAMIR headquarters and I spent the better part of that night on the satellite phone with Jules in Amsterdam. There was heavy shelling in the city as I outlined the situation and we planned for the next few days. It wasn't possible to plan any further.

We returned the next morning to the Faisal Hospital. Our nurse, Efke, moved out the people living in the operating room and arranged to get it cleaned and ready for use. Within hours, Eric and Giovanni started surgery on the most severely wounded. From among the people living in the hospital, Efke found those with medical experience to help. I went into the operating room to assist Giovanni and Eric with a difficult patient. A tall Rwandan woman stood by the operating table, and when she saw me she started to cry. "It's you, it's you, Dr. James." It was Thérèse, the nurse I had known in 1988. We embraced. Now we were both crying. Thérèse had been separated from her Tutsi husband and her children. She didn't know if they were alive or dead.

Over the next week, we established the Faisal as a functioning hospital. People were moved out of wards and into other rooms, the wards were cleaned, and pediatric, post-op and adult wards were established. Jacques was responsible for the adult wards, Eric and Giovanni for the surgery and post-operative wards, and I was responsible for the children's ward.

There were some eighty patients on the children's ward. Giovanni had operated on some of them, but most were suffering from malnutrition, diarrhea or untreated malaria. My first patient was a three-year-old boy with a massive abscess in the space between his lung and chest wall. It had developed around shrapnel embedded in his chest. After cleaning out the shrapnel, I put a chest tube in to drain the pus. Most of the children

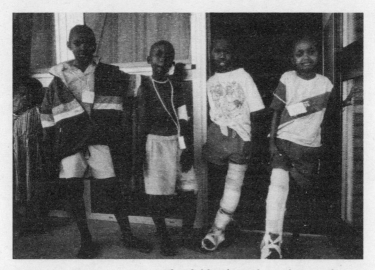

The children's ward, Faisal Hospital

had relatively minor injuries from machetes and clubs, which I stitched and dressed.

Eli, a seventy-year-old Hutu man, organized some of the women living in the hospital to feed and bathe the children. Eli limped slightly and had sad, bloodshot eyes. He had been a cleaner at an MSF clinic in Kigali before the genocide started. I would know nothing more about him, except that he always wore a white lab coat that he had found somewhere, and that he was the only person who had a kerosene lantern. I watched him from afar early one morning as he attempted to re-tape the piece of wood I had taped behind a child's elbow to keep her arm extended for an IV line the day before. He soothed the child as he worked. He was not a nurse, but he tried. Someone had to. I trusted him. He was the self-appointed guardian for the children—and a good one—especially at night. No one got on the ward except through Eli.

Shelling and mortar fire around the hospital was a major problem, so we created bomb shelters around heavily reinforced concrete pillars between the floors and around stairwells. We vaccinated all children in the hospital against measles and tetanus, and established an orphanage on the top floor for those without parents and who had no serious medical or surgical needs. With the help of the Red Cross, we set up a water system for the entire hospital. By the time it was finished, the multiple hoses connecting bladder tanks on each of the four balconies and on the grass of the hospital grounds looked like a family of very large spiders crawling up the side of the building. Despite this progress, though, we were running short of medical supplies, as was the Red Cross. The airport was still being shelled. No UNAMIR flights could get in.

Every morning I attended the UNAMIR "morning prayers," the daily briefing with General Dallaire and his command team. Before or after the meeting I would meet with Colonel Yaache, a Ghanaian who was first in charge, or Don MacNeil to coordinate our movements and, when possible, to plan beyond a three-day horizon. I would also talk with the fifteen journalists, all of whom were living at the UNAMIR compound, to give and get information, or with Maj. Frank Kamanzi, the RPF liaison officer to UNAMIR. I never met with any RGF officials, as they refused to post anyone at UNAMIR.

The international campaign by MSF and others was having some effect. In early June, MSF argued publicly that doctors could not stop a genocide and demanded UN protection of civilians. On June 8 the Security Council had voted to expand UNAMIR and authorized it to establish and protect "secure areas" for civilians inside Rwanda. But rhetoric, no matter how fine the words, does not change much. Dallaire was still waiting for the first soldiers of the 5,500 reinforcements promised in the May 17 UN resolution. The UN, and most especially the Americans, still refused to recognize genocide. Two days after the May 17 resolution, the U.S. State Department insisted that "although there have been acts of genocide in Rwanda, all the murders cannot be put into that category." They were playing word games to avoid the legal obligation to intervene forcefully and immediately.

At morning prayers, reports were read from UNAMIR military observers who were on the borders and around the country, describing RGF and RPF troop movements, advances and losses. There were now an estimated one and a half million displaced people in Rwanda, and a minimum estimate of half a million refugees in Tanzania. Tutsis were moving into northeast Rwanda from Uganda, as displaced Hutus moved west towards Zaire. The RGF was openly hostile to UNAMIR, firing on its vehicles and blocking any effort to exchange Tutsis and Hutus trapped in the city. In the face of the UN's decision to not stop the genocide, the RPF had decided to stop it themselves and worked to keep UNAMIR out of the way. It restricted UNAMIR's movements around the country, and insisted on controlling aid in the regions the RPF held. With continued shelling at the airport, UNAMIR's overland supply routes were sporadic at best. Uganda blocked the UN from monitoring arms movements to the RPF from across its border. In the early days of June, UNAMIR had only a few days' worth of food and water left, and at one point, only two days' worth of fuel for its force of 470. And like that force of 470, our MSF team was now living on expired UNAMIR rations of beans, sardines, canned sausages and cherry pound cake from Germany.

Major massacres and all planned exchanges of Tutsis from one site for Hutus from another were reported at these morning briefings. The political gyrations of the UN and the international community were described every day. One day, we learned that the UN Human Rights Commission was sending an envoy team to Rwanda to determine if in fact a genocide was taking place. After this announcement, an officer leaned over and whispered to me, "No shit, Sherlock. Where the fuck have they been for the last two months?" The local and international media were also monitored. The daily reports of UNAMIR's repeated demand for the UN or others to jam the hate radio of RTLM had become farcical.

On one occasion it was announced that the UN Department of Peacekeeping Operations support team in Nairobi would not authorize more food and water for UNAMIR because the requisition forms had not been filled out according to procedure and, anyway, UNAMIR was short of cash. Staff in Nairobi would seek advice from New York on Monday, but probably wouldn't get an answer until Tuesday, as the contact person was going to be away. It might be Wednesday. Dallaire immediately stood up and bellowed, "Who the fuck are these people? Don't they get it? The Interahamwe works on Sundays, and so do we."

The situation was not good. No incoming flights, an inept UN peacekeeping administration, political malfeasance at and around the Security Council, shortages of fuel, food, water and reinforcements—UNAMIR was living on borrowed time. And for all practical purposes, with or without UNAMIR, so were we. I had the MSF team prepare to leave at a moment's notice.

I met with Dallaire in his office to discuss the evacuation of the French MSF expatriates at the Red Cross hospital. Dallaire was firmly in command of his troops, and clearly respected. He was trim, well groomed, obviously tired and absolutely focused. He was sombre and listened carefully as I described the situation at the Red Cross hospital. He knew it well. Gaillard had been right: Dallaire would get them out. "The key is to not wait until it is too late," he said.

"Have we not already passed that point?" I asked.

"Look, I want them to stay," Dallaire said, "but if and when your team goes is up to you. You tell me. As long as I am here, I'll move them, even if it gets beyond 'too late.' That I promise you."

It was nearly impossible to move around the city. Snipers

were everywhere. The RPF were disciplined, bold and unwavering. They used guerrilla warfare and shock raids to advance through the city. They shelled and infiltrated RGF strongholds at night, and returned heavy fire during the day to hold the positions just won. Slowly, inexorably, they were wearing down their enemy.

About 50,000 people remained in Kigali. Of these, an estimated 25,000 were hiding in the attics of houses, in the pits of latrines, or in the brush and ravines that cover the city. Getting to them was nearly impossible. People drank sewage water and ate tree bark or what foliage they could find if they dared venture out at night. Most didn't dare; everyone starved and many died.

One afternoon I managed to get to the CHK. It had been ransacked and was deserted. I was afraid to go too far inside the grounds. I lit a cigarette and summoned the courage to go in to my old pediatrics ward, near the front of the complex. Blood splatters covered the floor and the yellow walls. I heard a noise, the sound of something big moving farther inside. I was scared; my hands sweated and I could feel my heart pounding. The sound was coming from the ceiling. I called softly, "Est quelqu'un ici? Quelqu'un? Je suis un médecin avec MSF." More noise, and then a few moments later, two men, a father and his teenage son, came in from the next room. They were clearly starving. They had been watching me from a hole in the ceiling tiles.

"Vous êtes seul, Docteur?" the father asked.

"Oui," I replied. "How long have you been here?" I asked in French. He looked at me quizzically. His son's lips quivered as he held on to his father's arm and stared at me with eyes nearly wild with fear. His father's were the saddest eyes I have ever seen.

"I can't remember," he answered.

"Are there others?" I asked.

He didn't know. "We stay only here, up there," he said,

pointing to the ceiling. He looked to his son, and then to me, and asked, "Quelles nouvelles?"

"Ça continue," I said. They wouldn't leave with me—they were too afraid. But the father asked me to return with food. I told him I would try but that I couldn't promise. He said he understood. He asked me for a cigarette. I gave him my pack.

UNAMIR was in constant negotiations to arrange temporary ceasefires along the roads and through the Interahamwe checkpoints. Even then, vehicles were often fired on. When we could get through to the gathering sites, we could do little more than bring a few medical supplies and some food, and assure people that they were not forgotten. Dallaire frequently sent media on these "drop-ins," if only to remind the Interahamwe and the RGF that the world was watching, and that these particular people at this particular site were now known to exist.

One late afternoon I went to College St. André, a church and school in the Nyamirambo district of Kigali, to try to give medical care to a group of children trapped in the compound. I went in an APC with Luc Racine, a UNAMIR military observer for Kigali. We weren't sure whether we would be able to get there. I couldn't see much through the slit in the APC door, nor could I hear what was going on over the sound of the engine. I could see the faces and muscled arms of men as we stopped and started through each Interahamwe checkpoint.

When we got to St. André, only a few Interahamwe were scattered on the road outside the compound wall. Inside, the children were in a terrible condition. They had little food or water. They were all at least partially malnourished, and all had scabies and torn, stinking clothes. Many had malaria or pneumonia if not both, and some had knife or machete wounds and injuries from beatings. All had timid, scared eyes. They huddled together in small clusters in the row of open-door rooms and around doorways, afraid to go out into the compound or anywhere near the wall or its gate.

I went into the priest's small room. He sat on a bed clutching his crucifix, holding it tight to his chest as he mumbled a prayer, his eyes open. He was a white Frenchman who looked about forty-five years old. He was emaciated, his hair shoulder length and unkempt, his black beard nearly down to his chest. His feet were dirty and bare, except for thick leather sandals. I tried talking with him, but he wouldn't interrupt his prayer. I stayed for a few minutes and waited. I looked at a picture of Jesus on his wall opposite the small bed. It was the only picture in the room. When I eventually started to leave, he stopped me. "Merci, merci, merci pour l'arrivée." He could tell by the stethoscope around my neck that I was a doctor and he said in French, "We need medicines for the children. The children are sick. We need medicines for the children." I asked him his name. "Medicines, we need medicines for the children," he replied and then went back to his prayer.

The priest had stayed with hundreds of children at St. André. Slowly, they were being culled. The Interahamwe would kill at night outside the church and throw bodies and severed limbs back over the wall so that the living would know what they would face. The children were butchered systematically, but only a few at a time—sometimes five, sometimes thirty, sometimes more, whatever the killing squad's alcohol and weed would allow for each night. We tried to persuade the RGF commander that the children needed to go to the Faisal Hospital. We would return with trucks to move them. I said they needed to be quarantined because of an epidemic of measles. I asked him if he had children. He was a father of four, he told me. "My children are out of the country, for now," he said. "But these here are not children, they are Tutsi *inyenzi*"—cockroaches. "They will be crushed like insects." We kept talking with the commander, but it was late. We had permission to pass on the road until 6 p.m. It was now 5:30, and we had to get back through the Interahamwe checkpoints. We left.

The next day I went to the Sisters of Charity Orphanage, down the hill from the Ste. Famille Cathedral and run by the Sisters of Mother Teresa. The sisters hadn't left their walled compound. Since Jules had told me about the orphanage, where more than 140 adults and 200 children lived, I had been able to get there a number of times. One of the sisters I often met was an Indian woman, another an African. On this day, children were laid out in rows of cots, one cot touching the other, some with two or three children on a cot. The room was dark; little light came through its small windows. I examined the sickest of the children and said I would try to return with medicines and try to arrange to take at least the sickest to the hospital. I returned several times with supplies but was never able to move anyone.

One day I went to St. Paul's with a UN peacekeeper. St. Paul's was another religious compound in Kigali, this one below the hill not far from the Red Cross hospital. There were hundreds of children there, just like at St. André. Again, like St. André, we tried to persuade the RGF commander to let us take the children to the Faisal, and again, we were refused.

The next day, we returned to St. Paul's with some medical supplies. We got out of our vehicle and walked towards the compound gate. The militia, a few more than the day before, were scattered along the road outside. They taunted us, jeering and laughing. I crossed the ochre soil of the parking lot. I looked down and saw what I thought were small sausages sitting in pockets of pasty brown-red mud. I thought they were very small for sausages and that someone must have dropped them. And then, as the militia continued to jeer, it became clear. They weren't sausages, they were fingers—children's fingers. The night before, a group of children had been butchered, and now lay covered by a blue plastic tarp, a heap of limbs, clothes and blood. Inside the compound, there were fewer children than the day before. A boy sat against a wall. He was about seven years old. His ears had been cut off and he had a machete wound over his right eye. He was paralyzed on his left side. As I examined him, I wondered what it would take to hold a child while he screamed in terror? What kind of rage would it take to do this to him? How could anyone see an insect in the face of a child? I felt my own rage and I felt fear. Rage for what I knew, and fear for what I could not answer.

We drove out of St. Paul's up the hill to the main road. Men were milling about. They were Interahamwe. We drove past them without difficulty. Some stood in pairs talking, some alone, some milled about drinking beer. The atmosphere was nearly festive. They were taking a break during a hard day's work. One man, a few years older than me, wearing a red T-shirt with cut-off sleeves, caught me looking at him. He stared back in at me, taking my measure. We looked at each other. Then he raised his veined hand that held a machete, smiled at me and tipped his hat with the end of the blade. I kept looking at him. This is not some collective psychosis, I thought. It's deliberate murder delivered with rational cruelty. Fuck you, I thought. Fuck you.

Later that week, Luc Racine had returned to St. André and had again tried to take the children out. He had gone this time with a journalist, and the visit sparked the rage of the Interahamwe. Shots were fired. A bullet hit the journalist in the buttocks, but the men escaped. Racine brought the journalist to me at the Faisal. The bullet had gone in one side and out the other. Giovanni and Eric removed damaged tissue before the journalist was evacuated.

I was often very afraid when I left the UNAMIR HQ or the Faisal Hospital. But I had to try. Others were trying. I had doubts, confusions, uncertainties about what we were doing, about the risks we were taking. Sometimes I was so afraid that I hoped that it would be impossible to leave the compound or the hospital. I hoped that others would stop trying, so that I could. Every time we went out it made it more difficult to go out again, but even more difficult not to at least try.

Over the next week, the RPF advanced, and the Faisal was now in RPF territory. When the RPF had taken control of the perimeter around a key roundabout leading to the Faisal, the team moved from the UNAMIR compound into the hospital, where there were eleven Tunisian UNAMIR troops. The move meant the patients would get better care, and, for me, that I could go the children's ward more often. By now the hospital was more organized, and more children were recovering from malarias and pneumonias. The care was definitely improving.

The night we moved into the hospital, I stepped over people living in the hallways and stairwells. Some were asleep, but most were not. I went to the pediatrics ward to check on a number of the sicker patients. Eli had his lantern and was singing with the children. I stood at the door and watched. Though antibiotics had treated his fever, the three-year-old boy with the chest tube hadn't eaten for a week. The tube was still draining pus, and his body needed nourishment. Eli had been trying to feed him, and was encouraging his sister to try to feed him as well. I had seen the boy at least once every day that week, and every day, all day, he cried for his mother: "Mama-we, Mama-we." His twelve-year-old sister guarded him on their small patch of floor, turning every few minutes to wrap him in their blanket. The boy now sat quietly beside his sister, his arm draped across her outstretched leg, his eyes swollen from tears. He was losing weight rapidly, and without food would soon die. Eli had left the boy's plate of gruel in front of him, long after the other children's plates had been collected.

His sister had only one leg. Giovanni had amputated what was left of the other one a week before. She had stepped on a grenade while running away at night from the shed behind her house where she and her brother, with his shrapnel wound, had hidden for a day. Somehow someone got them to the Faisal. Their entire family had been killed by the Interahamwe. Only she and her brother escaped.

I watched from the door as she tried to feed him. She held the spoon to his mouth, but he turned his head away. She tried again and again. Each time, he turned away. She put down the spoon. Now she was crying too. She stretched her arm out behind her, her hand open, then she swung her hand full force, cracking it into her brother's face, and started screaming at him. The other children stopped singing. The boy screamed "Mama-we! Mama-we!" His sister picked up the spoon. As Eli approached, the boy opened his mouth to the spoon. He took a mouthful of food. Whimpering, he took another.

UNAMIR engaged in endless discussions with the RGF and the RPF in an effort to exchange Tutsis and Hutus. Hutus and Tutsis would have to be carefully counted, documented and verified, militias and commanders informed, trucks arranged, routes mapped and road clearances granted from both the RPF and the RGF before any exchange could happen. To attempt otherwise would mean certain death. It could take hours and more often days to get agreements in place, and even then these were tenuous. As the RPF advanced in Kigali and westward across the country, the government was in turmoil. The RGF struggled to maintain its positions, and the Interahamwe split into factions. An uninformed sniper or a rogue militia or military man could turn a planned transfer into a disaster.

UNAMIR's most immediate limitations were a lack of armoured vehicles and a lack of fuel. At one point, stores were down to 2,000 litres of diesel fuel, less than a day's supply. Sometimes transfers were stopped not because UNAMIR feared it would run out of courage but because it feared it would run out of gas.

The casualties were getting heavier, and both hospitals were seriously lacking in medical supplies. Gerry McCarthy, a gregarious Irishman and the only UNICEF person in the country, knew everyone and could make a deal with anyone for anything.

He knew of some medical supplies, and we worked out a deal. But still, these weren't enough. MSF had stores at the airport and at abandoned warehouses in the city. Both Pepijn Boot and Jonathan Brock were very able logisticians and were determined to get what we needed. But first we needed vehicles and fuel, which we "borrowed" without permission from among a few trucks that we found sitting unused at the Kigali airport. Vehicles from the UN and the Red Cross were acquired in the same way. Jonathan and I made our way to an old MSF warehouse in what is known as the Rwandex district of Kigali. Getting supplies out was not easy. Inside, rats scurried over looted boxes of drugs, and the RGF had left land mines and grenades to deter people like us. In addition to drugs, dressings and IV lines and fluids, we found a box of toys for the orphanage. We made it safely out of the warehouse, but as we approached a roundabout near the Faisal Hospital, a sniper started shooting at us. I was driving the borrowed truck and had never driven anything like it before. While I struggled to shift from second to third gear, Jonathan crouched on the floor of the cab. He lit me a cigarette as we drove through the sniper fire.

We took the toys back to the children's ward. Like other people in the surrounding neighbourhood, a group of prostitutes who had worked at the local Kigali Nights Bar—one of the most popular hangouts for whites—had fled to the Faisal in the first week of the genocide. They had organized their group to cook for the children in the orphanage and on the pediatrics ward. The three-year-old boy was especially enjoying the food, and by now, more than a week after I had first put one in, I had taken his chest tube out.

I split my time among the Faisal, the UN compound, the Red Cross hospital and the stadium, bringing whatever supplies could be found. In the morning I would do a quick round of the pediatrics ward before going to UNAMIR. Carl Wilkins, an American, sometimes showed up at UNAMIR's morning prayers. People called him Master of the God Squad. "Momma Poppa One, this is Carl. How y'all doin'? How d'ya copy, over?" Whenever his southern accent came over the radio, a collective groan would erupt from those listening. He was a Seventh-day Adventist pastor who had been living in Kigali with his family when the genocide started. He sent his wife and children to Nairobi, but he remained. "I do what I can—gotta do something," he told me. "Can't just walk outta here, can ya?" And he did more than anyone else I know dared. Alone, he drove around the Kimihurura district, trying to help people who were trapped. One morning his car window was shot out by "some real crazy Hutu boys." He knew some people thought him crazy, but he didn't care. "I'm with the Lord, and as long as he keeps after me, I ain't leavin.'"

Carl asked me for a lot of help and asked a lot of questions, but never really waited for the answers. He'd tell me what he needed and when he would pick it up. One of the first times he came to me, he needed medical supplies for a family who were hiding in an attic. They had been there for weeks, and one of the boys was sick "with some fever from something or other—could it be malaria? What d'you think, Doc? I'm goin' back there today—that boy's some sick—so any medicine you might have would sure be appreciated. Say, I need some bandages and whatnot too. Some of them folks got a few injuries. One of them looks infected—s'got some pus an's all red like. I'll swing by your hospital—nice work you folks are doin' there—boy, it's some needed 'round here—I'll be by say 'bout 'n hour from now?" We didn't always have the supplies Carl needed, but we always gave him something. He gave me something too—something I can never forget.

MSF was stepping up its international campaign, lobbying hard for a UN military intervention. (Even the Red Cross, for the first time in its 130-year history, was breaking from its traditional neutrality, though it never went so far as to call for an intervention.) MSF took out full-page ads in *Le Monde* and worked to get articles in other papers and to do television and radio interviews around the world. UNAMIR was not alone in monitoring the international press; we knew the RGF and Interahamwe were doing the same.

Everyone listened on portable radios to RTLM, the government propaganda machine inciting and instructing genocide. The radios at Interahamwe checkpoints could be heard in the Red Cross hospital and at the Faisal. In RGF areas, MSF and UNAMIR were now open targets. RTLM broadcast "cash rewards for Dallaire's corpse and for the arms of whites." As I left the hospital for the UNAMIR morning briefing, I was warned by a man waiting outside my room that my arms were worth $50 each. UNAMIR radio monitors had heard the same broadcast, and Dallaire ordered extra protection for the hospital and for my vehicle. "Be goddamn careful, for Christ's sake," he warned me that morning.

At one point, as I was driving through the city, a wild dog lunged at my open window. I hadn't seen it approaching as we slowed at a roundabout, and now I saw a pack of wild dogs tearing at a corpse in the grass by the roadside. They looked up at us as we drove by. The dogs were fat, bold and vicious. They were not moving from their mound of flesh. The dog that had lunged at our four-by-four returned to its pack, growling, baring its white teeth, and held me in its stare.

The city was littered with bodies. "Jesus Christ," the driver, an Austrian UNAMIR soldier, said in crisp English, looking over to me as I lit a cigarette. "You'd think they'd at least hide in the bushes . . . Fucking dogs . . . fucking war . . ." He paused and then added as an afterthought, "For a doctor, it is very surprising you smoke." How Austrian, I thought. I threw the just-lit cigarette at one of the dogs, who sniffed it quickly before returning to the corpse. Then I lit another.

I spent at least two hours of every day in communication with MSF offices in Europe, giving and getting information and trying to coordinate the team's activities in Kigali. Pepijn was doing all that he could at the Amahoro Stadium, the Faisal was performing up to thirty surgeries a day, and the team at the Red Cross hospital continued to work even as the front line continued to shift around them. We all worked between sixteen and eighteen hours a day. Our sleep was often interrupted by emergency calls about new patients or from the wards. At the Faisal, we were running short of morphine and had to ration our stock. Patients often screamed in pain, especially at night, when there was little to distract them in the long hours of darkness.

About 10:30 one night, I had just finished assisting with an amputation, the eleventh surgery Giovanni and Eric had done that day. I was learning how to perform amputations because there were so many to do. So many of the patients brought to the hospital, lying in the wards, in the corridors, under the stairwells, had blast injuries, or such brutal damage done to their limbs by machetes that amputation was the only option. Eric and Giovanni had gone to the surgical ward to finish their evening rounds. I had yet to return to the pediatrics ward for my own final rounds. After leaving the OR, I stopped on the second-floor balcony, just a few feet away from a group of people cooking their evening meal.

They heard my walkie-talkie and turned towards the English voices barking through the static. A man had a pot of tea that he was pouring for others sitting in a small circle. A few in the circle smiled at me, but most just stared. By now I was a familiar face, a familiar authority, and as is the custom in Rwanda, all defer to authority. They did not interfere with my obvious effort to steal a moment of privacy. There were no nurses or staff nearby, and I buried myself in the corner darkness, away from the usual questions and problems that the staff needed addressed. It was a moment to be alone in what was certain to become another twenty-hour day.

Cool night air had fallen on the city. Lines of smoke from

the cooking fires below the balcony floated into a silk-like blue blanket. The stars were beautiful. I took the last cigarette out of my pack; I fumbled for matches, reminding myself how it was bad for my health to smoke. But here, in this place, it was bad for my health to not smoke. I heard people talking, a transistor radio somewhere nearby, and dogs howling in the hills of the city.

Every few minutes the sky lit up with shell blasts, and then, seconds later, the crash and muffled thud of an explosion would be heard. Sometimes the balcony shook, but as long as no bricks fell, nobody moved or stopped their conversation. No one looked to see where the stranger had fallen. Just a pause to let the vibrations pass. The hospital was shelled several times. Mortars landed in the grounds within metres of the main building. These were apparently strays, aimed by the RGF at the hill behind the hospital, a hill where the RPF had set up mortar sites to shell Nyamirambo, an RGF stronghold.

Sometimes the well-aimed bullet of a sniper would find its way into the hospital grounds. Other times bullets arrived through the staccato burst of machine-gun fire. And still other times stray bullets would come, shot into the air from some far-off place by some far-off finger attached to some far-off body. These were random and unwelcome visitors, prompting a few moments of caution, a few moments of scurrying on a floor that bruised the knees, a few moments of penetrating fear. And then the moment would pass. Someone would get up and look over the wall, and gradually things would return to normal.

I smoked my cigarette. It was a strange place I was in: a building, sometimes a hospital, most times something else. By now Lulu, the young Métis boy, had become a regular friend. His mother, Sylvie, had discovered a large broom closet beside my room at the hospital, accessible from the second-floor balcony walkway through an open window. She had moved her two children, Lulu and four-month-old Vanessa, to the closet, where they slept at night. Every morning I would get up early, prepare a list of tasks for the day and then go to the children's ward. Lulu would often come with me to the children's ward, insisting on carrying my stethoscope. Eli fed him, and he would play with some of the other children.

That morning before going to the children's ward, I saw Sylvie. She was on the balcony bathing Vanessa in a blue plastic bucket. The water splashed the baby, and the sun caught the water on their skin. I felt like a doctor then, and the building felt like a hospital. Lulu had already been bathed and was sitting on the balcony. The older boys were waiting for his mother to leave so that they could start their daily torment. A Métis is never fully welcome anywhere, I thought, least of all here. Beneath the surface calm of this hospital, everyone was afraid of everyone else. The minority of people in the hospital were Tutsi and afraid of what the Hutus around them might do. And the Hutus, the majority at the Faisal, were afraid of the RPF outside the hospital and what they might do.

The man with the teapot got up from his circle and walked carefully in the darkness towards me. "C'est pour vous, Docteur," he said as he leaned forward, giving me a cup of tea

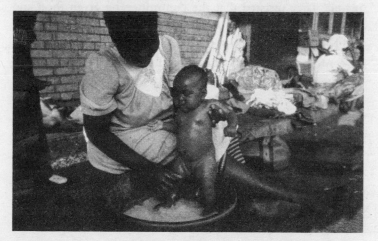

A mother bathing her child at Faisal Hospital

before turning back to join his group. I drank my tea and finished my cigarette. I went back to the pediatrics ward to check on a few patients. Most of the children were sleeping. Eli had his lantern and sang with those who couldn't.

One morning Don MacNeil and I spent a few hours meeting with the hospital's self-proclaimed Committee of Intellectuals. A few days before, I had received a three-page handwritten letter from them. It was the first I had heard of them. I didn't want to waste time meeting, but now I had no choice. The day before they had delivered a second note, a one-page meeting agenda, the last item of which was "The Cutting Off of Rwandan Arms and Legs by MSF."

We sat around two tables, one short, one long, facing each other. The committee sat at the long table—a group of twelve men. MacNeil and I were at the other. Some of the committee members wore suits. They were all dishevelled, but far less so than the other six thousand people at the hospital, and far better fed. They had convinced themselves that MSF was unfairly distributing food in the hospital, that MSF was, for some reason unknown to them, withholding water and blankets from the people. They insisted that the committee be given food and relief supplies that they would distribute themselves. All this had been outlined in their three-page letter.

After a long introduction in polished French, the committee presented the last agenda item from their second letter. It was an explosive issue and the reason that I had agreed to the meeting. After noting how much the work of MSF was appreciated, one committee member referred to alleged rumours running through the hospital that MSF was killing the people of Rwanda. Another committee member wanted a count of severed limbs so that it could be checked against the number of wounded brought to the hospital to ensure that there were no "extras." I thought of the RTLM broadcasts and my own $50 arms.

I sat and listened. MacNeil turned to me and whispered,

"Are these fucking eggheads serious?" The truth was that dogs were digging up buried limbs that we had surgically removed from wounded patients. I had seen a dog with a piece of leg in its mouth that very morning. The committee then outlined the other agenda items.

MacNeil was impatient. "These fuckers have to understand that this is the way it is: take it or leave it." But we couldn't ignore them. We had a hospital with six thousand people living in it, nearly 350 in-patients, and more wounded coming in every day. Like MacNeil, I knew we had only a five-day food supply, and that supply routes were uncertain at best, despite the hopeful rhetoric from the UN.

The committee had decided on what message would be carried as the "voice of the people"—a collective they defined, represented and spoke for. I smiled as I listened. The committee then opened the floor for discussion.

I was not going to give them a single bean or blanket. But I couldn't insult this potentially dangerous group. So I talked. And I talked some more, and more still. I posed questions that "would be discussed in more detail at the appropriate time." In the end I made it known that one member of the committee who was at the meeting was being paid by MSF to dispose of the surgically amputated limbs. He was to burn them in the incinerators that we provided. It was not a pleasant task, but a necessary one. I was grateful that he was willing to do this and very happy to be paying him to do so. I suggested that perhaps the committee member, in a generous effort to share the money, had paid others to do the work. Perhaps he hadn't supervised his employees to ensure that the limbs were incinerated and not buried. I apologized that MSF had not made it clear to him that he needed to do the job himself, and that we had failed to offer proper supervision. I did not say that he was selling the fuel we provided and was paying someone else to bury the limbs, or that he was using his surplus cash to finance his black-market food business within the hospital, or that I knew this through my own network of hungry storytellers. Instead I thanked the committee for bringing the issue to my attention and asked them to find a solution to the problem. I concluded that until this small matter, embarrassing to all, could be resolved, we could not responsibly consider any other issues.

"Are you sure you're a doctor and not a fuckin' diplomat?" MacNeil asked before I excused myself.

The next day, I crossed the front line to bring some supplies to the Red Cross hospital and to talk with Gilbert Hascoet. The RPF was advancing rapidly in Kigali. Among those living at the Red Cross hospital were some extremist Hutus who were now holding secret meetings where lists of Tutsis, both patients and Red Cross national staff, were being drawn up. Given MSF's campaign for immediate UN intervention and the calls for the arms of MSF workers on RTLM radio, I assumed that the MSF expatriates would be on those lists. Gilbert knew this as well as I did, and had discussed it with the team. I wanted the team to leave immediately, but Gilbert said that the work was too important just now, there were far too many sick and wounded to be abandoned. His team was not prepared to leave, and besides, he said, he had friends among the Hutu staff who would warn him if something was going to happen. "It is our decision," he said. "We are not ready to go."

On the way back, I saw the corpse of a murdered priest in the street. One of his feet had been cut off by a machete. His hands, clasping a set of well-worn wooden rosary beads, were petrifying in the heat. One of the beads was split along the woodgrain. Not all the priests were dead. There was the French priest at St. André, and the one I would soon meet very briefly at the Ste. Famille Cathedral.

It was late in the day, and Jacques, a UNAMIR peacekeeper, and I had stopped to try to deliver medical supplies to the people who had sought refuge in the cathedral. I was sweating in the hot sun as we pulled in. There were no Interahamwe in the parking lot that day. We entered the brown-brick cathedral. Nearly two thousand people were inside. Some sat on the pews; others lay on them under a piece of cloth or plastic tarp. Triangular coloured flags, the kind one would see at a sporting event or carnival, hung high across the width of the church. Blue smoke from nearby cooking fires outside filled the space but could not cover the smell of feces and unwashed bodies. Blades of light came in through the long, narrow windows. Nobody moved when we entered, no one talked, no one approached us. I could nearly smell the fear.

Everyone stared as I walked to the altar at the front of the church where the clinic was supposed to be. I gave some medical supplies to a woman. I saw the priest as he quickly walked away with a group of men. He was wearing pants and his clerical collar. He had a potbelly. He nodded to me, his expression stern. He was wearing a bulletproof vest. It was military-issue green.

I would later learn about Father Wenceslas, the Hutu priest who was in charge of Ste. Famille. I met a Tutsi survivor of Ste. Famille, Léondre Cyusa. He was nineteen when he fled to the church. Initially, there were about six thousand like him in the cathedral, Hutus and Tutsis alike. Most Tutsis were eventually murdered by the Interahamwe. "Father Wenceslas was a terrible, horrible, evil man," Léondre told me. The priest decided who would live, how many would die, and when. Father Wenceslas chose among the young Tutsi women, letting the most attractive live so that he could rape them at his leisure. Léondre told me that everyone was terrified of the priest. If they were seen talking to anyone who came to the church, they would be killed. He told me that "the means we had to speak was to write something." Léondre wrote a note: "Dear UN: there is massacres here in this church. People are killed here. There are a lot of bodies here. Help us please." He slipped the note into the side pocket of a UN soldier's flak jacket. Léondre said he felt better after this, that at least he had been able to do something to try to save himself and the others. One day soon after, Father Wenceslas came into the church with an RGF commander, the mayor of Kigali and some Interahamwe militia. One of the militiamen recognized Léondre as a schoolmate. "You are a Tutsi! We have not done our job well!" A few moments later, as Father Wenceslas had tea with the mayor and the general, the militia started shooting inside the church. Léondre ran outside and managed to escape into RPF-held territory.

It was late and we had to leave before the six-o'clock curfew. We walked out of the Ste. Famille church into the parking lot and towards our Hilux pickup truck. A girl of about eleven was crouched by the side of the church. She got up, calling, and walked towards us, holding out her hand as if to shake mine. I stopped and took a step towards her. She took my wrist and gently directed me to the gutter alongside the cathedral. She let my wrist go and bent down to lift a printed shawl. She had placed rocks on the corners of the cloth to hold it over her mother, who lay in the gutter. Her mother's eyes and mouth opened and closed to dissuade the flies that swarmed around her face. She was too weak to use her hands. She lay sweating among several corpses that had been thrown out of the church. She was covered in vomit and diarrhea. She was delirious, emaciated and barely alive. Her chest heaved, the skin rising and then falling back between her ribs with each breath. Jacques was now screaming at me to get in the truck. "For fuck's sake! It's five to fucking six!"

There was no choice, no thinking. I just did it. I picked up the girl's mother and carried her to the truck. For Jacques, there was no choice either. He put the girl in the cab and showed her how to stay down below the dashboard. If Interahamwe saw her or her mother on our way back to the hospital, we would all be dead. I lifted her mother into the back of the pickup and lay her out on the flatbed. I got into the cab and Jacques took off. "We've got three minutes," he said, "and then someone's gonna take a shot at us." I lit a cigarette as he drove at full speed. The girl's mother rolled around with each pothole.

"She's going to fly out of the flatbed," I said.

"We've got two minutes. I'll stop and you climb on top of her and hold her down," said Jacques. He pulled over and I climbed into the back of the truck as I threw away my cigarette. Just as I was lying down and Jacques was putting the vehicle in gear, I heard a whizzing sound beside my left ear, and then the crack of a rifle shot. "Fucking lie down!" Jacques screamed as he hit the gas.

The girl's name was Thérèse, and her mother had dysentery and likely TB as well. She died two days later. During those two days, Thérèse never left her mother's side, washing her, holding her hands and trying to feed her. When her mother died, Thérèse went to the pediatrics ward to help Eli.

The killings and massacres continued. UNAMIR had suffered casualties, and even though it now had an extended mandate, it still didn't have the means to fulfill it. UNAMIR's survival both politically and practically was uncertain as the RPF extended its hold, day by day, piece by piece, into the city. Around the country millions were displaced, hundreds of thousands had already moved across the borders to Tanzania and Burundi, and at least a million were now on the move westward towards Zaire. Millions needed assistance. No matter what happened politically or militarily, the humanitarian needs were immediate. They were already overwhelming, and they were growing by the day.

I had been in Rwanda for two weeks. I stood on the second-floor balcony, looking out into the night. I was coughing from too much smoking. Except for the nurse Thérèse, who had found me, I had not been able to find anyone I knew from 1988.

MSF's four French expatriates were all but trapped on the other side of the front line. RTLM broadcasts grew ever more desperate, and the RGF and the Interahamwe were increasingly undisciplined as the RPF advanced towards the Red Cross hospital. I was scared for my team, scared for myself.

Rwanda existed in a state of exception—a black hole in the community of nations where the law against genocide existed but could not be applied because genocide would not be said to exist. There was no possibility of organized humanitarianism. Ours were individual acts of kindness, sometimes possible in the face of what we knew was happening around us, most times not.

MSF and others stepped up their demands for immediate support for UNAMIR and a UN Chapter 7 intervention allowing for UN soldiers to use force to protect civilians. MSF France ran more full-page ads in *Le Monde*, applying enormous public pressure on the French government to supply the logistical and financial means. In France, public outrage that the government could be implicated in a genocide was growing. Meanwhile, the UN Security Council remained deadlocked over the use of the word *genocide*, still blocked by American reluctance to allow it. Both the United States and the United Kingdom stifled efforts to support UNAMIR. MSF lobbied the UN and Washington directly for the United States to supply the promised APCs and to support a Chapter 7 mandate. Amnesty International, Human Rights Watch and Oxfam were doing the same. Jules told me that there were rumours in Europe that the French government might be planning to send troops.

On June 17, Bernard Kouchner appeared suddenly at the UNAMIR headquarters. I knew nothing about the visit from UNAMIR, nor from MSF in Europe, which had been pretty good at informing me of which diplomats were on their way to where.

I had gone to the UNAMIR compound that afternoon for a

meeting with Colonel Yaache and Don MacNeil. Kouchner had arrived hours before as an official representative of the French government and had met with Dallaire. Now, MacNeil told me, Kouchner urgently wanted to meet me. MacNeil didn't know why. I thought it must be about orphans. Kouchner had been in Kigali a few weeks before and had returned to France with a planeload of children who had lost their parents. He had come as president of Médecins du Monde, the French NGO he had founded after breaking with MSF. The fifty children had been flown to a waiting French military hospital aircraft in Nairobi, and from there to France, where they arrived in time for maximum media exposure.

I waited for Kouchner in the third-floor MSF office, but I had patients waiting at the hospital, and more wounded had just been brought in. He came just as I was closing my office door to leave. I started to reopen the door. "No, no," he said, "that will not be necessary. This will be very brief. I am Bernard Kouchner. Of course, I know MSF very well." He tilted his head as he made eye contact with me. He didn't ask, nor did he leave space for me to tell him, my name. He was a short man, confident in his olive-green safari vest and chino pants. For all I had heard of him, I expected him to be bigger. Kouchner informed me that he would be going to the MSF Faisal Hospital with media. He instructed me to facilitate the visit. "There is not much time," he said.

"Well," I said and paused. So much can go on in the mind at one time. I knew that the French government might be planning to send troops, but when? To do what? To support the RGF? To create safe havens? It didn't matter. If they did come they would be suspect the moment they crossed the border. I knew in my gut that to be even minimally effective in the coming months, MSF would need to distance itself as much as it practically could from any French intervention. Kouchner being photographed at an MSF hospital filled with wounded

Rwandans before the French forces arrived would not help us or the hundreds of thousands needing assistance—though it would go a long way towards moulding French public opinion in support of intervention.

"That is not possible," I said.

"What do you mean? I need to be there as soon as possible. I am ready. The journalists are waiting."

"I will not allow it."

He looked at me, then to the floor, and then to me again. His face swelling with anger, he screamed, "You are a fucking fool!" His veins bulged in his neck. He pointed one finger into my face and his other arm gesticulated wildly as he moved from foot to foot. I stepped back from him. "You fucking know nothing . . . nothing!" he screamed.

"It is simply not going to happen," I repeated slowly.

Kouchner stormed down the hallway and down the stairs. I opened the office door and called Jules on the satellite phone.

That night, the French government announced that in the interests of humanity, it would lead a "Franco-African humanitarian intervention" to provide safe havens and allow for humanitarian assistance in Rwanda. Chad, Niger, Mauritania, Senegal, Congo and Togo—some of the same countries that had French-speaking troops now in UNAMIR—pledged support for the French initiative. Its domestic and international reputation badly tarnished, the French government wanted legitimacy for its intervention and would work for the next five days to get UN authorization for its plans. The intervention was to be completely separate from the UNAMIR operation. I later learned that Kouchner had arrived in Kigali as the French government envoy to both Dallaire and Kagame, charged with officially informing them of the coming initiative. UNAMIR, the very force that could have stopped the genocide had it the means to do so, was being thwarted by the government that had continued to arm the RGF throughout the genocide.

The next morning, fresh French flags flew at every checkpoint. Their morale boosted by the French announcement, the RGF and Interahamwe went on an invigorated killing spree, cheering and singing, "Nos frères français viennent! Les français viennent pour nous sauver!" (Our French brothers are coming! The French are coming to save us!) There were more killings at the checkpoints, and more slaughters at churches and orphanages. At the same time, Radio RTLM denounced the presence of MSF anywhere in Rwanda.

The next day I was coming back from the Red Cross hospital when I heard over the radio that one of the peacekeepers had just been shot on a nearby road. Ours was the closest vehicle. I radioed MacNeil, telling him we were going, and the UNAMIR driver sped to the scene. We pulled up behind the other vehicle and, afraid of more sniper fire, ran hunched to it. The peacekeeper was lying on the seat. We pulled him out and into the back seat of our four-by-four. Havoc followed on the radio. MacNeil called: "Momma Poppa One to Momma Poppa Nine-James. Status? Over." I called Eric at the Faisal: "Momma Poppa Nine-James to Momma Poppa Nine-Eric, prepare operating room for UN gunshot trauma. How do you copy? Over." Like everyone else, the UNAMIR Bangladeshis were listening: "Momma Poppa Bangladesh, is everything all right? Over." MacNeil answered them: "Momma Poppa One to Momma Poppa Bangladesh, stay off the radio. How do you copy? Over." I examined the peacekeeper as best I could as we sped through the front line to the Faisal. His flak jacket had taken the bullet that had come through the door of his truck. He was stunned, his flank area swelling rapidly. He was a Russian with a Polish name and he took some comfort that I had a Polish name too. "We are brothers! We are brothers!" he repeated. I called to answer MacNeil. "Momma Poppa Nine-James to Momma Poppa One. Patient is stable, repeat stable. Get evacuation going. Over." Again, the Bangladeshis radioed:

"Momma Poppa Bangladesh, is everything all right? Over?" MacNeil answered me. "Momma Poppa One to Momma Poppa Nine-James, well copied. And fuck off the radio, Bangladesh. That's an order, asshole. How do you copy? Over." Then Eric at the Faisal answered me: "Momma Poppa Nine-Eric to Momma Poppa Nine-James, OR is ready for peace-keeper, and perhaps for asshole too. Over." We got to the Faisal. The Russian had a small amount of blood in his urine from severe bruising to his kidney and flank, but otherwise he appeared uninjured. The airport was still closed, so he would have to wait until the next day for an overland medical evacuation to Nairobi. I saw him later at the UNAMIR compound. He was drinking heavily. We raised our glasses in a toast, and his vodka spilled onto the table. "You doctor, my friend forever."

The day before, UNAMIR had been fired on by the RGF during a transfer of Tutsis. The RPF then fired on UNAMIR as it retreated into RPF territory. One peacekeeper was killed and another badly injured. The incident provoked a melee at the UNAMIR compound, with a delegation of RPF soldiers attempting to "arrest" a delegation of RGF there to discuss political issues with Dallaire.

In the wake of the French announcement, with its peace-keepers openly targeted by both the RGF and the RPF, UNAMIR's military observers were unable to move in the city. All transfers were called off. With no reinforcements, nearly out of supplies and attacks coming from all sides, it looked like UNAMIR would have to fight its way out of Kigali. I checked their evacuation plans and had my MSF team check our own readiness to go with them.

That night I stood on the balcony, cigarette in hand, listening to the dogs. I leaned on the railing, and my stethoscope hung from my neck, its cold bell now brushing against my bicep. I could smell burning eucalyptus wood, its scent seeping up from the cooking fires below.

I watched the people who sat around their fires. The

horizon danced with the silhouettes of those who ventured beyond the safety of the hospital grounds for firewood. It was safer at night; there were fewer snipers.

As I watched over the hospital fence, I saw a small child bend over to pick up some wood. I inhaled from my cigarette. I watched her hand reach to the ground. As I exhaled, she collapsed. A split second later the ring of a sniper's bullet echoed through the night air.

A woman rose and walked in the direction of the fallen girl. Her pace quickened, and she started screaming her child's name. She ran towards the fence, then she fell to the ground as another sniper's shot rang out. My heart raced as she crawled. Another shot. It's too dangerous, she must have thought, for she turned around and crawled back, screaming at the men around the fire, turning again, screaming her child's name, then rising, a few steps towards the men, more screaming, a few more steps, more screaming. And then she waited.

The people who lived on the balconies of the hospital were standing now, looking into the nighttime blackness for the cause of the panic. The mother stood, her hands to her mouth. Some men from around the cooking fires ran hunched over towards the fence, pausing briefly and furtively behind bushes. They moved forward looking for the girl, looking for the sniper, looking only by the light of the stars.

If they found her, if she was still alive, I knew I would see her. She would be another casualty, there would be another surgery, another series of dressing changes and another chance that a patient would die of infection or some other complication. If she were dead, I wouldn't see her. She wouldn't be brought to me, and her mother would remain anonymous, another face in the morning among the thousands who lived in the hospital. Fuck it, I thought. I took in the blue-smoke calm of nicotine. I had another cigarette, threw the butt over the balcony and made my way back to the pediatrics ward.

The battle for Kigali intensified. Even with a boost in morale, the RGF was losing territory and the Interahamwe were increasingly undisciplined as they were pushed farther back. In the uncertainty that followed the announcement of the Franco-African intervention, the RPF targeted all French-speaking African peacekeepers. Dallaire was forced to evacuate them. Canadians were now the only French speakers on the UNAMIR force, and all Canadians—including me—were being openly targeted by the RTLM hate radio.

A UN force—UNAMIR—had been abandoned by its political masters, the same ones who were now considering a Chapter 7 intervention by the French, the most volatile intervening force possible. The RPF feared that the French were going to try to save the perpetrators of the genocide, and were adamant that if they encountered the French, they would fight. This wasn't just bluster. If any African army was willing to take on the French, it was the RPF. There were unconfirmed reports that the French already had reconnaissance teams in Zaire, along the Rwanda border. Dallaire feared that the French would seek to divide the country, as Cyprus had been. The RPF was determined to take Kigali and as much of the country as they could before the French arrived. No one knew if the French planned on moving to Kigali. If they tried, it would be another bloodletting in a seemingly endless spiral of genocide and civil war.

We were caught in the middle. MSF met with RPF officials in Europe to try to convince them that MSF was against France's unilateral intervention, that it supported instead a UN intervention to stop the genocide. MSF had called for anything but unilateral French intervention. The problem was that only the French had declared their intention to intervene. I wasn't sure that we could create new humanitarian space for our work. Other than reporting on and dealing with events on the ground, I had nothing to do with internal MSF deliberations and debates on how to respond politically, but I would have to respond to the consequences in Kigali.

I had my MSF team prepare our own evacuation supplies and map out three separate overland routes that we could try without UNAMIR. I confirmed the routes with Jules, but did not tell UNAMIR or ask the RPF for a guarantee of safe passage. I didn't want to send any worrying signals unless it became absolutely necessary. It wasn't clear that any of our plans could get us out safely. At this point, it was best to stay put, wait for an opening, and take it if required.

—

On June 21, Philippe Gaillard called me: "Come now, immediately, with all of your doctors, with everything you have." The Red Cross hospital was overrun with casualties. "There are hundreds. Hundreds! You must come now." I called MacNeil. He had heard the radio call and had already sent an APC to pick us up at the Faisal. MacNeil said the fighting was intense, and it was not clear that we could get across the front line, even in an APC. There was heavy shelling and mortar fire from both sides, some of the roundabouts were now openly contested, and snipers were everywhere, some with rocket-propelled grenades.

Eric and I made our way in the closed box of the APC. We could hear shelling, mortars and heavy machine-gun fire. The UN soldiers were nervous, and I was too. We made it through the roundabouts and two checkpoints. As we lumbered up the last hill, I looked out the door slit to see a group of RGF soldiers and Interahamwe about a hundred metres away from the hospital. It wasn't clear what kind of weapons they had. We proceeded up the final stretch of dirt road to the hospital. The APC stopped just inside the hospital gate.

People all around us writhed and screamed in pain. Others lay dead as relatives and friends wailed. Some wounded walked alone, and others were helped; still others were carried, some conscious, some not. There were hundreds of casualties, and scores of national Red Cross staff struggled to make order out of the chaos. Among the injured were RGF soldiers; young men, some of whom were Interahamwe; and many women and children. There were people with gunshot wounds, machete blows, shrapnel and blast injuries. There were women and girls who had been raped. The fighting continued around the city and near the hospital. The wounded came in wave after wave. We inserted chest tubes, tied off bleeding arteries and closed eviscerated abdomens on the roadside. Blood flowed like streams of water, and the red-ochre soil soaked it up.

There were so many, and they kept coming. Patients were taped with a 1, 2 or 3 on their foreheads: 1 meant treat now, 2 meant treat within twenty-four hours, and 3 meant irretrievable. The 3s were moved to the small hill by the roadside opposite the emergency room and left to die in as much comfort as could be mustered for them. They were covered with blankets to stay warm, and given water and whatever morphine we had. The 1s were carried by stretcher to the emergency room or to the entrance area around it. The 2s were placed in groups behind the 1s.

We were overwhelmed. The dead could not be moved fast enough. The wounded could not easily be carried over the dead bodies to the ER, the operating room or the wards.

I was on my knees on the dirt road beside a patient who lay on a tarp slowly bleeding to death from multiple lacerations. I started an IV line and pushed fluids into her. I examined her carefully, identifying slow bleeders on her head, torso and legs. I quickly tied them off with sutures as I went. Her body trembled. She was conscious and afraid.

A nurse called me to go to the next patient. "Maintenant! Tout de suite, Docteur!" The woman moaned and winced as I stitched. And then her hand reached to touch my forearm. I looked up to her face from the small bleeding artery I was sticking on her chest. She looked at me, and only then did I understand what had happened to her.

She was slightly older than middle aged. She had been raped. Semen mixed with blood clung to her thighs. She had been attacked with machetes, her entire body systematically mutilated. Her ears had been cut off. Her face had been so carefully disfigured that a pattern was obvious in the slashes. Both Achilles tendons had been cut. Both breasts had been sliced off. Her attackers didn't want to kill her; they wanted her to bleed to death. They knew just how much to cut to make her bleed slowly. She lay on the road, a 1 taped to her forehead, and now we were looking at each other.

"Je m'excuse, je m'excuse," I said, apologizing for the pain my pinching forceps gave her. She blinked once, slowly, to let a wave of pain pass. She held my forearm. I felt a wave of nausea as I looked again at the pattern someone had cut in her face. I turned from her and vomited for the first and only time during the genocide.

She waited as I spit out what was left of the bile in my mouth. Then she touched my forearm again. I looked into her brown eyes. "Ummera." I wasn't sure if she was saying it to herself, but then she continued. "Ummera-sha." *Sha*, I thought, it means my friend. She was speaking to me. "Ummera, ummera-sha," she repeated. I tied off the bleeding arteries where her breasts had been. The nurses were calling again, "Docteur, le prochain, le prochain! Vite, Docteur!"

The woman was one among many, among hundreds. She knew there were so many more. Again she reached to touch my forearm. She didn't hold it this time. She nodded, looking at me. "Allez, allez . . . Ummera, ummera-sha," she said in a slow whisper. "Go, go. Courage, courage, my friend." It was the clearest voice I have ever heard.

I got up off my knees and went to the next patient. He was a soldier. At least eight feet of his small bowel spilled out in loops from a gash across the front of his abdomen. He was fully conscious, sitting up on the road holding his guts into himself and crying. "S'il vous plaît, aidez-moi . . . Je tombe de mon corps . . . s'il vous plaît, aidez-moi, je tombe, je tombe . . ." Does the humanitarian treat a soldier? The doctor looks for the wounded, not for uniforms. I lay him down. Using sterile gauze to gain traction on the slippery loops of bowel, I carefully tracked it foot by foot back into his abdomen. I put in some temporary holding stitches. He was carried to the lineup for the operating room. I moved on to the next patient.

On and on it went, for hours we worked, one patient after another. The ground shook several times from heavy shelling nearby. The gutters ran red with blood. I stepped over bodies laid out on stretchers. In the doorway to the emergency room, one girl lay in a fetal position. I saw her several times, her mouth opening and closing in pain. She will be next, I kept thinking, but there was always another.

An hour later I stepped over her dead body as I carried an injured girl up the outdoor stairs to the pediatrics ward. As I walked, heavy machine-gun fire rang out. It was so close, my ears rang and I fell instinctively to the cement stairs, trying not to crush the girl. There was one more burst of machine-gun fire before I went back down to the ER to find Gaillard.

The high-calibre gunfire had stopped, and the shelling seemed more distant. Philippe and I agreed we had to keep working. He informed Dallaire and protested to the RGF and RPF commanders about the attacks on the hospital. Philippe was now in the emergency area carrying patients himself, encouraging his staff, bringing supplies from one room to another. "We must keep working," he said. "This is what we can do." He repeated it, more loudly still. "This is what we can do! On doit le faire, on doit le faire!"

We ran medical supplies through the front line from one hospital to another, using an APC or the Red Cross armoured ambulance. We ran the emergency and operating rooms as the shelling continued into the night. I returned to the Faisal that night to collect what I could—chest tubes, plasma expander and blood—to take back to the Red Cross hospital the next morning.

That day, June 22, the UN Security Council declared that "a multinational operation may be set up for humanitarian purposes in Rwanda until UNAMIR is brought up to the necessary strength." It was a Chapter 7 mandate for the French, allowing their troops to use "all necessary means"—diplomatic speak for the use of force to achieve its end—for a maximum of sixty days. The vote was 10–0, but with five abstentions it was by no means unanimous. The five abstainers were China, New Zealand, Brazil, Nigeria and Pakistan. No mention of genocide was made in the resolution, and MSF slammed it for that reason.

The French were coming. It was the beginning of their Operation Turquoise. The news came as I was at the Red Cross hospital on the pediatrics ward. I had been asked to see two brothers with tetanus. They lay like stiff boards in their beds, their abdomens rock hard, their shoulders pulled up, their limbs extended, their hands turned into their thighs. They screamed in fear as I examined them. Both were somewhere between twelve and fifteen years of age and had extensive blast injuries to their legs. Both had had surgery.

Somewhere in their past, the vaccination campaigns against tetanus had failed. They had the lockjaw and facial spasms characteristic of the disease. Over the last two days a spastic paralysis of the neck and limbs had set in. As tetanus neurotoxin spreads, the spastic contractions can be so powerful that they tear the muscles or cause compression fractures of the neck vertebrae. Stiffness rapidly develops in the chest, back, abdominal muscles and sometimes the laryngeal muscles, which then interferes with breathing. In normal circumstances, without treatment, one out of three infected people will die. Here, the odds were worse. We had penicillin, but no tetanus immunoglobulin. The Red Cross hospital had run out. The best we could do was give the boys IV diazepam—Valium—as a muscle relaxant.

When I heard about the Security Council vote, I left immediately for the UNAMIR compound. If things were bad now, they were only going to get worse, and worse still if the French tried to enter Kigali. The RPF had written a letter to the UN Security Council insisting that UNAMIR leave, as the RPF could not guarantee their safety. And the RPF was openly hostile to the French, reiterating that it was prepared to fight. The four French MSF workers at the Red Cross hospital were surrounded by RGF and Interahamwe, and the RPF was advancing. I was desperate to ensure their safe passage out of the hospital. I first met with Dallaire. Again he said, "Just tell me if and when. I will do everything I can to get them out."

I next met with Maj. Frank Kamanzi, the RPF liaison officer. He told me he would ensure the safety of the MSF workers if they left the country immediately: "And tell your MSF European friends that MSF can have no French nationals anywhere in the country." If we accepted this demand, the RPF would effectively be defining our operations, and infringing even more on our independence and our already wilfully and rightly broken neutrality. I discussed the situation with Jules. When I met Kamanzi again the next afternoon, we talked and talked and talked. Eventually we agreed that he would guarantee safe passage of the MSF French expatriates through RPF territory whenever they were ready to leave, and that we would resolve the nationality of future expatriates on a case-by-case basis, according to situational demands. In other words, we dealt with the immediate issue and put off the other.

I returned the Red Cross hospital. No one knows exactly

how many we treated in those few days. Hundreds of the people died after we marked them as "irretrievable." Many died despite treatment, and many died later of infections or other complications that we could not adequately treat. Hundreds lived.

On June 24, the French government dispatched 2,200 paratroopers to Goma and Bukavu in Zaire, the two towns with airstrips closest to Rwanda. From there they began to enter with reconnaissance patrols into western Rwanda, but they were not yet fully deployed. The motives of Operation Turquoise remained murky at best. Even with the UN resolution, it still wasn't clear what the French would actually do.

Inside MSF some thought that in the face of genocide, the priority had to be to stop the killings. Some said anyone but the French, while others recognized Operation Turquoise as the only option that had come to the table and were glad that the call for intervention had been heard. I wanted the killing to stop, by any means necessary. MSF said publicly that it would be watching the French and was prepared to denounce the actions of Operation Turquoise if it strayed in any way from their stated humanitarian intentions.

With the RPF determined to take Kigali and the RGF trying to hold on, the battle for the city raged over the next twelve days. The shelling around the city became intense, and the two hospitals were hit repeatedly. That first night, the ER of the Red Cross hospital was hit, despite the twenty-by-twenty-foot Red Cross flags meticulously tied to the roofs and outside walls of the school. A pandemonium of calls in and out of Kigali followed. Journalists, families and friends who had heard news of the attack were calling. I couldn't get through to Gaillard. I had to call Jules to call others to find out if anyone on my team or the Red Cross team had been injured or killed. It turned out they were all safe, but seven patients had been killed and four more injured. The emergency room had been destroyed. At the Faisal, high-calibre bullets hit the balconies and exterior of the building. One came into the operating room just after a patient had been moved out. At the Red Cross hospital, the situation was far worse.

The next day I returned to the Red Cross hospital, to see Gilbert and to deliver some dressings and antibiotics, as well as diazepam for the two brothers with tetanus. We passed a large group of Interahamwe and RGF about two hundred metres from the hospital. Most of the Interahamwe were drunk, waving their clubs, machetes and French flags as we passed.

I couldn't find Gilbert, so I went to check on the two brothers. As I entered the pediatrics ward, bricks started cracking in the wall opposite the entrance. High-calibre machine-gun fire sprayed across the outside of the building. The children instinctively crawled out of their beds to the floor. A nurse yelled at them to come over to the side of the room if they could. The children dragged themselves and each other across the floor. Their screaming was made worse only by the look on the faces of those too scared to scream. More gunfire, and more bricks started to crack in the wall. The brothers with tetanus lay stiff in their beds. One screamed; the other stared, his terrified eyes shifting repeatedly from the nurse to me and back again. We crawled to them and pulled them from their beds first to the floor and then to the group huddled against the opposite wall. The machine-gun fire stopped. The children stopped screaming, looking to the nurse and me with open eyes. Some whimpered, some were silent.

Philippe Gaillard and his team had no plans to leave, at least not yet. I tried to persuade Gilbert and the other MSF expatriates to leave with me in the APC. The night before, Gilbert had spent hours discussing the situation with the team and with operations people in Paris. It was no longer up to MSF, he said. It was now a personal decision. They knew the risks and for now they were staying. I told Gilbert that I understood. I told him I respected his team's decision, that I would try to get to the Red Cross hospital as necessary, and that I would continue to call him and to always be available by satellite phone. I told him that my heart was with him and the team. I told him I was honoured to know him. I got into the APC and we drove back across the front line. I lit a cigarette. The APC crew didn't care, and if they did, I didn't.

That night on the balcony I smoked too many cigarettes. The dogs howled, some patients wailed with pain, and for a few moments, I cried. Then I went to bed.

As the RPF pushed forward from the east, the RGF resisted but was moved west towards Zaire. Two and a half million Hutus were now displaced and moving west in front of the RGF, fearing RPF reprisals. As they moved, the RGF and the Interahamwe massacred all Tutsis and moderate Hutus in their path.

Sniper fire continued around the Faisal. Several mortars landed within metres of the hospital. They were getting far too close. The people living in the hospital were terrified. The shelling was so close that some windows shattered with the blasts, even though we had taped all the windows. We had set up bomb shelters inside the hospital grounds, but there wasn't nearly enough room for everyone.

There was no way to identify snipers, but we knew the mortars were coming from the RPF. In their eyes, MSF was now linked to the French, even though none of the MSF expatriates on their side of the front line were French nationals. Were they trying to intimidate us? Did they want us out? I met again with the RPF liaison officer, Major Kamanzi, to protest.

"Since when does a doctor advise us on military tactics?" he asked.

"I know nothing of military tactics," I answered, "except their consequences, and when their aim is off."

Kamanzi smiled, as did MacNeil, who was at the meeting. I reminded Kamanzi that firing on a hospital was a violation of the laws of war, and that MSF expected them to be a bit more careful with their aim.

He smiled again. "Accidents sometimes happen," he said but agreed to take care of it.

"As a small reminder to you," I said, "I have written an official letter." I handed it to him.

The mortars continued, but their aim improved. Heavy shelling from both sides persisted throughout the city as the RGF tried to stave off the steady advance of the RPF. Snipers kept taking shots at whatever moved out on the roads.

I stood on the hospital balcony having a cigarette. I had just gotten off the satellite phone with the MSF supply team in Amsterdam. For weeks we had listened to the nighttime screams of people in pain. We needed morphine. I had called the MSF medical department, then the logistics department, then the medical department again. Each reminded me that morphine was supplied in limited quantities in the standard MSF surgical kits. "You will have to cope with what you have in your surgical kit. It's our standard system."

"Well, it's not fucking working for my standard patients," I screamed into the phone. I called Jules. He promised the morphine would be on the next possible cargo flight into Kigali.

I could feel the cold night air. I could feel indifference creeping into me. I needed to escape, to find a reprieve. I was tired beyond what I thought I could bear any longer. I felt beaten by the waves of suffering, of killing, of screams, of silent stares, of terror, and waves of not just political indifference but malfeasance.

Before I went to bed, I wanted to check on Vanessa, Lulu's four-month-old sister. I had forgotten about her until that morning, when Sylvie had knocked on my door around five-thirty, just as I was getting up to start my rounds. She was nearly desperate. "She has lived this long," she said. "I have tried to keep the children clean, away from all the germs and killers in this place. Please, Dr. James, you must help us."

Vanessa had a fever and was breathing rapidly. I listened to her chest with my stethoscope and could hear the rattling sounds of an early pneumonia deep in her chest. I brought her some antibiotics from the children's ward. I had told Sylvie to find me or one of the doctors if Vanessa didn't improve within a few hours. Now, more than sixteen hours later, Sylvie was calm. Vanessa was breathing better, and her fever was improving. I examined her and went to bed somehow happier. I slept well that night.

With the French deployment now a reality, the RPF's attitude towards it changed. As long as the motives of the French were clearly humanitarian, and as long as the French stayed within an agreed-upon zone while UNAMIR built its strength so that the French could soon be phased out, the RPF would not object to the intervention. The task now was for UNAMIR to define the French zone of operation. With this, the battle for Kigali raged. The RPF continued its advance west, and the flow of casualties did not slow.

The RPF allowed UNAMIR reconnaissance teams through its territory once again. UNAMIR was preparing to receive reinforcements, and spirits at its compound were better. There was now a sporadic overland supply line from Kampala. The Red Cross managed to get a truckload of medical supplies in, but there was no morphine with it.

The Red Cross hospital was overloaded with patients. UNAMIR was sometimes able to arrange temporary ceasefires along the front line and through the various checkpoints to transfer patients to the Faisal. MSF also managed to get some of our own supplies in from Kampala, including morphine and antimalarials. We urgently needed both. There was an increase in the number of malaria cases, among them Gerry McCarthy of UNICEF and Frank Kamanzi. I treated both.

As well as wounded civilians, wounded RGF soldiers were

also brought to the Faisal. We treated them as we would treat anybody else, though they were on a separate, locked ward. The RPF was aware that enemy soldiers were in the hospital, and it began to make surprise inspections of the hospital, armed and without permission, demanding to interrogate the wounded. It also wanted to "inspect" the people living at the hospital. The RPF said that at one of its checkpoints it had discovered hand grenades on the civilians transferred from the Red Cross hospital. It suspected soldiers or Interahamwe were among them.

During one such unannounced visit, the RPF took medicines and supplies, including antimalarials. It also wanted to remove the RGF soldiers. I met with MacNeil and protested to Frank Kamanzi, insisting that the Geneva Conventions on the treatment of POWs be observed. MacNeil proposed that the people living at the hospital eventually be transferred to a displaced person's camp, and that a weapons inspection take place then. We also agreed that the RGF soldiers would remain housed as POWs on a separate, locked ward guarded by the UN, and that the RPF would enter the hospital grounds only with prior notice, unarmed and with a UN escort. The RPF agreed not to take MSF stocks or supplies. It returned what it had taken and stuck to the agreements.

The fighting across Kigali was intense. At one point, a journalist, while standing on the roof of the Meridien Hotel, was shot by a distant sniper. He had a bad leg wound, which Eric and Giovanni attended to, but nothing as serious as what others were suffering. The journalist was worried that his family would be terrified when they heard the news over the wires and he asked me to call them. Their fear, despite my reassurances, reminded me that each of us outsiders had family and friends who had no way of understanding what we were living. As I hung up the phone I thought about the fears of my own family, and if I would ever be able to explain to them what had happened here.

Nearing the end of June, the formal zone of operation for

the French had yet to be defined, and it was still not clear what the French would try to do. The RPF continued its advance, taking all but a final strip of the western region. The RGF still hoped for French support from the west of the country through to Kigali, and there were rumours that the French were planning to parachute into Kigali. The French met with the RGF leadership at the Meridien Hotel in Gisenyi, the heart of Hutu power in the northwest of the country. The French brought supplies for the RGF generals, and were greeted with garlands from crowds of schoolchildren mobilized by Radio RTLM. At one barrier a member of the Interahamwe, wearing a straw hat painted the colours of the French flag, posed for the camera with his machete in front of a sign that read, "Vive la France." After the meeting, the RGF generals announced that they would begin a major counteroffensive.

The French began deploying their forces into Cyngugu, in southwestern Rwanda. Again, they were greeted and garlanded by crowds mobilized by RTLM, which had told people to dress their girls in frocks to welcome the French. When they went beyond Cyngugu, ten French soldiers were ambushed by the RPF and held hostage for a few hours in the Butare region. Another French soldier was injured in Kibuye. The RPF was deadly serious when it said, "We will fight" and "We can handle more body bags than Paris."

On July 1 the UN Security Council moved to establish "an impartial Commission of Experts to examine and analyze . . . grave violations of international humanitarian law committed in the territory of Rwanda, including the evidence of possible acts of genocide." By then bodies were stacked in stinking piles at the Red Cross hospital. Thousands of people were still afraid to leave the compound, and more tents had to be set up between the buildings. At the Faisal, thousands waited, for what we did not know.

One morning I found myself sitting in the morgue, looking, waiting. I had carried a child's body from the pediatrics ward down to the morgue the day before. Eli had wrapped it in a piece of cloth. She was an infant, three months old. She had been born only days before the genocide began. How her mother kept her alive, I don't know. They had been in the hospital only a few days. The infant had an IV antibiotics line that kept falling out. The mother kept trying to nurse her. The baby had eventually succumbed to the pneumonia that followed her starvation. The morgue was full, so I left her on the floor, beside a row of similarly wrapped adults. The next day I passed the open door and noticed movement at the head of the infant's body. I went to take a closer look and saw a rat's tail scurry away. The shroud had been chewed around the eyes. I sat down on the floor behind the door. First I wept, then I smoked. The sun shone in, and dust particles danced in the cool basement air. I watched the rats watching me with their little black eyes, waiting for me to leave. A bird sat on the windowsill, looking in at me. It was a black-crowned finch, with red speckles on its grey wings, wide free eyes in a clear, living face. It looked like a fledgling, just out of the nest, and I wondered what she saw.

I found a letter for me on the table in the hospital office. It had been brought in with the MSF supplies from Uganda that day. It was from Father Benedict—he had probably heard the CBC Radio interviews I had done by satellite phone to Toronto. It was as though a dear but forgotten friend had shown up at my door. I put the letter in my pocket and I felt it there for several hours as I finished my rounds on the pediatrics ward. Later that night, after more surgery and a smoke on the balcony, I opened it. Benedict has a slight palsy that makes his writing difficult to read, but the letter was simple. "Dear James: a small and important thought." What followed were a few lines from a poem by Gerard Manley Hopkins that Benedict had carefully copied out for me. I read the shaky blue writing:

> *Generations have trod,*
> *Have trod,*
> *Have trod;*
> *And all is seared with trade;*
> *Bleared, smeared with toil;*
> *And wears man's smudge and shares*
> *Man's smell: the soil*
> *Is bare now, nor can foot feel,*
> *Being shod.*
>
> *And for all this, nature is never spent;*
> *Their lives the dearest freshness*
> *Deep down things . . .*

He signed it, "With all good wishes, Benedict." I looked out to the cooking fires below and listened to the dogs howling beyond the fence. The poem was like discovering a coin in the deep forest—interesting, but of no use here. I lit another cigarette. I was alone in this hell. Even Benedict did not understand. He couldn't, and how could I ever explain to him what Rwanda had become? What I knew others to be, and what I knew I could be?

The next morning, after my briefing with UNAMIR, I returned to the hospital to finish my rounds. It was around midday, and the sun was at its brightest and hottest. I had sent Giovanni and Eric by APC to the Red Cross hospital, and I was the only doctor at the Faisal. A nurse asked me to go to the operating room to see a boy who had just been brought in.

The boy was crying, lying on a gurney in the outdoor hallway of the operating room. His mother stood with him, holding the side of the gurney, guarding all that was on it. Her shawl—a cheap synthetic material with a gaudy yellow floral pattern—was not African. Probably from a secondhand clothing market, I thought. Her eyes inspected me with the same care that I inspected her son's wound. I noticed her

239

headscarf, dirty from weeks of wear, stained with blood. I could feel her assessment of me: "uncertain, but my son's only chance." She adjusted her shawl, pulling it tight around her, as the nurse wheeled the gurney into the operating room.

The boy was fourteen, his lower right leg destroyed by a land mine. What was left of his foot hung from his calf like severed wires that made a gnarled web capturing bone, bits of flesh, a piece of a shoe. The explosion had happened two or three days before. He was febrile, and already infection was tracking up towards his knee. It would have to be an above-the-knee amputation, the first amputation I would do alone. I was afraid that I might cut an artery, that I might kill him. The nurse, Thérèse, could see my anxiety. We anaesthetized the boy with ketamine; it does not cause respiratory depression, so a good nurse can monitor vital signs while the surgeon attends to other matters.

I could feel sweat beading on my back, around my eyes, gathering in my gloves. My fingers were wet, and the powder inside the gloves turned to paste. I was looking for arteries in the maul that was his leg. Thérèse opened a new pack of sterile gloves for me. Eric Vreede had brought a small Walkman with speakers to Rwanda and had left it in the OR. Thérèse put on Ry Cooder's Chicken Skin Music, Eric's favourite. We laughed for a moment about the parties we had back in 1988 and about the great dancing at Susan Allan's place behind the Centre Hospitalier de Kigali.

I cut, irrigated and tied off the arteries. In the last six weeks, Giovanni had broken all of the surgical saw blades. Now we were using a sterilized hacksaw. I sawed through the bone, and then cut, shaping and stitching the tissue, leaving a flap that we would close later just above his knee. In thirty minutes, I had sawed off his leg. It would take a lot of sweat to cut off a leg with a machete, I thought; it would be hard work. If the angle was right, though, less work to cut off a foot at the ankle, and even less just to cut the Achilles tendon. And with the right blows, it takes seconds—and very little sweat—to kill. The Interahamwe had figured this out. *Yes,* I thought, *it's different with a machete.*

Thérèse took the severed limb and put it in a bucket on the floor at the end of the operating table. It stood out of the bucket, like a bent flagpole, dripping blood onto the floor. My shoes had another layer of blood on them.

Then she pushed through the operating-room doors. One door slammed against the wall, the other swung closed. His mother screamed, "Mama-we! Mama-we y' nola" and louder again "Mama-we y' Nola!" as she lunged towards her son, one hand outstretched, the other clasping her yellow shawl. She held him and stroked his forehead. The light came in through the windows, making the sweat on his brow glisten, and making the yellow of her cheap synthetic shawl yellower still. His leg was in a bucket, and he was alive—an imperfect offering. She held him around his head as he quietly whispered, "Mama-we, Mama-we." They were beautiful to me. And I saw what Benedict had wanted me to see.

The next morning the city was noticeably quiet. It was July 4, and there was no shelling, only sporadic machine-gun fire coming from Kimihurura district. As I left the hospital to go to UNAMIR HQ, an RPF unit moving artillery stopped me. There were no longer snipers around the roundabout. At the morning briefing, UNAMIR people were elated. The RGF was fleeing. The RPF was moving into its abandoned positions around the city; it had conquered an all but empty capital. A few thousand civilians were still in hiding. Half of Kigali's original 300,000 inhabitants had fled, and the other half had been massacred. Kagame's Kigali victory was complete, but the war continued elsewhere in the country.

We had drinks that night at the UNAMIR compound.

Philippe Gaillard told me about a poem that was carved in the windowsill of his summer home in Switzerland. He recited it word for word. I can't remember it, but I do remember thinking it was as beautiful as his courage. He left Rwanda the next morning.

Roméo Dallaire brokered a clearly demarcated area for the French zone of operations. The French called it the Humanitarian Protection Zone, and it would effectively become the main route the RGF and Interahamwe would use to escape to Zaire. The only other route that remained for the RGF was a small sliver of land in Rhuengeri, the historical stronghold of Hutu power.

Unannounced, that afternoon the RPF brought a truckload of about thirty TB patients to the Faisal. They were dumped on the front steps of the hospital, nearly thrown out of the back of the flatbed truck. An old man lay coughing up blood. A nurse gave him a piece of cloth. He wiped the dripping, bloody phlegm from his lips. As the truck drove off, we began organizing a TB ward.

That night, I listened to the chest of the old man, who insisted on smoking his clay pipe. He could not walk on his own. We sat together on the balcony floor, low enough not to fall in the sight of snipers still shooting from pockets of resistance around the city, but high enough to see the stars. I admonished him for smoking when his chest was so bad. "C'est la guerre, Docteur. Le RPF sera le nouveau chef. Il y a toujours des chefs. Pour le moment, je dois rester confortable."

I offered him one of my cigarettes. He thanked me in French: "I'll enjoy it. Tomorrow I will have to walk. We'll see how things go, Doctor, we'll see how things go." I looked down at my bloodstained shoes and thought, *Yes, we'll see how things go.*

The next morning I went by APC to St. André Church. The militias were gone. The children were no longer herded into their rooms. They looked out the gate, still afraid to leave. The French priest's eyes winced in the bright sunlight, his long beard whisping over his pale skin and bony shoulders. He had stayed with the children for three months. He was filthy. His feet were brown with dirt worn deep into the skin under the heavy leather sandals he wore. He was walked out of the church supported under his arms by two UN soldiers.

He broke away from them and staggered back to his room. He emerged a few moments later with a crucifix, the one that he had clutched the first time I met him some four weeks before. He came with me to the hospital, and I arranged for him to have a meal, some hot water for washing and a clean room to himself. He had bad back pain and couldn't sleep. I examined him as he sat stooped over the edge of the bed. He was frail, his muscles wasted from starvation, and he flinched at the touch of my hand on his back. I gave him some Valium and made sure he took it.

The priest stayed with us for about five days. He never ate a full meal, only a few mouthfuls at each sitting. Even as he walked, he mumbled constantly, praying, looking down to something on the floor. When he sat, he pulled at his fingers, and his toes opened and closed as he was if trying to scratch against the soles of his sandals. I heard a few of the staff in the dining area mocking him. "That beard, those sandals, who does he think he is? Jesus Christ?" I looked around at the smirking faces. "After what he has done, as far as I am concerned, he is Jesus Christ," I said. A few days later, he was flown to France.

New patients arrived in the days that followed. People who had spent months in hiding were starving. As they came out of hiding, some were wounded by unexploded land mines and grenades that were littered about the city. I tried to stop a group of children from throwing rocks at an unexploded rocket-propelled grenade, while someone else picked it up and threw it into a ravine, where it exploded.

I went with Jonathan Brock one morning to an RPF-designated collection site for people who had been trapped in the city over the past three months. We walked into the seminary compound. There were at least fifteen thousand people there, with more arriving by the truckload all the time. They were all Hutus. There was no sign of weapons, no militia or RGF uniforms, but there were many well-muscled young men in clean clothes. I was nervous. I wasn't in a vehicle looking out at the faces of young men; I was standing in the dirt among them, closer than I had ever been. I was scared, and they can smell fear, I thought. I couldn't figure out where we had just come from, where our vehicle was, which way was out. I tried to take notes about the buildings as we walked.

Jonathan looked at my scribbles. "We're lost, aren't we?" he said.

"Just keep walking . . . and look confident," I told him.

After about a minute of more wading through the dense crowd, Jonathan took me by the elbow. "It's this way, O great fearless leader." We walked towards some RPF soldiers standing by their military vehicle. I was relieved to be with them. I got my bearings and calmed down. We found several people with some medical experience and located sites where bladder tanks of water could be set up. We returned later that day with more supplies and saw a truckload of young men in clean clothes being taken away by the RPF.

Many RPF soldiers had lost their entire families to the genocide, and no amount of military order could contain their rage completely. Not far from the Faisal, one RPF soldier was executed on the spot after his senior officer discovered that he had raped a woman. The RPF continued its mop-up and slowed or stopped our movement around the city. At new checkpoints, they inspected our vehicles, checked the nationality of all expatriates, and either let us proceed or turned us back. Elsewhere in Rwanda, the RPF was not as disciplined as it sometimes appeared in Kigali, and it was still fighting the RGF in the west of the country.

At the request of Frank Kamanzi and Colonel Yaache, I went by convoy with UNAMIR to what Kamanzi said was an orphanage outside Kigali. He had suggested media travel with the convoy, and Henry Anyidoho, the UNAMIR Deputy Force Commander, led us in three four-by-fours out of the city and over dirt roads. It wasn't necessary to take APCs as the visit was by RPF invitation and we would be going to what was now uncontested RPF territory.

We drove slowly for just under an hour along some very bad roads. As we entered the countryside, we could see no living people. I remembered that just six years before I had had the sense of never being alone. It was different now. I could hear wild dogs fighting among themselves in the distance. They had already eaten the flesh from the roadside corpses. Fresh greenstick branches browned by the sun slapped onto the windshield, yet even with the dense undergrowth, bodies were visible in the grass and underbrush along the road. They were at least a few weeks old. Sun-bleached white bones stuck through petrified leather skin that had been cut by machete, or torn by dogs. Women lay on top of their children. They had probably been forced to watch their children be butchered before being cut themselves. Other women lay on their backs; their knees and legs spread apart, sticks thrust into them, their arms covering their faces. The sun blared down. I felt smothered. I opened my flak jacket and lit a cigarette.

When we got to the site, it wasn't an orphanage but an abandoned boarding school where a group of psychiatric patients had somehow collected. Perhaps they had been left there; perhaps they wandered there and stayed. They were all men, and all of them were psychotic. I had seen many psychiatric patients in 1988 at Mugonero. Many Rwandans hold to the traditional belief that "worms" have taken over the minds of those suffering from psychiatric illnesses, and that spirits in the form of birds talk to the possessed. Now, here, all were starving.

Some walked endlessly in circles, some talked to themselves. One man stood talking to the birds in a tree.

"These are just crazy people. The children are inside," a well-dressed RPF man in civilian garb said. He seemed utterly unconcerned about the men, and I was immediately suspicious.

The media forgot the crazy people. They wanted to see the children. I wandered around the grounds, followed by a man who kept smiling and waving at me. I found a storeroom at the end of the covered outdoor walkway in front of the row of rooms. It had a locked wooden door with a small grille in its upper half. I looked in and saw sacks of maize and flour, at least several tins of cooking oil and some taped, unmarked boxes.

I made my way to the children. Inside their room was a row of beds, each with five or six infants and toddlers. Some older children about age three or four sat on the floor, staring at the collection of people with cameras and flak jackets standing before them. Many of the children were crying, all were filthy and afraid, and the smell of diarrhea mixed with clothing that had not been changed for weeks was overwhelming. There were about forty children in all. I looked at the group and examined some of the children, as the RPF man explained to the journalists that malaria did not only come with the rains.

The children were starving. Some had fever, and some had enlarged spleens, likely from malaria. Many were lying in at least a day's worth of diarrhea. Someone had been feeding them something, that much was clear. Without food and water the infants and the sick ones would have been dead already. "Who has been looking after them?" I asked.

"They are not here right now, but the children are being looked after," replied the well-dressed RPF man.

In an interview he said that the children needed food and medicine—"especially medicine for malaria. The doctor will agree, I am sure." The cameras and journalists immediately shifted to me. I knew that the RPF needed antimalarials. I answered their questions while walking out of the room and down the hallway to the storeroom. The journalists followed.

"Food may not be the problem," I said. "If you look inside here, there are several bags of maize already here. But of course, let's check. There may be other supplies already here."

"I don't have the key," the RPF man said, "and the caretaker is not here. Even still, the children are obviously sick, and it would be a travesty to not treat them for their malaria. What are you going to do, Doctor?" he asked.

"Some of the children may have malaria," I said, "but they have a lot of other problems too. They need proper medical care. I will take them to the Faisal Hospital."

"You can take more pictures while we discuss how best to approach the situation," the RPF man told the journalists as he took me politely by the arm and walked with me into the open compound. "No, the children cannot be moved," he said. "RPF orders. You can give the medicines to us, and they will be cared for here." I explained that we did not work that way. At least some of the children needed to be treated in hospital. All of them needed to be treated for malnutrition and bathed and cared for properly. None of them were getting that here. "The children cannot be moved," he repeated.

"I am not sure how you will explain to the journalists that even the sickest children cannot be taken to hospital in a convoy that is here, waiting and willing to take them," I said.

I knew we didn't have enough transport to move them all now. An agreement was reached that allowed Henry and me to take the sickest children and the infants back to the MSF hospital now. We agreed too that the other children would be taken when adequate transportation could be arranged. "And what about these men?" I said. "They also need to be brought to the hospital where we can give them proper care."

"We will bring the crazy people to you," he said. *The* crazy people? *The whole fucking country is crazy,* I thought. As we drove away, the smiling man waved at me until we passed behind the undergrowth alongside the road. That night I made my daily call to Jules.

"The RPF are not exactly Boy Scouts, are they?" he said.

A few days later Eric Goemaere, a general director of MSF, arrived in Kigali unexpectedly. He had come from Butare, now RPF territory, where MSF was establishing aid programs. He told me that the RPF was ordering the movement of people into organized regroupment camps. Medical staff were being intimidated, patients were disappearing at night, some Hutus were being singled out and killed. In the northeast, where MSF was now also working, the situation was not much different. I wasn't surprised.

In their Humanitarian Protection Zone, the French would not disarm the retreating RGF and Interahamwe, but pledged to prevent further massacres of Tutsis from taking place. They were not always successful. Some French officers were so disgusted with what their force was doing and not doing that they saw themselves as accomplices to a genocide they had been told did not exist. After discovering a group of eight hundred starving Tutsis who came out of the southwestern forest, three hundred of whom had survived being macheted or shot, one officer said, "We were manipulated [by our government]. We thought the Hutus were the good guys and the victims." For those French officers, after what they had seen, there was no doubt.

That night at the Faisal, Eric and I were called to attend a mother about to give birth. The generator had been turned off, so we used an oil-fuelled lantern as we made our way among the people who still slept in the hallways, on the stairs and in the doorways. Most were Hutus and were afraid to leave the hospital grounds. Some were awake, and were anxious to know why we were up at 3 a.m. Even though the RPF denied it, their soldiers often came through the fence during the night and took people away for interrogation. "Il n'y a aucun des soldats," I said, "Tout ça va calme."

The labour was obstructed, the mother was exhausted, and the baby would not deliver beyond a slight showing of its head. An old Rwandan woman who had presided over the birth while smoking her clay pipe, a privilege reserved only for the most senior women in Rwanda, laughed phlegmatically from deep in her chest. Her eyes squinted as she handed her pipe to a younger woman while I examined the mother. The old woman was a bony figure with a deeply wrinkled face and leathery skin. She spoke in a cackling, confident Kinyarwanda, and a younger woman translated for her. The flame was flickering and smoking. There wasn't enough fuel for a full light. A mortar exploded somewhere in the city, and the night crickets stopped singing for a while. I reached for a Vonteuse extractor, a rubber vacuum device placed on the head of a child and then pulled to extract the baby. I could smell the tobacco on the old woman's breath as she leaned into the mother's legs. I pulled on the extractor. "If it's a boy, the killing will continue," the old woman said as she watched me pull. "If it's a girl, it will stop." I forced the head out of its mother, and its body came easily. The baby boy cried. "Soon," the old woman said, "there will be a girl."

I wrapped the newborn in the same way I would wrap a newborn in Toronto—swaddled in a blanket that allowed the baby to breathe comfortably while keeping it warm. The old woman took the baby from me. As she rewrapped the baby in the traditional Rwandan way, she said, "You helped okay, but the baby lives here, not where you come from."

In those days after the fall of Kigali, new NGOs and UN agencies flooded into the city. MSF dispatched a British surgeon, three new nurses and a logistician to us, as well as a new head of mission who would soon take over from me. A sufficient and safe supply of water was the priority for the UN agencies. For us, there were new medical priorities for the city, and we had to plan how to hand over the hospital to new Rwandan authorities that had not yet been identified. I helped the new MSF team as best I could, but I couldn't easily leave the place where I had been.

On July 13, the RPF captured Rhuengeri. On July 14, Gisenyi fell. It was the final stronghold of the RGF. The next day, displaced Hutus began walking over the border to Zaire, heeding rumours of RPF reprisals. At the same time, farther south, six thousand people an hour, including Interahamwe and interim government officials, among them thirteen cabinet ministers, flooded into the French protection zone. The French would not arrest the accused leaders of the genocide, nor did they disarm the RGF. Instead their tactical general staff "initiated and organized" the escape of the genocidal government into Zaire.

Within two days, more than a million people had crossed the border into Zaire. It was the largest and fastest movement of refugees across a border ever recorded. They joined 500,000 refugees in Tanzania and 200,000 in Burundi. The RGF took its military hardware, and former government officials made sure that every removable object was looted and carried into the camps. Entire factories were disassembled; every computer and pencil, every piece of medical equipment or tablet, every vehicle and every hammer was taken from Rwanda into the camps. In Zaire, the mass of more than a million people was now herded together between Goma and Bukavu in Kivu province, just inside its border with Rwanda. They had no shelter, clean water, medical care or food. Rain and diarrhea washed around them. MSF and Oxfam started to distribute clean water, but people were dying of cholera and dysentery, epidemics that would run in deadly waves through their numbers in the coming days, killing thousands.

Hundreds of journalists flooded in too. CNN, BBC, ABC and every major television and wire service in the world were now there. While the genocide had been taking place in Rwanda, the number of reporters never rose above fifteen. In the camps, "genocide" was quickly replaced by "refugees." Complicated differences between Hutus and Tutsis, accomplices and bystanders, victims and perpetrators, hostages and kidnappers, government and rebels were obscured and effectively erased in fifteen-second sound bites that said it all. Now there was "a cholera epidemic in a humanitarian crisis," or "this child with diarrhea who has suffered the trauma of war." America and the world could not stand by. President Clinton said, "A child is dying every minute." In the coming days, four thousand American troops with very big guns would pump clean water to a million people, joining French troops and thousands more troops from other countries to assist the UN agencies and NGOs in delivering aid. No troops went to Rwanda, except of course, the French. In addition to offering assistance to refugees with cholera, French soldiers also delivered ten tons of food to RGF troops now in Zaire.

UNAMIR still had no secure water supply and no secure stocks of food or fuel. The APCs and trucks promised to UNAMIR by the May 17 UN resolution would begin to arrive in late July without radios, without repair equipment and without machine guns. The troops also promised in May began to arrive around the same time. Most didn't have the right equipment; some had none at all.

On July 18 the RPF declared the civil war over, established a transitional government, and outlawed the use of Hutu-Tutsi identity cards. That night, Jules asked me to go to Zaire. One million Tutsis had been killed in the Rwandan genocide. Hundreds of thousands were injured or sick. Millions were displaced inside Rwanda, and at least two million refugees were now pushed outside its borders by what was left of their genocidal government and army. During the fourteen weeks of genocide, UNAMIR had saved about thirty thousand lives in Kigali and lost fourteen of their own. MSF had lost hundreds of national staff. The war was over, and another was waiting to begin. I was smoking at least a pack a day. I had had a fever for the last two days and was coughing up bloodstained phlegm. Mycobacterium bronchitis or pneumonia—I wasn't sure. I was taking antibiotics and starting to feel better. Maybe not the right diagnosis, but the right treatment: that was better than the other way round, I thought. I was spent. I had nothing left to give. I told Jules I was going home.

I stood on the balcony, having another cigarette. The French MSF team had left the Red Cross hospital a few days earlier. It was complete luck and not by any shrewd strategy of ours that they were not killed. I knew that the meaning of their choice to remain would stay with me always. I thought of the crazy men and the children at the boarding school. They were never brought to us. I thought of the woman who called me her friend. Ummera-sha. She had helped me find my courage. I never saw her again. I finished my cigarette. Sylvie was awake in her broom closet, and Lulu and Vanessa were asleep in a blanket on the floor. I gave Sylvie some money and told her I would see them tomorrow.

Then Eli came. He wanted me to examine a girl brought to the hospital earlier that day. She would not speak, and he didn't know why. She sat in a corner of the children's ward. She had been bathed since arriving, but there were no clean clothes for her. Her blue school tunic was torn and stained. She was uninjured and silent. I sat on the floor with them. Eli stroked her hand, talking with her. Eli translated for me as she started to speak.

She said that she had escaped being killed by the Interahamwe. "My mother hid me in the latrine. I saw through the hole. I watched them hit her with machetes. The men were angry and strong. I watched my mother's arm fall into my father's blood on the floor and I cried without noise in the toilet." I listened to her and watched her lips quiver as her words came at a slow, staccato tempo. I watched her brown eyes look away as tears dropped to her cheeks and I could not stop my own.

At that moment, I felt both despair and rage. Despair that she knew intimately our capacity for the most extreme rational cruelty; that she was alone. Animals could never do this. Animals can be brutal, but only humans can be rationally cruel. We can choose anything, we can be anything, we can get used to anything, I thought. Only humans can be evil. Only humans can make this choice. I felt my heart pounding and I wanted a gun. I wanted to kill the men who had done this to her. I wanted to pull the trigger again and again and again. My heart was racing; I was fighting my tears, gasping for air, for freshness, for something other than this. Then Eli clasped my arm with his strong hands. I felt an overpowering despair for the little girl, for myself, for all of us—that we can be alone, trapped in our passions, in our reasons, in our minds, in our politics, that I and those men could be so angry and strong.

It felt like something was broken that could never be fixed.

I couldn't sit any longer. Eli turned to the girl, and soon I was embarrassed by my tears. I walked down the stairs and went back to the balcony for a smoke. I had three. The next morning, I packed, then I said goodbye to the team. I looked for Sylvie, Vanessa and Lulu, but couldn't find them. I left Kigali that afternoon on a UNAMIR flight.

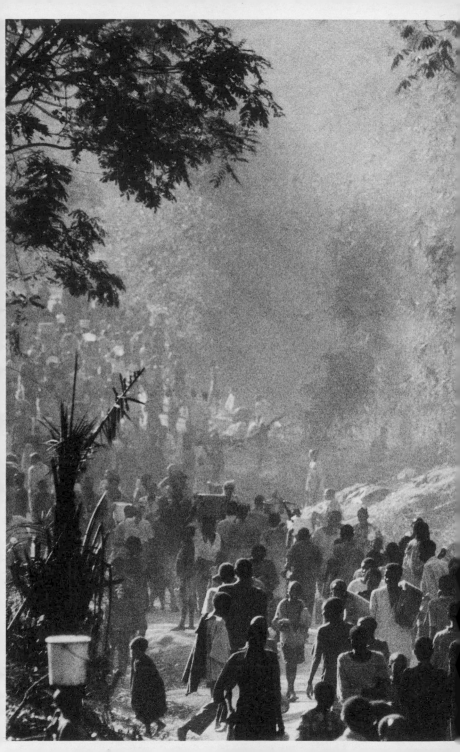

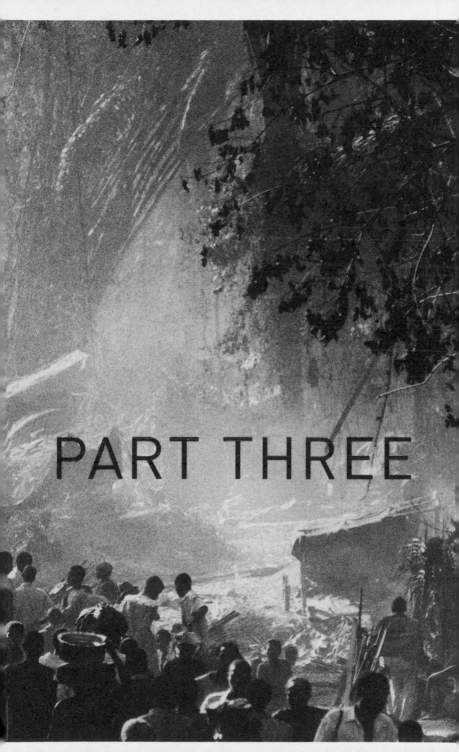

PART THREE

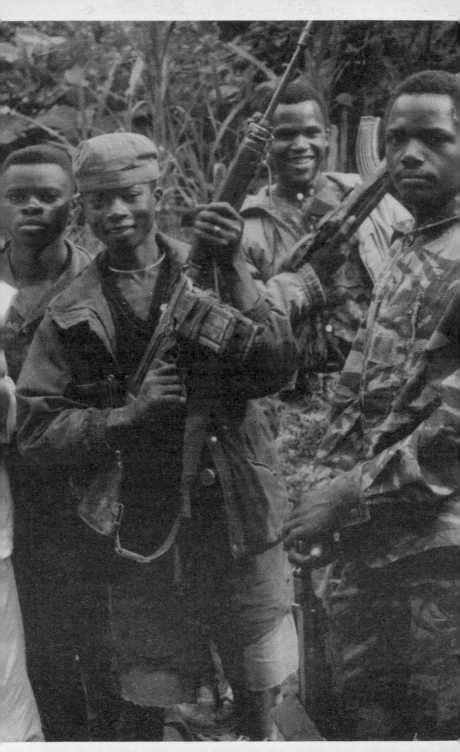

REFUGEES IN ZAIRE:
FEAR OF WHAT THEY KNOW, FEAR OF
WHAT WE CANNOT SEE

I was driving along Highway 401 in Toronto as a blue Mazda Miata passed me. It was the same colour as the plastic tarp that I had been dreaming about for months without knowing why. Instantly, my car filled with the sweet smell of freshly killed flesh and blood. I saw sausages and then children's fingers in the red soil around the tarp. I veered as I tried to open the windows. The bumper scraped the guardrail as the car came to a full stop. I sat in the car, the smell and sausages gone. It was snowing outside. The wipers kept rhythm but I had fallen out of time. The world had not changed—I had. I sat there, counting pieces of roadside garbage and debris, and then I just drove for a while. I arrived at my parents' house three hours late.

Canada was a world away, blissfully ignorant of what I had witnessed in Rwanda. On July 31, 1994, the country's largest newspaper, the *Toronto Star*, had interviewed me for a front-page article that ran with the headline: "Doctor Calls Events in Rwanda Genocide." I had lost weight in the eighteen months since I had returned. I was smoking too much, not returning phone calls. I continued as vice-president of MSF Canada and was doing emergency-room shifts. I was pursuing a master's in medical epidemiology. Something about the logic of statistics calmed me, but I couldn't completely escape what I knew. I was possessed by what I had seen in Rwanda, trapped between rage and despair.

Over dinner my parents engaged in small talk, probing rather than being direct, trying to take the measure of me. Rwanda was never mentioned, but it surrounded us like its heavy humid air. After a long silence, the kind where you begin to count the ticking of the clock in the other room, my mother started to cry. "You should have never gone back to that place. You're not the same." My father reached across the table and rubbed her shoulder. My mother shook her head as she cried into her hands. "You can't just lie down in the snow, James," my father said. "Do you hear me? You can't just lie down in the snow. You've got to get up. You'll find your way."

I went to bed and dreamt of the white blanket of lime covering the bodies at Auschwitz and of the beautiful eyes of the shoe-store man on St. Laurent. I could see now why those eyes were beautiful. They were beautiful because they were ready to die and yet chose to live; beautiful because he had made life with the same slow deliberateness with which he and his wife removed one shoebox from between others. He smiled at me, and I felt his hand on my neck.

A few weeks later, I went to see Benedict. Neither of us said a word as we walked through the snow for more than an hour. When we returned from the woods he said, "Sometimes it is good to be silent: to be as we are, free to choose in the space between what we know and what we feel." We talked into the night about Rwanda, and I thanked him for sending me the poem when he did. I went outside for a smoke and took in the blue hue of the moon lighting the midnight snow. Over the next few months, I saw a counsellor, and soon I was

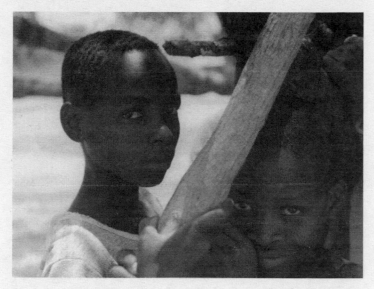

Zambia, 1996

asking myself, "Why would I want to see the world any other way than the way it is?"

I met Rolie Srivastava, my future wife, at an MSF party in Toronto. She was a friend of a friend and knew nothing of MSF's world of dilemmas. With her freshness, I felt a thawing. Sometimes opposites are best. I could breathe again.

In August 1996, a friend at the Canadian Public Health Association called me. Someone had cancelled, and they desperately needed a doctor to do an evaluation of their programs in Zambia. A few days later I was on a plane. I spent the next ten weeks travelling the Zambian countryside, inspecting clinics and latrines, tabulating childhood immunization rates and eating fresh chickens with village chiefs and elders. And for that time I was all but cut off from international news and MSF. Then, on November 17, while I was writing my final report in my hotel room, the phone rang. It was Jules. "I have been trying to reach you for weeks. By the

259

way, your parents send their regards," he said. "It's Rwanda again. Well, not exactly Rwanda."

"Don't tell me. Zaire. I'm watching it on CNN," I said.

"The RPF have attacked the refugee camps," Jules told me. "MSF has called on the UN to send in a force. It's not entirely clear what's happening. I need you in Goma. What are you doing tonight?" I had to go back, I thought. The story was not over, and nor was mine in it.

For two years, even with its hundreds of other projects, MSF was, like me, possessed by the Great Lakes region of Africa. On behalf of the organization, I had been lobbying Canadian government officials on Rwanda. I had travelled back and forth to MSF's office in Amsterdam many times, editing lobbying documents and debating operational dilemmas. We had hundreds of expatriates trying to provide humanitarian assistance in a post-genocidal political crisis that was getting not better but worse.

Since taking power in July 1994, the new Rwandan government led by vice-president Paul Kagame, who was also the country's minister of defence, had struggled to maintain order. Besides moralizing rhetoric on the "never again" of genocide and the need for justice, the international community was doing little to deal with the Rwandan reality. The World Bank demanded interest payments on outstanding loans made to the former genocidal regime before it would advance loans to the new government. In late 1994, I met with officials from the Canadian International Development Agency and urged them to support Rwanda's justice system, something less appealing to Western publics than humanitarian assistance but no less vital to Rwanda's future. Two years later, the justice system was still little more than a phantom, getting paper, pens and its only vehicle from Rwanda's Citizens' Network, an NGO set up by MSF Belgium in the months following the genocide. The country had only five judges—all the others had been murdered or were in exile. In November 1994, the UN Security Council passed a resolution establishing the International Criminal Tribunal for Rwanda to bring to trial those accused of genocide. But none of the Security Council members had given money to actually create the tribunal. By 1995, the only financial support had come from the Swiss government, and that was a paltry 100,000 Swiss francs—enough to buy a Mercedes-Benz with an empty gas tank. Meanwhile, in the former Yugoslavia, $1 billion a year was being spent on UN peacekeeping.

In Rwanda, more than 100,000 people were in prison, having been denounced by their neighbours as *genocidaires*, and their numbers were growing daily. The conditions in the country's numerous prisons and *cahotes*, or interrogation camps, were deplorable. Prisoners were so tightly packed that they could sleep only in shifts while sitting down, and most had foot rot from standing in excrement and waste. Many needed foot or leg amputations because of spreading gangrene, and one in eight prisoners were dying of diseases like malaria and pneumonia. A few days after I arrived in Kigali, in late November 1996, one distraught MSF doctor would tell me that HIV/AIDS was spreading like wildfire in the prisons. The doctor had seen a fourteen-year-old boy who complained of stomach aches. The prison had been designed for four hundred prisoners but was holding seven thousand men and boys. The boy had vomited in front of this doctor. The boy had been forced to give fellatio to so many prisoners that he was vomiting semen.

The Kagame regime continued to be anything but Boy Scouts. When the French left the country in August 1994, dozens of camps for displaced people in Rwanda had been established in the former French-controlled humanitarian zone. Some 400,000 Hutus were living in the camps that came under the supervision of UNAMIR—the UN Assistance Mission for Rwanda, itself now under the command of Canadian general Guy Tousignant—while other UN and private humanitarian agencies worked in them. The Rwandan government wanted the camps closed, and insisted it was safe for the displaced people to return to their homes. But many people stayed, fearing retribution at home. Those who did want to leave were often beaten or killed by the Hutu Interahamwe militia, who remained an armed guerrilla force inside the camps. On April 22, 1995, a year after the genocide had begun, the RPA—as the RPF became known with the declaration of the new Rwandan government—attacked the Kibeho camp inside Rwanda, killing at least four thousand Hutus. They were massacred over some five hours of unrestrained fire with machine guns, rocket-propelled grenades and anti-tank weapons. The Zambian UNAMIR commander repeatedly asked his Kigali headquarters for permission to counterattack, and repeatedly he was told he could only watch and assist the wounded. Several days before, the RPA had surrounded the camp with some 2,500 reinforcements, cut off food supplies and destroyed and burned people's shelters. The massacre was witnessed by MSF and UNAMIR, and both gave similar initial estimates of the number killed. Individual UNAMIR soldiers then leaked an internal document that reported the RPA were removing thousands of bodies from the massacre site at night. UNAMIR officially fell silent, denying the report. Under intense public pressure from MSF, the RPA government launched an investigation that concluded that undisciplined soldiers seeking revenge for the murders of family members during the genocide had killed just over three hundred people at Kibeho. As security incidents and harassment of MSF teams across the country continued, MSF was so vociferous that thousands had been massacred in a planned attack on the camp that by the end of the year, the Rwandan government had expelled MSF's French section.

As well as its public condemnation of the Kibeho massacre, MSF lobbied hard and publicly on the need for the international community to support a viable justice system to bring the perpetrators of the genocide to justice and the need to offer financial support to the new Rwandan government. We drew attention to the conditions inside the prisons and to other massacres that had occurred around the country. But MSF pushed hardest on the intolerable situation inside the refugee camps in Zaire and Tanzania. The camps had become places of totalitarian rule by the Interahamwe militia and the former Rwandan government army, now known as the ex-FAR, or ex–Rwandan Armed Forces.

Eighty thousand refugees in the camps had died of cholera and other diseases during the summer of 1994. Two years later, upwards of 1.2 million people were crowded into the camps in Zaire, less than seven kilometres away from the border with Rwanda. There were 750,000 refugees in camps in Tanzania and another 250,000 in Burundi. They were being held as human shields. The camps had become rear bases from which guerrilla incursions into Rwanda were being launched, and where the ex-FAR and the Interahamwe were openly preparing for what they called Operation Insecticide, a plan to invade Rwanda to "finish the work of genocide."

Despite a UN embargo, arms were still being delivered to the ex-FAR and the Interahamwe via the Goma airport in Zaire, and many of these arms could be traced to French sources. The French government offered political support to President Mobutu Sese Seko of Zaire, who had been abandoned by his Cold War patron of thirty years, the United States. Mobutu had been a long-time ally of the Habyarimana government in Rwanda, and now gave the Hutu forces that controlled the camps virtually free rein in Zaire's Kivu region. The military, political and administrative structures of the former Rwandan state had effectively been used to establish mini-states inside the camps in both Tanzania and Zaire. Boys as young as ten were being forcibly recruited into the Interahamwe and the ex-FAR. Those refugees who wanted to return to Rwanda were raped, beaten or executed publicly.

The UN High Commissioner for Refugees and various UN agencies, MSF and roughly two hundred other NGOs were working in what were now the largest refugee camps in the world. Since the summer of 1994, more than $2 billion in aid had poured into the region. The power of the *genocidaires* was fuelled by the massive diversion of this aid, including the more than $1 million a day that UNHCR was spending there. Aid workers faced constant open death threats and intimidation. Attempts to conduct a census to accurately determine the needs of the refugees were obstructed. Even with the huge amount of aid going into the camps, at least 10 percent of the children there were malnourished.

MSF, a few other NGOs and the UNHCR made direct appeals to the UN Security Council for a security force to disarm the ex-FAR and the Interahamwe and to separate them from the refugees. Platitudes were offered in response, but nothing was done. The Security Council had characterized the genocide as a humanitarian disaster rather than a political crime. Now it was doing the same with the crisis in the camps. And most NGOs played along, claiming an apolitical humanitarian neutrality and avoiding any confrontation with the international community. Many of these same NGOs were funded by the Western states that refused to act. For all concerned, it was a convenient humanitarian alibi.

In the face of the Security Council's inaction, the impossible choice now facing MSF was to knowingly provide material support to a totalitarian army intent on finishing the genocide it had started, or to abandon the refugees. It was a dilemma that had to be confronted without retreating into notions of neutrality. Again and again MSF insisted on a UN force and threatened to withdraw from the camps if it did not come. With great difficulty, we organized some other NGOs to join us. It was not an easy choice for anyone. After months of nearly bitter internal debate, and the failure of a concerted humanitarian resistance strategy, MSF began to withdraw from the camps: first MSF France in November 1994, then MSF Belgium in the spring of 1995, and finally MSF Holland in August. Faced with reduced funding from donor states, few NGOs followed MSF's lead. MSF Belgium continued to work inside Rwanda, delivering medical care to hundreds of thousands of Rwandans and challenging the government on conditions inside the prisons, and MSF Holland continued to work outside the camps in the surrounding Masisi district of Kivu, Zaire, on the border of Rwanda. With the refugee camps having been in existence for more than two years, the Kivu region—the country's poorest and most densely populated—was ready to explode.

The ex-FAR and Interahamwe were forcing Hutus, whose ancestors had lived in the Kivu region for hundreds of years, to join in their effort to create a "Hutuland" from which they would launch an invasion of Rwanda. Other indigenous Kivu groups that had lived in the region for centuries—like the Hunde and Tembo tribes—were being played one against the other by Mobutu, who allowed his own undisciplined army to rape, rob and pillage at will, and allowed the ex-FAR to do the same. At the same time, Zairean Tutsis, whose roots in Kivu went back more than three hundred years, were being terrorized by the ex-FAR and Interahamwe, as were other Tutsis from Rwanda who, since 1959, had escaped to the region after anti-Tutsi pogroms. All the Tutsis of Kivu were now the targets of a violent harassment campaign by both Hutu militias and Mobutist forces. Their cattle were raided, their crops were burned, women were raped. Entire villages were massacred, and a campaign of ethnic cleansing saw Tutsis driven out of others. As a result, in addition to the more than one million Rwandan Hutu refugees, there were now more than 250,000 Zairean people displaced from their homes and living in the hills and farmers' fields of the Masisi region. But they were residents of Zaire, not refugees, and despite MSF's protests, the UN was not interested.

Some Tutsis from Zaire joined the Rwandan RPA. By early October 1996 they were organized by Rwanda and Uganda into a rebel army, the Alliance of Democratic Forces for the Liberation of Zaire, or ADFL, led by Laurent Kabila, a former Marxist rebel and diamond and gold smuggler. Based in Kivu, the ADFL opposed Mobutu, whose thirty-year kleptocracy had left the country in ruins and made him one of the richest men in the world. Mobutu was in Europe for cancer treatment, his regime was crumbling from within, and Zaire was ripe for change. The ADFL seemingly came out of nowhere, but would soon be everywhere.

In late September, the RPA and ADFL rebels started attacking the Zaire Armed Forces, or FAZ, in South Kivu. By mid-October they were attacking the refugee camps in the region, and then those camps around Goma in North Kivu. All the UN agencies and NGOs in the camps drastically reduced their teams. As the violence continued, the remaining one hundred aid workers retreated to the UNHCR compound in Goma before being evacuated into Rwanda. The fighting escalated as the ex-FAR joined the FAZ against the ADFL rebels, and, even though the Rwandan government wouldn't admit it, Rwandan troops crossed the border into Zaire to support the ADFL. Some journalists reported that in response to the attacks, the ex-FAR and Interahamwe militias inside the camps herded the refugees together and ordered them to move west, away from Rwanda and into the Zairean jungle. Other journalists reported that anyone who resisted was killed with machetes, and that in many cases entire families suffered this fate. Later accounts by surviving refugees say that many willingly followed directions from the ex-FAR and Interahamwe militias for fear of what they would suffer under the ADFL rebels and their RPA and Ugandan allied forces. By November 1, half a million refugees were trapped in the jungles around South Kivu, and about 600,000 had fled north towards the Mugunga refugee camp just outside Goma.

Hundreds of journalists swarmed to the area. MSF flew in 180 expatriate volunteers and tons of medical supplies. However, the Rwandan government and the ADFL rebels closed the border and blocked anyone from returning to Kivu. For nearly a week in North Kivu, and two weeks in South Kivu, there were no aid workers and no journalists to actually see what was happening. MSF feared the worst—that the crisis would develop into a bloodbath for the refugees and the civilian population—and said so publicly. On November 4, MSF called for a UN military intervention to protect civilians and refugees from the fighting, and to break the hold the ex-FAR had over the refugees. Twenty minutes later, Laurent Kabila declared a unilateral ceasefire, saying that the ADFL would allow the refugees to return to Rwanda. MSF waited while clamouring for access at the border. The fighting continued inside Zaire, and the borders remained closed.

From experience, MSF predicted that 13,600 people could already be dead from cholera, malnutrition and other diseases, never mind from violence. MSF kept up the call for UN intervention, and was joined in this by the UNHCR, regional African governments and a coalition of other NGOs. Even the usually neutral Red Cross said that it "was time to act" and that it would not object to a UN military force. Apparently at the urging of Prime Minister Jean Chrétien, who had been watching the crisis unfold on television, Canada began rallying other governments to the cause and offered to lead an intervention force itself, though only with a UN mandate. Political pressure intensified, and the European Union's Commissioner for Humanitarian Affairs described the Security Council's slow response as an "international scandal."

Mobutu's army was losing badly to the Rwanda-ADFL alliance and agreed to a UN force, while the Rwandan government strenuously objected. Pressure continued to build. The Rwandan government eventually admitted to assisting the

ADFL, but reiterated that the ex-FAR and Interahamwe in the camps were a threat to Rwandan security and maintained its objection to an intervention. Kabila categorically insisted on a "neutral" force with no French or French-allied troops. Kabila then allowed a select number of journalists to be taken on strictly controlled tours of Uvira city in the south and Goma city in North Kivu.

To assuage mounting political pressure, Kabila held more conciliatory press conferences and gave permission for a tele-vised NGO aid convoy to drive into the stadium at Goma. The world would then see that aid was getting through to the camps. Once in, the supplies were unloaded and the NGOs were told to immediately return to Rwanda. The ADFL announced that it would allow the NGOs to return to Kivu once they had been reg-istered and screened for their "impartiality." In the meantime, the ADFL seized the humanitarian supplies and claimed it would distribute them. The journalists moved on to Kabila's next press conference, where he shared his reaction to President Bill Clinton's stated willingness to send 1,000 American soldiers with a Canadian-led intervention. Clinton's press secretary, Mike McCurry, had said that while a final decision was pending, "our interests are largely humanitarian, to save lives." For nearly three weeks no journalists and no aid workers had actually seen what was happening in Kivu.

On the night of November 14, ADFL rebels attacked the Mugunga refugee camp near Goma. Only hours before, the Security Council had finally passed a resolution authorizing a UN force, not to separate the refugees from the ex-FAR or to protect them from the war between the ADFL and the Zairean army but simply to safeguard humanitarian aid. Within hours of the UN resolution, the Rwandan border was opened. Over the next three days, hundreds of thousands of refugees streamed through Goma into Rwanda. Journalists and aid organizations were then allowed back into Zaire, but only into certain parts of Goma and only into abandoned camps. The rest were "too insecure," the ADFL said.

It was the strong and the fit that had walked across the border carrying their possessions on their heads. Some were exhausted, but the Rwandan government would allow MSF only to set up temporary water and first-aid stations along the road to Kigali. The RPA seized vehicles from MSF and other aid agencies to move the returnees more quickly. RPA soldiers pushed a line of people thirty kilometres long through the border crossing and into carefully prepared reception sites. Some of the returnees were arrested on suspicion of having participated in the genocide, but most were resettled in their home communities within a span of just three days. The press declared the operation orderly and well planned. Many observers suggested that the refuges would all soon be home, their return precipitated by the proposal for an intervention.

On November 23, the day before I arrived in Rwanda, a few days after Jules's call, the Americans held what would be described to me as a "whiz-bang" press conference, complete with electronic slides, graphs and images taken from their satellite and Orion aircraft reconnaissance flights. They argued that the original number of refugees in the camps—according to UNHCR figures, 1.2 million—had been overestimated and that between 600,000 and 900,000 had already returned. The Americans claimed to have identified clusters of people in Zaire which, by nature of their movement and other clues, the Americans argued, could be assumed to be the ex-FAR and Interahamwe and their families. Let them be damned, was the implication. The refugees were coming home in relatively good shape, all things considered, and the world was witnessing it on TV. The Americans now questioned the need for an intervention. The Rwandans and the ADFL had done what everyone else had failed to do: they had solved the problem of the camps. Even with as many as half a million people unaccounted for, these were exceptional circumstances, and it had been an African solution to an African problem.

Those who had been left behind were lost in the story of those who had returned.

I arrived at the Kigali airport just as many journalists and aid workers were lining up to leave. In the pillars inside the terminal there were bullet holes dating back to 1994. Arjan Hehenkamp, my friend from Somalia, who was now MSF's head of mission in Rwanda, met me at the airport. We drove past the Amahoro stadium. Even in the twilight I could see that it had been freshly painted. Nothing could cover over what I remembered. We stopped briefly at the MSF compound and then went out for dinner. There was a fleet of air-conditioned Land Cruisers outside the Cactus restaurant overlooking the hills of the city. Inside, UN officials, aid workers, diplomats and American soldiers talked loudly through their meals.

Over dinner Arjan and I talked about the numbers—they didn't add up. The UNHCR had estimated that in the first three days after the November 15 attack, 450,000 refugees had crossed back into Rwanda. Since then the flow of those returning had slowed to fewer than 10,000 a day, and the numbers were falling. Nevertheless, journalists had expected to see the apocalypse. Instead, said Arjan, "all they have been allowed to see is empty camps and hundreds of thousands of well-fed refugees returning to a well-planned welcome in Rwanda." I asked about those left behind. They were still without any protection and faced the immediate risk of being murdered. "Welcome to the land of deceptions, where everything is only as it appears on CNN," said Arjan. "In a game of delays, lies and half-truths, perception is everything."

MSF continued to press for a UN intervention, but its credibility had been damaged. The press challenged MSF on its predictions of a cholera epidemic and accused MSF and other aid agencies of crying wolf and inflating the numbers of dying refugees to boost fundraising. Press commentaries pointed out what everyone could plainly see on their TV screens: the refugees were returning plump and well fed on humanitarian assistance delivered over two years of highly effective humanitarian fundraising campaigns.

What were we doing now? I asked Arjan.

"We are looking for between four and five hundred thousand people who seem to have been airbrushed from history. They are somewhere in the jungles of Kivu being forced forward by the ex-FAR/FAZ and chased by the ADFL Rwanda Alliance." Were we sure of the numbers? "Not a hundred percent, but sure enough that we're going to look and look hard. The press isn't interested. The Canadians have an advance military team here, but the multinational force seems to be falling apart. It's all smoke and mirrors. Information is coming from highly controlled access to Kivu. The Rwandan government is hostile to us," he explained, "but they have to be seen to be 'humanitarian.' We are finding unexploded hand grenades thrown into our compounds, the RPA government is constantly changing the rules for visas to slow us down, and they are 'requisitioning' our vehicles and trucks. We are trying to do our own overflights of Zaire to try to figure out what is going on and to find the refugees."

We finished our meal and walked in darkness down the hill to our vehicle. I was back in Rwanda and it felt like I had never left.

I slept on the floor that night with some thirty other expatriates. The next morning Arjan and I met again in a tent set up at the back of the MSF compound. Maps were taped to the canvas, day-old coffee was spilled on the table, cigarette butts littered the dirt floor and journalists hung around in search of a story. "Got any more predictions on the refugees?" one asked. "Just that we'll find them," Arjan replied.

Arjan and I drove to the border. The few remaining journalists were taking pictures of not thousands, not hundreds, but scattered groups of people who walked silently along the road, moved on by RPA soldiers. Civilian faces stared blankly from passing trucks driven by soldiers back into Rwanda. I transferred to another MSF car waiting for me at the border and crossed over into Goma, where I met the head of mission, Marc Gastellu-Etchegorry, whom I was to replace. The MSF team of eighteen in Goma was extremely frustrated, having been denied access beyond the ADFL checkpoints that were everywhere in and around the city. Marc knew there were refugees just out of reach, as some had broken through or been delivered to us by the ADFL. Marc had also been told by Father Laurent Balas, an expatriate Belgian priest who had worked in Masisi for several years, that villagers were reporting massacres of refugees in the forest. There were shell-damaged buildings around Goma, and soldiers, artillery and other heavy weapons were everywhere. Groups organized by the ADFL were clearing the city of debris. It was the first time in more than thirty years anything like street cleaning had been attempted, and it was taken by the international press as evidence of the orderliness of the new rebel regime.

Marc took me to an abandoned warehouse where MSF had set up a temporary field hospital. It was designed for 250 patients; inside there were only 34. The hospital was a model of what MSF facilities should be and it was practically empty. Leslie Shanks was the doctor in charge, and she explained that most of the patients were afraid to talk. Some did tell her of being forced out of the camps by the ex-FAR, and then of being attacked by ADFL rebels. As we talked, one woman sat on the plastic sheeting on the floor and stared at the warehouse wall as her child tried to feed on one of her breasts. Leslie explained that the woman feared for her husband and other children who had fled into the forest when their camp was attacked. Marc and Leslie knew that there were thousands more families like this woman's in the jungle.

The MSF team was solid but tired, and a good number of members were young and inexperienced. "You will have to watch each of them closely," Marc said. "Give them breaks in Kigali when you can." Others on the team had friendships with the national staff and local leaders. Some had been evacuated during the attacks in October and early November. They were impatient with the pace of what they were able to do, which wasn't much. "We aren't reaching the outlying areas, and we are blocked everywhere," said Marc. "They are only letting us see what they want." The few refugees who came out of the forests were screened by the ADFL before being delivered to the UNHCR and to us. We would treat the sick, and then the UNHCR would shuttle them in trucks to the Rwandan border. Areas were opened up to us only after the ADFL had "secured" them. We were expected to provide food, medicine and water to whomever was left. Marc showed me a temporary cholera treatment centre designed for 150 patients; we had 14. "They are all people from the city of Goma," Phil Clark, a British MSF logistician, told me. "There are no refugees here, I'm afraid. Apparently, they don't actually exist." Members of the MSF team, especially the medical staff who were treating patients coming from the camps and forests, seemed stunned by what they were experiencing. "It is too hard for them to see such fear, to know that here, the only justice is what you dream," said Marc. Morten Rostrup, a Norwegian MSF doctor, said to me, "It's criminal and no one knows what to do."

Water systems had been destroyed in the last weeks of intense fighting in Goma, and MSF was supplying water to several areas around the city. Now the fighting had moved west, north and south into the hills and jungle surrounding the camps and into the densely populated countryside. Marc warned me of the dangers we faced and suggested that before

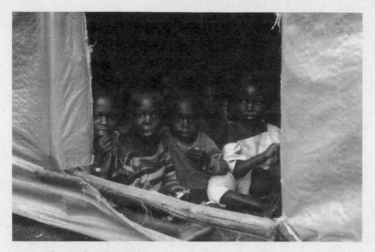

Sake Feeding Centre

sending anyone into any new areas, I or other experienced people should go there first. "Try to go west to Masisi," he told me. "We think there are about 200,000 people moving in that direction. Try to go north too, towards Bunia, but be careful—the ADFL is not as strong as it pretends, and the FAZ are repositioning to take it back. Of course they have the help of the ex-FAR and Interahamwe, and there are more rumours that they have French government support and are hiring mercenaries," he said. "Then try to connect south with our teams in Bukavu, just past Sake."

We drove through several heavily armed checkpoints along the twenty-five-kilometre road to Sake, south of Goma. The three main volcanoes of the Virunga jungle loomed over us in the distance. A minor volcano had erupted days before and rumbled as we passed the site of the former Mugunga camp. We stopped at the edge of the thirteen-kilometre-long camp, but were immediately forced back into our vehicle by an ADFL patrol. Only weeks before, the camp had held 400,000 people. Now it looked like a ghost town of rags, bamboo sticks, blue plastic tarps, covered pit latrines and shelled vehicles that had been blown over in a passing tornado. It smelled of rotting flesh, and the only things that moved were the wind and the rats. I would later learn that as we passed that day at least five thousand bodies were being collected in the camp, and thousands more were cleared from the covered pit latrines in other camps.

We drove farther, looking out on eucalyptus and banana trees and mango and bamboo stalks that lined the border between the camp and the jungle. We came to a roadblock. A stone-faced soldier about thirty years old walked up to our vehicle. He ignored our efforts to talk with him and just stared at me and Marc. Our nervous driver opened the rear of the Land Cruiser, and the soldier looked in. The soldier waved his hand at two of the six other ADFL rebels, who quickly moved the red and yellow plastic beer crates placed across the road. As we drove on we nearly hit a boy about four years old who was sitting in the road. He didn't move as we approached, honking. We stopped. He sat in a daze, his deep brown eyes looking up at the white men standing over him. After speaking with bystanders who said he was an orphan, I took him with us to the feeding centre MSF had set up a little way down the road. He had a bad cut on his face and the fine red hair and swollen hands and feet of a starving child. He was wearing an adult's T-shirt that hung on him like a dress. It was so worn that holes were tearing in its decomposing fabric. He smelled of diarrhea. There were 130 people at the feeding centre, mostly women and children who had come from the outlying villages. There were no refugees.

Marc left that night, and the following morning, Graziella Godain, a French MSF nurse, and I tried to go west to Masisi. On every road we tried that day and every day in the weeks ahead, the ADFL would not let us pass. It was the same story in the South Kivu. José Antonio Bastos, a Spanish doctor, was the MSF coordinator in the south. Since early November he had pressed at the border with his team. It had taken them twenty-three days to be allowed to cross into Zaire from Rwanda. Once in Bukavu, their movements were extremely restricted by the ADFL, and they were able to do less than we were doing in the north.

Arjan was in constant contact with other MSF teams in the Great Lakes region and Europe, with other NGOs, and with me in Goma and José in South Kivu. When it could get airspace clearance, MSF was doing its own flights, sometimes with the Red Cross and the UNHCR, sometimes alone. Based on all the information we could gather, we knew of groups of refugees ranging in size from 10,000 to 100,000. We also knew of smaller pockets of people who had broken away from the larger groups that had been attacked by the ADFL as they fled west. Our plan now was to try to get our teams into other parts of Zaire, to "meet" the refugees where they were thought to be heading. Our efforts to get to them were thwarted by the war, the continual movement of troops, and rumours and obstructions in both Rwanda and Zaire.

Our program in Goma, such as it was, continued. I didn't want to close the cholera centre or the temporary hospital in case we had an influx of refugees. We started offering training courses for Zairean nurses and doctors on cholera and epidemic management. At our nightly meetings, team members expressed deepening anger and frustration that was fed by the fearful and incomplete testimonies of fewer and fewer refugees. I felt exactly the same. I had seen the worst in Rwanda and now feared for what I could not see. No one knew what was happening in the villages and jungle beyond Goma. There was a curtain of darkness behind the roadblocks with no clear way through. It was becoming more obvious by the day that we were little more than a mop-up crew for the ADFL alliance.

Later that week I had some luck. Not far from the feeding centre in Sake, I got through to an unguarded back road that would lead us west to the Masisi road. My driver and I drove through the dense jungle, radioing back to the MSF compound every fifteen minutes. At one point we stopped to urinate. I walked a few feet into the bush and saw the face of a dead man staring up at me. Beside him were two other corpses, not more than a day old, partially eaten by wild animals. They were young men and they had been shot in the back of the head. In the face of the rumours of massacres, I didn't know if the corpses I was looking at were the victims of an isolated incident or remnants of a much bigger problem. We continued up the road. In farmers' fields were the remnants of a vast camp for thousands of people. It looked as if the occupants had walked away suddenly without packing. They had camped long enough to set up makeshift shelters of blue plastic tarps, but these and the possessions that people had carried with them for two years had been abandoned. The fields and the roads were thick with cooking pots, tins of cooking oil stamped "Gift of the People of the United States," clothes, school textbooks. Jerry cans were pressed into a trail tilled by the feet of thousands. I looked down at a lone red plastic sandal half buried in the mud. The strap was broken: "Made in China" was stamped across its sole. We passed villages that had been looted and burned. Some had been abandoned. We could see a few people standing in the hills. My driver was afraid to stop. These are not my people, he explained. He was Tembo, and they were Hunde. We made it about twenty-five kilometres through the hills, but a landslide across the road forced us to turn back. I spoke with Arjan that night, and he told me that Gen. Maurice Baril, the Canadian leading the UN multinational force, wanted to be briefed by MSF.

I met General Baril across the border in Gisenyi at the four-star Meridien Hotel. We sat in the outdoor restaurant under the thatched roof of a stylized African hut. He came with a bevy of advisers and was a friendly, humble and direct man. Using maps I gave him the most up-to-date information MSF teams had gathered from the air and on the ground about where we knew the refugees to be. I told him about the road I had been on the day before and the abandoned villages I had seen. The next day, December 8, he and the UNHCR travelled 17 kilometres along the same road I had taken. Then they returned. Afterwards, in an interview with the BBC, to my astonishment, he said that where he had travelled life appeared to be normal. He had not seen any refugees himself but acknowledged that there might be smaller groups in the forest and the hills. He was confident that these refugees would be able to sustain themselves by living off the land. He said that the access aid agencies had to the refugees was improving and that he was reassured that the rebels would increase it further. He said intervention had been required because aid agencies could not freely enter and move about Kivu, but the situation was now changing and further assessment would be needed.

In other words, the UN intervention by a multinational force was dead. There was some talk of food being airdropped in time for Christmas television, but it was clear that even this was not going to happen. For weeks after, MSF and others tried to talk to any journalist who would listen. However, as our past predictions about refugee mortality from cholera now appeared to be false, we were talking to the skeptical. In the interviews I was able to give, I insisted that without a multinational intervention hundreds of thousands of refugees would remain in a precarious position: they would continue to be coerced by the ex-FAR and Interahamwe militias and chased through the Zairean countryside by rebel forces. I referred to recent MSF surveillance flights that had found 50,000 refugees near Walikali, another 48,000 at Shabunda, 30,000 near Hombo and 20,000 near Masisi. I said that the refugees who were delivered to us told us of many more who were wounded and sick, but the ADFL prevented us from getting to them. Together with others from MSF, I said a lot, but it didn't matter. The ADFL and their allies continued to move forward, battling south, north and west, visiting a massive revenge upon hundreds of thousands of unseen refugees.

The battle was going well for the ADFL, but not as well as planned. As the rebel army advanced, they encountered the Mai-Mai: men and boys, some as young as ten, who invoked traditional beliefs to fend off armed attacks on themselves, their villages and their ancestors buried in the land. They believed that through rituals that invoked the life power of water, they would be invincible. They were fierce fighters, and the mere mention of Mai-Mai could empty a village. I provoked screams, wild dancing and anger when I offered a cigarette to a naked fourteen-year-old Mai-Mai with a machine gun he could barely hold. I put the cigarette on the ground. The boy sprinkled some powder on it and then smoked the cigarette.

The alliance of convenience that the Mai-Mai had first formed with the ADFL to fight off the ex-FAR and FAZ had broken down. The Mai-Mai were increasingly resentful of the rebels, whom they saw as interlopers from Rwanda and Uganda, though both countries continued to deny that they had troops in Zaire. At Sake, Mai-Mai had taken over the checkpoints.

One night a priest came to see me at our office. He was a white Belgian who had been working in Kivu for years. He asked me to send MSF doctors with a group of Boy Scouts he wanted to lead into the jungle around the city to find refugees. I said, "Not now." For the time being, I judged it too danger-ous. Two days later a group of Boy Scouts were attacked in the jungle by Interahamwe and the ex-FAR.

Using the back road that had been open just days before, I tried again to go west. The rainy season had started, and the mud roads through the hilly jungle were nearly impassable. The mudslide we had encountered earlier had been covered over with logs by the advancing ADFL. Farther ahead my driver and I cleared fallen trees and abandoned minibuses. We covered mud pits with logs and dug our way out of mudslides using jacks, winches, picks and shovels. We went as far as we could, but the story remained the same. At one village, people came slowly out of the hills as my driver called to them. I asked them about houses that were still smouldering. The people were afraid and would only say that the ex-FAR had pushed the refugees through the region, that the ADFL had followed, that many people in their village had died, that there was "still much fighting." Farther down the road we saw evidence of what must have been an intense battle. Green Rwandan buses, "Gift from Japan" painted on their sides, lay overturned and mortar damaged in a ravine by the side of the road. Military vehicles of the ex-FAR had been forced over the cliff, and I looked at the destroyed UNHCR, MSF and other NGO vehicles that had been stolen by the FAZ in October and November. In the fields and along the road there were the abandoned possessions of hundreds of thousands of people who had moved west. There were no bones, no flesh, no human beings living or dead.

I had just called in to the MSF compound by radio when we spotted an unmarked brown Land Cruiser heading towards us. I

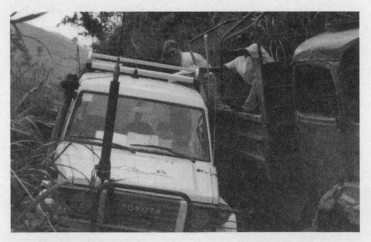

Stuck in the mud

immediately turned up the volume on our radio so that anyone nearby would know that we had one and that we were likely to have used it. The vehicle stopped and a heavy-set white man about forty years old got out from the driver's seat and approached us.

"James Orbinski, with MSF," I said. He introduced himself as Dave Kyzner from the American embassy. I was surprised and suspicious to see a lone embassy official driving through smouldering villages. I asked him what he was doing in the area. "Oh, you know, human rights and all that stuff," he replied. With map in hand, he advised me that the roads were impassable and that there were ex-FAR and Interahamwe patrols. He told us to turn back. I told him we would turn back once we had tried to deliver the medicines we had with us. He drove off back towards Goma, and we drove on. We made it to the village. I found a male nurse in the burned-out MSF clinic. He was surprised to see me and had the look of a hunted animal that had survived. No one would tell me anything, except that things were bad and I should go. A patrol of ADFL soldiers in black rubber boots came into the clinic. They had new AK-47s and ordered us back to Goma.

We stopped at the village of Mweso. We saw more people, mostly women and children, trembling and silent. A woman sat alone by the roadside, her shaking hands clasped over her groin. She stared blankly at the deep brown mud. I asked what had happened, but nobody answered. Smoke billowed from the smouldering houses around us. There was blood drying on the wrap that covered her. She got up. Her face twitched as she walked, limping and stooped over with pain. I helped her towards a group of other women sitting farther down the road. They had also been raped. Two women got up and helped her sit among them. Who was doing this? I asked my driver. "The rebels or the ex-FAR—it is not clear," he said. "No one will speak and they will only stay in the bush. Some people think we are animals. But you know we are human." We made our way back through the mud in silence.

Night was falling, and we stopped at the feeding centre in Sake. Mothers sat with their children waiting for food. A fat Zairean woman, her hair in spiky pigtails, was mixing a huge vat of gruel, and the smoke from the charcoal fire filled the air inside the tent shelter. She was in charge, the "Mama" of the centre. I found the boy whom we had nearly run over a few weeks before. He had gauze taped to the side of his mouth, and a green discharge from his nostrils was collecting over his lip. He smiled at me, and I touched his head. "Comment tu vas?" I asked him. The Mama translated for me and she laughed, slapping her knees, at his reply. "He says he is waiting for his mother. It was raining last night, that's why she didn't come. Tonight God will put the stars to stop the rain from falling down. He says she is coming tonight." She held the boy warmly. I smiled at him and touched his head again. "God! Hah! Heh! Where is God here?" she laughed as she stirred the gruel.

We stopped at a temporary MSF hospital, where there were only ten patients. Most were local residents who couldn't afford the user fees at the regular hospitals, most of which had been damaged in recent fighting. Three had the dreaded African sleeping sickness, a parasitic disease spread by the tsetse fly. The doctor gave them an arsenic-based treatment that burns the veins as it is injected. One man screamed as the drug was administered; another woman, experiencing the psychotic symptoms of the disease, talked to a ghost. No refugees had been brought to the hospital that day, and only a trickle had come in the past weeks.

We were treating very few patients, but providing water for much of the city. We were running the temporary hospital and feeding centre in Sake. We were supporting groups like the Sisters of Mercy, as well as hospitals in the city and health posts in the small number of outlying villages that we could reach. We started gathering testimonies and witness statements from the refugees and villagers who would give them. Jane Little, the nurse who ran the Sake feeding centre, said to me one night, "I am scared, James." I told her that I was scared too and that I didn't trust anyone who wasn't. That night I wrote in my journal: "Fear, fear, fear: everywhere we are surrounded by fear of what they know and fear of what we cannot see. Fear: I feel my own. Stay focused."

A handful of journalists in Goma, along with the workers with MSF, UNHCR, the Red Cross and a small number of missionaries and other aid agencies, were the only foreigners in the city. Merlin, a British medical NGO, was leaving because it could not get donor funding. Western donors were concentrating their efforts on the refugees who had returned to Rwanda, and thus so were most NGOs. The UN had launched diplomatic initiatives towards peace talks. The ADFL alliance continued its offensive. Mobutu had returned from his cancer treatment in Europe, and there were rumours of a major FAZ counteroffensive to retake the Kivu. We reduced the team to our most experienced people.

With Mai-Mai on the road to Masisi

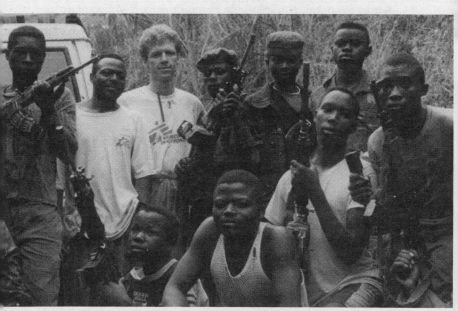

Late one night, the chief administrator for the Masisi hospital arrived at our compound. He was exhausted. He had walked sixty kilometres through the jungle to ask us to bring medical supplies. MSF had worked in the Masisi hospital for years, but in recent months had not been able to get there. The administrator was well known to our staff, and I said we would try.

Leslie Shanks and I drove with two Land Cruisers full of medical supplies on the road towards Masisi. We got farther than I had before, but then got stuck in some mud. We were digging the vehicles out when suddenly we were surrounded by heavily armed men and boys. I couldn't tell if they were ex-FAR, Mai-Mai or rebels. I was afraid that we were going to die. Then the chief pharmacist from the Masisi hospital emerged from the jungle with more boys and men. "MSF!" he said. He told us he was Mai-Mai. We signed over the medicines to him. They dug us out of the mud, and after insisting we take their photographs they disappeared into the jungle with his boys carrying the boxes of medicines on their heads. We had been stuck in the mud for several hours, and it was too late and too dangerous to continue much farther along the road. We went as far as Matanda, the next village, where MSF was well known and where we thought we would have a chance of being safe. It was surrounded by ADFL soldiers, who walked freely about the church complex where MSF had run a clinic. We found our way to the priest. He was a Tutsi from Rwanda and new to the post. He was friendly with the soldiers, who were at ease with him. Though he was surprised to see us, he invited us in to his living quarters. We were quickly shown to a guest room with a single bed, given some water and some food, and advised not to leave the room. I could hear the muffled sounds of English and Kinyarwanda as the priest talked with the soldiers. I stepped out onto the terrace. It was a cloudy night. There were no stars. Sometimes the night is so dark that even the stars are

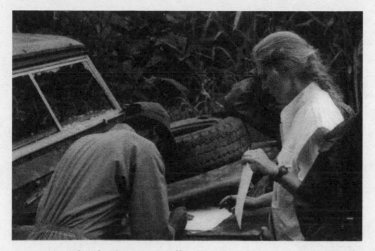

Dr. Leslie Shanks signing off medicines to Masisi pharmacist

afraid to come out, I thought. The priest returned to check on our comfort, and to remind me that we should not leave the room, even to go onto the terrace. "Don't worry, you will be safe," he said. I slept on the floor as the rain fell. It was one of the longest nights of my life.

On December 12, we heard new rumours that Mobutu's elite Zairean Presidential Guard had been dispatched to the Kivu region to repel the ADFL. Arjan told me that the MSF office in Kigali had been robbed during a military-style raid, and tear gas had been used. Other NGOs in Kigali that continued to press for answers on the whereabouts of the missing refugees, such as the American Refugee Committee, were also raided or robbed.

On Friday, December 13, General Baril's intervention force was officially disbanded, though hundreds of Canadian troops in Entebbe, Uganda, had begun packing their bags days before. By December 17, MSF, the Red Cross and UNHCR reconnaissance flights located some 200,000 refugees southwest of Goma. In the presence of the media, the rebels gave nominal consent for aid workers to assist the refugees, but on the ground we were denied access because of "insecurity." We kept up our political pressure in Kigali and capitals around the world. Occasionally we would be allowed to see the refugees, but only for a few hours at a time. The refugees were in a desperate condition. Baril had been only partially right: people had been eating roots and leaves since the camps had been attacked in October. Now those that had survived were starving; they were racked with malaria and diarrhea; they had swollen legs and lacerated feet. The ADFL continued to pursue them as Mobutu continued to arm the soldiers and militias that controlled them. Beyond these 200,000 sick, hungry and terrorized people, there were still hundreds of thousands uncounted, unseen in the jungles of Zaire.

In Goma the ADFL claimed that our relief supplies had been donated to the people of Zaire, and since the ADFL was now in charge of this part of Zaire, the supplies belonged to them. The ADFL accused us of working for the French, who were supporting Mobutu. "How do we know you are not spies?" the soldiers asked on their daily inspections of our office. In addition to the spies I knew the ADFL had among our national staff, they wanted our radios and communications equipment. In response to one officer's demand for the equipment, I threatened to withdraw from the city and insisted on a meeting with the ADFL commander for Goma, Colonel Kabongo.

The ADFL had wanted us there—we lent credibility to their humanitarian claims—but the situation was changing. Mobutu's forces were losing badly. He had hired Serbian mercenaries and was rumoured to have hired the South African mercenary company Executive Outcomes, whose attack helicopters were said to be coming any time. To the north, south and west of Kivu the Mai-Mai were breaking away from the ADFL. The refugees and the people of the region were caught in the middle. Our national staff was afraid the war was going to get worse. They sent their families away but stayed themselves because their MSF salary was the only income they had.

On December 18, I met with the head of mission for the Red Cross in Goma. The day before, six Red Cross workers had been assassinated in Chechnya. "They say it was robbers," he told me, "but they were shot by guns with silencers as they slept in their beds. It could be anyone from the Russian Secret Service to a disgruntled local commander." It was the bloodiest attack against the Red Cross in its 133-year history. In Zaire, the Red Cross was re-evaluating everything. "We are not able to do much here. Like you, our access is severely restricted and it is getting more tense with the FAZ, the ex-FAR, the ADFL and the Mai-Mai. The risks are too high. We are reducing our teams," he said, "and may well pull out until things change."

I had been trying to get a meeting with Colonel Kabongo, but he kept putting me off. Finally, an officer was sent to tell me a meeting had been scheduled for an hour's time. I went directly to Kabongo's hotel, the rebel command post, as I didn't want to be late. I arrived just as Dave Kyzner was leaving the hotel restaurant. I wondered why an American embassy official was meeting with a rebel commander. He was friendly, and we talked briefly about the security situation and the problem with the radios. After a three-hour wait, an officer called me in to see Kabongo. I walked into the restaurant where the commander was having lunch. In front of his table, CNN played on a large-screen television. He accidentally dropped his fork on the floor, and as a nearby soldier reached for it, the colonel picked up the meat from his plate and took a bite. He ignored me as I watched him wipe his lips and dripping hands with the napkin. The soldier put a clean fork on the table.

"It is unfortunate what has happened in Chechnya, is it not? The Red Cross are such kind souls," Kabongo said without looking me in the eye. "Accidents can happen anywhere. You have so many beautiful young and dedicated Europeans with MSF here in Kivu." I looked on in silence as he cut another piece of meat. I then raised the question of our communications equipment. We would not surrender our radios to the ADFL, but, I said, his soldiers were free to inspect them.

"Do not, dear doctor, tell me what I am, and am not, free to do." He took another bite of meat and chewed it carefully. I could feel my heart racing as I waited. "Don't worry, dear doctor, I am sure we will find a solution," he said softly. He waved his napkin.

A soldier approached. "Your meeting is now over," the soldier said.

In the parking lot of the MSF compound, I was stopped by a member of our national staff. He was a Zairean Tutsi and he told me that the night before, his house had been shot at and grenades had been thrown into his compound. He suspected Mai-Mai, but he couldn't be sure. His family had left for South Africa months before, and now he wanted to join them. However, the Rwandan government wanted all Zairean Tutsis to stay in Kivu. Then he told me there was a plot among members of our national staff to kidnap some expatriates. They wanted money so that they could flee. They had trucks ready and a plan in place. He didn't know if the ADFL was involved and he didn't know when it was going to happen, but he knew it *was* going to happen. He was afraid for his own life and wanted me to get him out of Zaire.

The rebels were advancing across Zaire. Our radios were being monitored and our emails intercepted. I passed through Sake. Mai-Mai were everywhere, and only those patients too sick to move remained in the feeding centre. There were fewer than twenty children and adults. The Mama in charge was gone, and so was the boy. I felt like I was trapped in a game I didn't know how to play. I went across the border to Kigali to talk with Arjan in person. We met with the Canadian, Dutch, French and American ambassadors in the capital. We wanted to know what they would do if we were trapped. "Don't get trapped," said the American deputy ambassador. She called her security officer to the meeting. In walked Dave Kyzner. Clearly uncomfortable at the sight of me sitting there, he offered garden-variety advice on security measures: be vigilant, maintain radio contact at all times, stay together, don't use unapproved roads, watch for mines. The message was clear: you are on your own. Later Jules, Arjan and I agreed that we had to get the team out, at least temporarily. Without attracting suspicion, we would try to move our vehicles and stocks across the border. Christmas was coming, and we would spend it in Rwanda with other MSF expatriates. I returned to Goma.

It is a Zairean tradition that in lieu of vacation pay, people are given a "thirteenth month" of salary. Over the next few days, I met with our national staff and told them they were going to get a thirteenth month and that we were going to spend Christmas in Rwanda with other MSF teams. If the war got worse and we were unable to return, it would be considered *force majeur*, ending their contracts, and they could use the thirteenth-month salary as security money for their families. Over the next few days, the expatriate team was moved out, one member at a time, and they took vehicles and stock with them. Other aid agencies did the same, and the Red Cross pulled out altogether from other parts of Kivu.

We spent Christmas, as planned, in Rhuengeri, Rwanda, not far from the border with Zaire. I had had so many meetings and made so many special arrangements, for people like the man who had told me about the kidnapping plot, that I hadn't slept properly for weeks and in the last two nights not for more than two hours at a time. On Christmas Day I slept for eighteen uninterrupted hours. The next morning we decided that, security permitting, a small, experienced management team would travel to and from Goma each day to monitor what was happening and to maintain our limited aid program. We did this for the next two weeks. I was to leave for Canada in mid-January. By then all roads from Goma, even to the few villages we had previously managed to reach, were completely blocked by the ADFL.

I spent my last night in Kigali on the balcony of the MSF compound with Arjan and José Antonio Bastos, who had come up from South Kivu, where his team's movements had also been severely restricted. The stars were out, and we were drinking heavily. "It's about as racist as it gets," said Arjan. "Hundreds of thousands of Hutu refugees are missing. Every Hutu is seen as a *genocidaire*, even the children. It seems it's a balance of payments, where mass extrajudicial executions are permitted by the international community. So much for human rights."

"Contrary to what some poets say, all is not fair in love and war," José said. "Even if it is impossible to help the refugees, we must keep trying, and find the truth of what is happening, and we must speak. Sometimes speaking is the only action that is possible. To not speak is to fail the possibility of humanity. No, all is not fair in love and war," he repeated. "If we are to remember or even discover what love really is, what peace really is, if there is to be real hope for any of us, we need to be reminded of this."

"You're a poet, José," I said.

"Well, I am Spanish." He laughed. "It's in the blood!"

"Everyone's?" I asked. He smiled. The three of us drank until the sun came up.

On January 20, I woke at home in Toronto to the newscast coming over my clock radio. Three Spanish aid workers with Médicos del Mundo—MDM—had been murdered in Rhuengeri. I later learned the assassins had gone first to the MSF compound where we had spent Christmas, but had been unable to get past the security guards. They had thrown a grenade over the compound wall, but it hadn't exploded. The assassins then went down the street to MDM. They beat the night guard and gained entry. They checked passports and then shot the three Spanish aid workers in the head. An American aid worker was wounded with a bullet to the leg. Half an hour later the RPA arrived on the scene and took the guard away. He was beaten to death in custody, though the official cause of death was given as malaria. The Rwandan government told UN and aid organizations that the Interahamwe had infiltrated the area, which they had, and that they were responsible for the killings. It was, however, never clear whether the RPA or the Interahamwe had killed the aid workers. A few days later, a Canadian priest, Guy Pinard, who had worked in Rhuengeri for more than twenty years, was shot four times in the back as he said Mass. Two weeks later, five UN human rights observers were murdered in the same area allegedly by the Interahamwe, the severed head of one placed on the seat of their UN Land Cruiser.

Rwanda appeared to be heading towards civil war, especially in the region bordering Kivu, the stronghold of Habyarimana's former genocidal government. The ADFL continued its advance through Kivu and into the mineral-rich Shaba province. Mobutu bombed Bukavu in South Kivu. The Red Cross, the UNHCR, MSF and a few other aid agencies struggled under security constraints to help Zairean civilians affected by

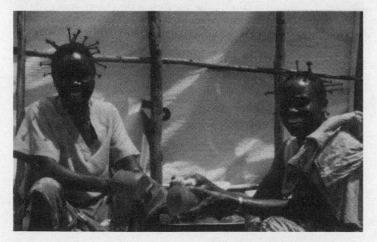

Sake Feeding Centre

the war and to keep searching for the refugees that nobody else wanted to find. At the same time, amidst heavy security in Kigali, and broadcast on public radio, the first trial of an Interahamwe leader charged with genocide got under way.

In mid-December 1996, thousands of refugees had been "discovered" west of Goma at Tingi-Tingi. By the end of January 1997, more than seven hundred of these people had died of starvation. Fighting and the now perfected ADFL game of "yes-no" meant that less than four days' worth of food had gotten to them. Thousands of people sat in virtually unstaffed and unsupplied clinics and feeding centres. As the Rwandan ambassador to the UN announced that there were no more refugees inside Zaire, the Shabunda group of refugees retreated into the jungle after ADFL attacks. On February 12, the Red Cross, MSF, CARE and Oxfam were invited to address the UN Security Council. Once again our message was clear: the refugees needed to be protected, the ex-FAR and Interahamwe needed to be separated from them, and humanitarian aid could not be a substitute for political action. Shortly after, the UN secretary general proposed reactivating a multinational intervention force. While France backed the initiative, the United States, with the support of the United Kingdom, killed it before the Security Council could send an unfunded political envoy to the region.

Over the following months, several facts would become known. Journalists found documents in the former camps that proved that the ex-FAR and Interahamwe had been planning a December 1996 assault on Rwanda, that they had Mobutu's full military backing, and that the French government was backing and arming Mobutu. It was clear, too, that the Rwandan government had organized ADFL soldiers and trained them in Rwanda over the summer of 1996. It was also clear that despite their denials, Rwanda, Uganda and Burundi had large numbers of troops fighting alongside the ADFL. Evidence emerged that

Dave Kyzner had not been alone in Kivu. American special operations forces had advised and trained the RPA inside Rwanda, and had provided additional logistical and material support to Kabila's forces during their advance. Covertly, the American Green Berets had crossed into Zaire with the RPA and had clashed with the FAZ in October. It was revealed that the United States had asked Canada in early November to lead the UN intervention force, though even as the U.S. suggested publicly that it might send troops for the force, it was also systematically obstructing diplomatic efforts to support it. The United States finally killed the intervention initiative at a November meeting of contributing countries in Stuttgart, two weeks before I had met General Baril. As one State Department official later put it, Mobutu had been a "useful tyrant" but he was now a "caricature of history" that stood in the way of a market economy, good governance and liberal democracy. It would also become clear that a Canadian and American mining consortium and other multinational mining corporations had made advance payments for mining rights to the ADFL alliance forces.

In late March 1997 the MSF team in Goma managed to get beyond ADFL checkpoints at Sake and discovered mass graves around some of the villages in the surrounding hills. At the same time, farther south, Canadian MSF logistician James Fraser went with the UNHCR to prepare rest stations within Zaire along the route to Rwanda for the dispersed Shabunda refugees who wanted to return home. After lengthy negotiations and intense media and political pressure by MSF, the ADFL had approved the tightly controlled trip. By the roadsides Fraser saw scores of freshly dug fields. Secretly, villagers told him they were the mass graves of refugees massacred by the ADFL. One white priest pleaded with him, "There's a Nazi-type genocide happening in the forest—you have to tell the world." As Fraser moved from village to village under ADFL escort, refugees, having seen the passing MSF car, came out of the jungle. Once out, women, children and men were massacred. Scared villagers secretly told Fraser this as he was escorted back several days later along the same route. One ADFL soldier admitted to him, "We can't reach the refugees in the forest. It's good to use the NGOs to pull them out." After this, Fraser was intimidated and his life was threatened. He secretly and meticulously recorded the information he now had: the precise location of graves, the number of people killed, and who had said what. "If they found my diary, I knew I was going to die," he would tell me years later. Fraser played naïve and managed to smuggle his notebook past the ADFL. It was the missing piece of the puzzle. Together with others from MSF he confronted Washington, New York, London and capitals around the Western world with evidence of the massacres and the "humanitarian bait and lure" tactics of the ADFL alliance. The ADFL countered with allegations of spying, or incompetence on the part of the aid agencies, all the while continuing its advance across Zaire.

The campaign of disinformation, murder of refugees, ethnic cleansing of villages and the intimidation of civilians in Kivu knew no bounds. With every public accusation, with every demand for access that MSF made, the safety of aid workers in Rwanda and Zaire came under increased threat. Over and over again, MSF people were forced to weigh their own safety against that of the civilians and refugees. Inside MSF debates about when to act, when to speak and when to remain silent, choices with life-and-death consequences, sometimes turned acrimonious and several times brought MSF nearly to its breaking point.

America Mineral Fields Incorporated met with Kabila in Goma in March 1997. Around the same time, it paid advances to Kabila for mining rights. A few weeks later, as the massacres continued, American Diamond Buyers obtained the right to open the first diamond brokerage in Kisangani.

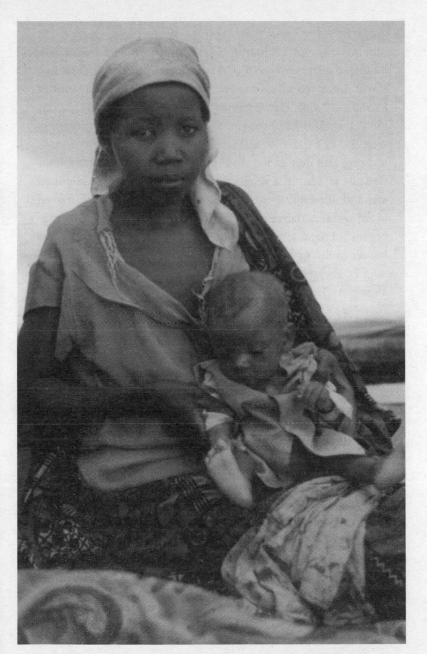

Sake Feeding Centre

At the end of March 1997 some 100,000 exhausted, wounded and starving refugees were located by MSF and the Red Cross along 150 kilometres of train track south of the city of Kisangani. People crawled along the ground for the food biscuits the aid workers had brought with them. A quarter of the group were too sick to move, and MSF insisted that they be given medical care and demanded their protection as refugees and their right of asylum in a third country. As ADFL radio condemned MSF and other aid agencies, violence and intimidation directed at aid workers increased across Zaire and in Rwanda, and after organized demonstrations, MSF and UN compounds and warehouses in Kisangani were looted.

Frustrated by the recalcitrance of the rebels and the apparent disinterest of members of the Security Council, UN Secretary General Kofi Annan charged the rebels with committing "murder by famine." He demanded unhindered access for the aid agencies and announced that he was sending a UN human rights commission to investigate allegations of massacres. The situation was becoming embarrassing for Washington, which now said that if the ADFL alliance sought good relations with the United States, they should "act out of humanitarian concern." But as before, the ADFL would publicly grant access to the refugees only to rescind it on the ground. When aid agencies were allowed through, they were greeted by the smell of rotting bodies, thousands of sick and wounded, and the sound of mechanical diggers burying bodies in the forest.

The United States sent its emissary Bill Richardson to help resolve the crisis. One American diplomat said that neither Washington nor Paris "has had a frank talk with Kabila or Mobutu in which their choices have been explained to them . . . but I think the time has come."[1] MSF again insisted on protection and asylum for the sick and wounded refugees, arguing that Rwanda was too unsafe for repatriation.

In Kigali, Kagame condemned MSF and blamed the UNHCR for being too "slow and incompetent" with repatriation. The next day the rebels blocked the distribution of food and water and started loading refugees into freight cars and transporting them to the Kisangani airport for repatriation to Rwanda. So packed were the freight cars that ninety-one people suffocated, and so sick were those forcibly repatriated that half of all people who were hospitalized upon returning to Rwanda died within forty-eight hours. At the same time, in a hospital in South Kivu, fifty child and sixty adult patients were removed by rebels and simply disappeared. And all the while there were hundreds of thousands more unseen refugees. In the first week of May, Emma Bonino, the EU commissioner for human rights, said plainly that eastern Zaire was a "slaughterhouse."[2]

On May 19, MSF released an analysis of events entitled "Forced Flight." It meticulously analyzed information gleaned from direct care, patient interviews, aerial and ground surveys, medical studies and the first-hand experience of our own volunteers. It detailed the systematic massacre, starvation and hunting and baiting of refugees by the ADFL alliance since October 1996, as well as the plight of indigenous peoples in Kivu. The next morning, in newspapers across the world, headlines read "MSF Accuse" and "ADFL Pursues Slow Extermination."

The timing of the report couldn't have been worse. On May 20, Kabila marched into Kinshasa, the capital of Zaire, and declared himself president. A week later, Bill Richardson, the U.S. emissary, said, "Let's give him a chance." France tried to maintain influence in the region by continuing to support Mobutu, incredulously and ineffectively looking for his *sortie honorable*, which meant negotiating a place for his men in the new government.

But the story of the missing refugees was not yet over. Some of those that remained in Zaire were chased over the border of Kabila's newly declared Democratic Republic of Congo into the Republic of Congo (a similarly named but different country). The ADFL forces had been witnessed firing indiscriminately on the fleeing refugees as they crossed the river, and were seen beating, shooting and attacking with machetes those who remained in the border jungles. An MSF survey conducted among the refugees who had been pursued for more than two thousand kilometres since the previous October revealed that only one in five family members had survived. All had been starved, beaten or raped along the way, and those that had died had been massacred or had succumbed to disease.

One survivor, a twenty-eight-year-old man, told MSF: "I got married in the Kashusa camp in 1995. It was attacked in September 1996. The people cutting wood in the Inera forest were killed. Then came the shells and machine-gun fire. We had a little corn, some clothes, and twelve dollars. We walked into Kahuzi-Biga forest, through the mud, without sleeping. Then we kept to a road with 30,000 others. We were held hostage by Zairean soldiers dressed in civilian clothes. About ten people who resisted the pillaging were killed. We lived on plants. Five to six thousand people were massacred at Shabunda. I found my father, two sisters and a brother at Tingi-Tingi. Then we moved on. One night, we stopped at Lubutu Bridge. When the bridge opened, some people fell in the water and drowned. I lost the bundle I was carrying on my head. I put my wife on my back and forded the river. We kept walking. People died of sickness and hunger. We had to give a pair of trousers to get across a river in a canoe. One group, including my father and brother, decided to go to Kisangani so they could be repatriated to Rwanda. We went in a different direction. My other brother had malaria and stayed by the side of the road. I heard that those who took Boede road were killed and I went back into the forest again. At Wendji, a pastor told us Kabila was coming. Some people turned back to cross Lake Tumba and go directly to [the Republic of the] Congo. We had no money so we waited for a free boat. [Later], the rebels arrived. There were 75 heavily armed soldiers in three vehicles. They fired Kalashnikovs into the refugee camp. I fled to the river. An old Zairean took us down the river, then we returned to see Wendji. About 20 people had been shot dead, almost all of them women and children. The rebels had gone. We found a canoe to take us to [the Republic of the] Congo. We paid with a blanket. In the forest I found a blanket, a Bible, and a handkerchief."[3]

Inside Rwanda, refugees who had been forcibly repatriated were returned to their communities as the ex-FAR and Interahamwe guerrillas infiltrated the western regions of Rwanda. There were no human rights monitors and no aid workers in the area. It was too insecure.

Early in 1998, Paul Kagame gave an interview to the BBC's Nick Gowing. In it Kagame said, "We used communication and information warfare better than anyone. We have found a new way of doing this. . . . I learned from the field that the media and NGOs would be a problem. For a specific amount of time these people have to be kept out. We managed to keep them out. They leaked information. They were very damaging . . . They are not neutral, as many claim to be. To allow a free hand will not bring us [Rwandans] the best results."

In March 1998, President Clinton spent five hours at the Kigali airport. He publicly apologized for American inaction during the 1994 genocide. He maintained that he and other world leaders "did not appreciate the full gravity of what was happening as Rwanda was engulfed in horror." I watched the clip on television and wondered what else he and other leaders would claim not to have known.

Nobody knows exactly how many were murdered between October 1996 and the ADFL alliance's triumphant march into Kinshasa seven months later. Somewhere there remain hundreds of thousands of unnamed, unseen refugees, living or dead. For them, justice is only what they dream.

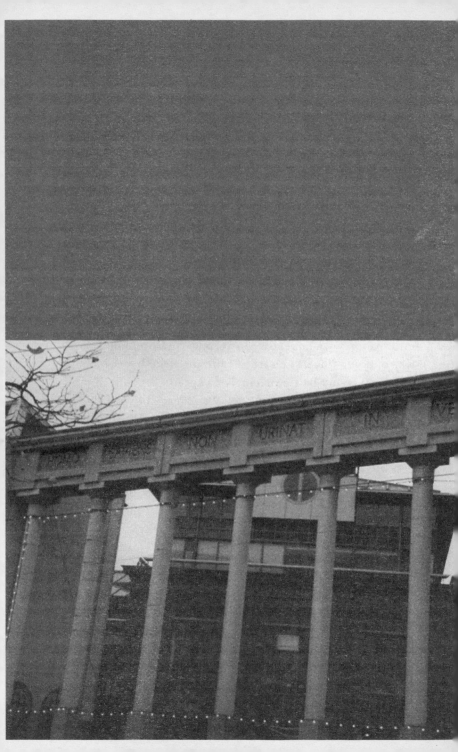

THE POLITICS OF BEING APOLITICAL: HUMANITARIAN ACTION IN NORTH KOREA, KOSOVO AND THE SUDAN

A few weeks after I returned from Zaire in January 1997, I went to see Benedict. "Justice is an illusion," I said as we walked through the woods.

"Not when you know what injustice is," Benedict replied immediately. "The victim is someone quite concrete. Justice only fails when we fail to imagine that it is possible. But like so many things, it depends not only on imaginings but on what we do." We talked about MSF and the dilemmas it had faced in Zaire—choices about when to speak and when to remain silent, when to stay and when to leave, unavoidable choices with life-and-death consequences for someone. "Sometimes we must struggle into a space that has no clear boundaries. It is the struggle for life between us and it is a good one," said Benedict. As we walked then in silence through the cold forest, I realized that what was broken and could never be fixed was my naive notion that I could remain completely outside of politics. I let it go.

I met Janice Stein, a professor of international relations, at a conference on global affairs, in Toronto. I had substituted for an MSF speaker who had had to cancel at the last minute. I spoke about the lack of humanitarian space in Zaire and the politics that impeded it. Janice heard my talk. Over coffee she said to me, "In politics you get what you fight for, and even then you don't always get it. But if you don't fight, you get nothing."

"Well, I love a good fight," I laughed. She laughed too and insisted I study with her for a year at the University of Toronto. I grabbed the opportunity, and while continuing to work emergency-room shifts and making the occasional trip to Europe, I spent the year deepening my understanding of politics and humanitarianism. I was most concerned with the question of how best to maintain humanitarian independence in the context of war, the importance of the question having been pressed so forcefully on me just months before in Zaire.

With the Cold War over and in the face of the global ascendancy of liberal democracy and free markets, a new type of activism was unleashed. International NGOs and other civil society organizations devoted to advancing a wide range of development, humanitarian and social causes grew in number and in size. There had been about 1,600 large and small international NGOs in the 1980s; by the mid-1990s there were at least 4,600. MSF itself had grown from a two-room Paris office to nineteen sections, or branches, around the world with a budget of $350 million and programs in seventy countries with 2,000 international and 15,000 national staff.

Many NGOs demanded that the international community act to address the root causes of conflict. There were strong calls to address impunity for those who violated the laws of war, and to impose onto humanitarian assistance efforts in war human rights norms such as gender equity as well as development agendas and conflict-resolution initiatives. At the same time state budgets for humanitarian assistance skyrocketed, from $2 billion in 1990 to nearly $6 billion in 1999. Human rights activists had led this "New Humanitarianism" and had achieved great things: international criminal tribunals had been established to try those accused of genocide, war crimes and crimes against humanity in Rwanda and the former Yugoslavia; international conventions to limit the use of land mines had been reached. In the long term these developments had the potential to deter violations of international human law and to limit the impact of violence on non-combatants in future wars. MSF had supported them all in one way or another.

The New Humanitarianism also pushed to make aid conditional on accepting a peace-negotiation process, thereby transforming humanitarianism into a tool for direct political change. For organizations like MSF and the Red Cross, practical humanitarianism in war was still concerned with the immediate relief of suffering and the struggle to create the space in which this could happen. When MSF denounced violations of the laws of war it did so not with a singular view to bringing violators to justice in the future, but with a view to affecting events as they were happening. MSF did not operate as a guardian, enforcer or architect of international law, though we did demand that it be respected. As Jean Pictet of the Red Cross had written, humanitarians in war have to "reckon with politics without becoming a part of it." We could not allow the need for humanitarian assistance to be ignored, abused or used by the political interests that surround it.

And of course politics was still politics and defined when and how the law would be applied. In April 1998 the UN Security Council voted unanimously to withdraw the UN human rights investigation team from Zaire. Under intense pressure from Rwanda and Uganda, Kabila had stymied investigators' efforts for months. On June 29, 1998, based on the evidence that the investigation was able to gather, the UN secretary-general wrote to the Security Council, "The killings by ADFL and its allies, including elements of the Rwandan Patriotic Front Army (RPF), constitute crimes against humanity, as does the denial of humanitarian assistance to Rwandan Hutu Refugees." Two weeks later, the Security Council called on the Democratic Republic of Congo and Rwanda to investigate allegations of human rights abuses and violations of the laws of war. In other words, the governments accused of war crimes would investigate themselves.

My year of study had been a luxury. I was ready to return to the reality of MSF, but how or where I was not sure.

In the spring of 1998, MSF's International Council was set to elect a new international president. In the past, candidates for the position had been drawn from among the sitting presidents of each of MSF's nineteen sections around the world. But the organization was still reeling from the crisis it had confronted in Zaire and the African Great Lakes region and was mired in disagreements about the structure and organization of the international movement. The council was deadlocked and could not choose from among the sitting presidents. It could agree only that it needed a full-time president for the International Council, the first in its history, and that it would look elsewhere in the organization for candidates. I got a call in early April from my friend Nicola Kaatsch, the president of MSF in Germany. "We think you can do it. Will you run?" she asked.

"Are you insane, or do you think I am?" was my initial response. I told her that I was more comfortable in the field or with operations research, and that I was a stranger to the high politics of MSF.

"That's exactly why we need you," she said.

"But my French is deplorable."

"This is not a problem unique to you," she said.

Nicola and others who wanted me to run called again over the next few weeks. Then they invited me to Europe. There, I spoke at length with Jean-Marie Kindermans, the international secretary for MSF. If I were elected, I would work with him every day. He had a solid reputation, and I liked his honesty and warmth. I talked with Philippe Biberson, the president of MSF France. More than anything, Philippe wanted debate. Despite the internal acrimony, I thought that what MSF had done or tried to do in the Great Lakes region was exactly right. We both agreed that the organization would continue to face dilemmas that could not easily be resolved, but if questions were exposed and shared, choices could be made.

Not long before I went to Europe I had met my friend Jonathan Brock for a beer. We had worked together in Kigali during the genocide. Since then Jonathan had finished medical school and had just returned from an MSF mission in Sierra Leone. We talked about why we were drawn to MSF, and at one point, while I was at the bar getting more drinks, Jonathan wrote down some of his reasons: "We suture, we record the events, we tell the world. We struggle daily with private thoughts of whether or not we make a difference. The ultimate solution may be political, anonymous and nebulous, in some remote teak conference room. But I have seen the blood, the people cry in pain and the people laugh with hope. And I know we need to be there." I had kept that piece of paper and I thought of Jonathan's words when I made the decision to run against two other candidates for the international presidency of MSF.

A year of thinking, studying and writing had made it clear to me that now more than ever MSF would have to fight for the language and space of humanitarian action. I saw the organization's strength in its focus on directly meeting medical needs, in its clear application of humanitarian principles, and most important, in its commitment to bearing witness. We needed to be as independent as possible. While many other NGOs received the majority of their funds from Western governments, in 1998 MSF raised 50 percent of its total funds from private donations. As a guarantee of operational independence, I wanted MSF to be even more independent financially. I was elected unanimously. That night, I sat in my hotel room looking out the window into

Place de la Trinité in Brussels. I lit a cigarette and thought, *What the hell have I done?* I had no office, no budget and no secretary. I would have to build from the bottom up.

Within weeks of my taking office, we held an intense internal debate about MSF's work in North Korea, a country where upwards of three million people had died of famine and its related illnesses in the preceding three years. North Korea was then and remains the last Stalinist state in the world. At the end of the Cold War, China opened its communist state to market reforms, while the collapse of the Soviet Union meant that it too abandoned the favourable trading terms that had so long supported North Korea's totalitarian government. The paranoid and cultish regime of Kim Jong Il then pursued its *Juche* policy of "structural self-sufficiency," which included building long-range missiles and developing nuclear energy and weapons. As North Korea could no longer rely on cheap food imports from Russia and China, *Juche* also included reforms in agricultural production—reforms that would prove disastrous. Two years of flooding over 1994 and 1995 damaged about 15 percent of the country's already inadequate food crops. There were reports of famine, but the regime kept its borders closed and its own statistics secret, so there was no way to measure how great the needs were.

In 1995, North Korea appealed to the UN for food assistance. The assistance came, but the regime insisted on tight control and restricted the movement of UN agencies, the Red Cross and the small number of NGOs—including MSF—that it permitted into the country. All expatriates required permission to travel inside the country and were accompanied by government officials at all times. Travel to certain areas remained forbidden. By 1996, North Korea's GDP had fallen by 50 percent since 1993, and the UN's World Food Programme—funded by the United States, the European Union and some other states—

launched what was then the biggest aid initiative in its history. By 1997, MSF was supporting over eleven hundred health centres and running sixty feeding centres in three of North Korea's twenty-four counties.

But all was not well. Seventy thousand North Koreans managed to escape from areas sealed to MSF and other organizations. The refugees brought news to the outside world of the catastrophe inside North Korea's sealed areas. The refugees crossed the river into China, where MSF was able to offer assistance to some and to collect their testimonies. One priest said, "I saw dead people in the streets, dead from hunger and cold. I saw seven children, one beside the other without shoes, who had frozen to death in a doorway. The army collects the dead at night. The violence is terrible . . . I saw children literally tearing bread from the mouths of smaller ones. I am told of cannibalism." Another man told of a "neighbour who had killed and eaten an orphan, and no one seemed surprised that this was possible." Escapees told us that the regime distributed food first to its military—the fifth largest in the world, with a standing army of more than one million—and then to those loyal to the state. Those considered "disloyal" seldom received rations. Large numbers of starving and desperate orphans were held in secret camps, named 6/29 Camps for the day that Kim Jong Il's father and predecessor had died, camps that did not officially exist.

Despite our repeated efforts, MSF had no access to half the country. Our teams saw large numbers of hungry street children at night who would disappear by day and whose existence the authorities denied. We did not see anyone older than about sixty on the streets. In secret we were told that the old were dying at home because they were giving their limited rations to their grandchildren to keep them alive. Other aid workers reported seeing kindergarten classes where children were too weak to stand. There were further reports of the army being called out to plant crops because farmers were too weak, and of people surviving on roots and leaves in the countryside. Bill Richardson, the U.S. ambassador to the UN, said, "The big concern we have is whether . . . the food assistance we are giving is reaching the average person. We know the military may be provided with the bulk of food aid."[1] North Korea had avoided war with the United States in 1994, when the regime agreed to inspections of its nuclear facilities and pledged to freeze and eventually dismantle its nuclear weapons program. As talks aimed at neutralizing a nuclear threat continued into 1998, the food aid program continued unchanged for fear of destabilizing the fragile politics of the regime and the region.

In June 1998, the North Korean government forbade MSF from conducting a nutritional survey, even in the few counties where we were allowed to work. Instead, it wanted us to provide raw materials for the manufacture of medicines. By remaining present, silent and without access to the most vulnerable, we were giving the impression that humanitarian action was possible and that the North Korean government respected basic humanitarian principles. It wasn't, and it didn't. By propping up the regime, aid was not only masking suffering but perpetuating it. We would not do what the regime wanted, and it would not allow us to do what was needed. That summer, we held internal debates with MSF doctors from North Korea. We knew millions were starving and that the government would not allow us to reach them. After three years of trying, it was clear that we had no other leverage but to use our voice. We would refuse to collaborate with a totalitarian regime in an abuse of compassion, an abuse that was forcing millions into starvation and some into cannibalism. And we would call into question the use of humanitarian aid as a political tool to contain a military threat. In August, the regime launched its first satellite in space and its first long-range missile over Japan.

On September 30, at a press conference in Hong Kong, MSF announced that we had effectively been forced out of

North Korea. Dr. Eric Goemaere, the general director of the Belgian MSF operational centre, said, "There are serious medical, nutritional and sanitation problems which need to be addressed . . . [But] we had no choice. We were forced out." He described the circumstances, saying that "aid cannot help the most needy unless it is freely distributed." Eric explained how MSF had arrived at our difficult decision: "It is not easy as doctors to pull out when so many people have died and when the health and lives of so many people are still in danger. But in the end, humanitarian assistance can only help those who need it when it is impartial and accountable. This is not the case in North Korea." He concluded: "Now it is time for the North Korean government to take responsibility for the health of its people and to allow direct humanitarian assistance." MSF called on governments to review their aid policies in North Korea. I later said that Western governments were using "humanitarian assistance as a form of political leverage . . . making humanitarian assistance conditional on political and not humanitarian objectives." In February 1999, North Korea allowed American access to its nuclear power sites in exchange for more food.

We continued to help North Korean escapees in China and South Korea and continued our appeals to allow independent, impartial needs-based humanitarian assistance to the most vulnerable people in North Korea. After our position was criticized by some aid agencies as "incomprehensible" and "unforgivable," some other NGOs stopped working in North Korea for reasons similar to MSF's. Nevertheless, the WHO, the World Food Programme, UNICEF, the Red Cross and some NGOs continued their work there.

In late 1998, I went to Nairobi for a meeting of MSF operations directors to discuss our work in Africa. It quickly became apparent that we had a major problem in Sudan. I met Marie-Christine Férier, the operations director for the Brussels office of MSF. A highly competent director, she was embarrassed about her poor English. We had the odd smoke together, and with my poor French we got along well. Marie-Christine explained that the UN's Operation Lifeline Sudan, or OLS, was not working.

Civil war had raged in the south of Sudan for sixteen years, leaving two million dead and the largest number of displaced people in the world in misery and at risk of starvation and disease. Civilians were bombed, raped, robbed and even enslaved by the Khartoum government and militias loyal to it. At the same time, the oil interests of Canadian, French, and Chinese corporations were protected by the Sudanese government. OLS had been set up by UNICEF in 1989 to bring humanitarian assistance to civilians affected by the war and to prevent famine or to intervene early if famine occurred. By 1998 it had become an administrative umbrella for several UN agencies and some forty-two NGOs, including MSF. Although effective in the beginning, nearly ten years and $3 billion later, OLS had become institutionalized and sclerotic. It was caught between the political and military interests of the government of Sudan in Khartoum and the rebel Sudan People's Liberation Movement in the south. The Khartoum government refused OLS access to vast areas of Sudan, such as the Equatoria region, where only MSF and a few other NGOs were working illegally to help hundreds of thousands of people. Where OLS was allowed access, it was limited at best. Flights bringing food aid were subject to the whims of the Khartoum government. Any aid that did get through was poorly monitored by OLS and too often did not get to the most vulnerable. The rebels who controlled much of South Sudan used the aid to feed their army and control the civilian population. OLS was failing the people it was supposed to serve, and because MSF was part of it, so were we.

In January 1998 the rebels had launched a major offensive to retake some government-held towns in the Bar el Gazel region of South Sudan. The Khartoum government responded by imposing a two-month ban on all OLS food aid flights as it bombed villages and relief sites in the rebel-held region. With continued fighting and without food, thousands of people were starving and forced to flee. MSF protested the lack of food aid, but OLS responded only after we smuggled in journalists to reveal the crisis. Eventually, under pressure from OLS, the Khartoum government allowed a few flights of food aid to a limited number of villages. The situation improved for some. However, supply lines and food airdrops were so limited that for days at a time MSF expatriates working in the feeding centres were without food themselves, and had to eat from the supplies that were meant to go to the starving Sudanese. In some areas, rebels stole more than three-quarters of the food that was making it in, but because OLS considered the rebels "humanitarian partners," little was done to halt this massive diversion. By July, in the town of Ajiep, with hundreds of tonnes of OLS food airdropped, more than 80 percent of the children were still malnourished while rebel-controlled food storage sites were full. By October, thousands of tonnes of food had been dropped into Ajiep and still half the children in the village were malnourished. Overall some fifty thousand people had died in the Bar el Gazel region while Khartoum maintained its tight control over aid and the rebels took what they wanted.

By the fall of 1998 the Khartoum government was politically isolated and targeted. On August 20, American cruise missiles had destroyed a pharmaceutical plant in Khartoum, the only one in the country. Sudan's government had allegedly supported al Qaeda, which was responsible for bombing American embassies in Dar es Salaam and Nairobi earlier that year. The Americans alleged that the Sudanese government was making biochemical weapons at the pharmaceutical plant (allegations that were later disproved by a UN investigation) and destroyed it on the same day that Monica Lewinsky was to testify before a grand jury set to indict President Clinton for

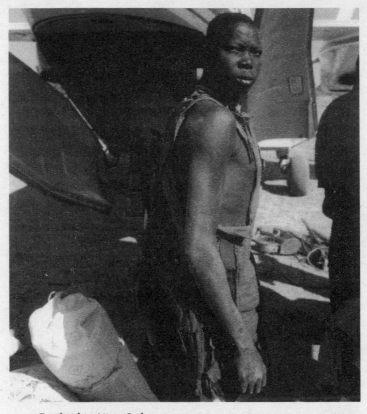

Food aid in Ajiep, Sudan

perjury. (Also that same day, Afghanistan was attacked with cruise missiles, in a failed attempt to kill Osama bin Laden, who had gone there, after allegedly going first to Somalia.) The tension between Khartoum and the United States, a major funder of OLS, resulted in tighter restrictions on aid. Khartoum became even more aggressive in the south, aggression that included bombing MSF hospitals.

Now, with the predictable famine season only months away, Marie-Christine feared that thousands more people would die needlessly. Through peace and war, MSF had been working in Sudan since 1978, and now had hundreds of expatriates throughout the country. In addition to offering famine relief in the south, in the past year we had vaccinated nearly three million people against meningitis in the north and had extensive health programs in some of the remotest regions of the country. At the operational meeting in Nairobi it became clear that we had too many inexperienced people in critical positions in Sudan, and that we had become trapped in the rules and bureaucracy of OLS. Numerous negotiated agreements over the years between Khartoum, the rebels, UN agencies, the UN Security Council, donor governments and NGOs had created a nearly impenetrable set of conflicting arrangements that meant everyone and no one was responsible and accountable for humanitarian aid. Jean-Marie Kindermans and I launched an internal review of our response to the crisis and an analysis of what our relationship to OLS should be. We knew that humanitarian issues had to be kept separate from political issues. OLS was a mix of the two, which left millions vulnerable not only to the politics of war between the government and the rebels but also to great power interests at play between the two sides. We didn't want to break OLS—we wanted to see it fixed. If our silence about the inefficiencies of OLS was a strategic choice, it had been a total failure.

I wanted to see what was happening for myself, and so I flew to Loki, the OLS operational headquarters on the Kenyan border with Sudan. In the ten years since OLS had been there, Loki had become a bustling UN town in the desert, with airstrips, airplane hangars and a control tower, and a perimeter fence. It was the semi-permanent home to hundreds of aid workers and their UN and NGO offices. Metal truck and train cargo containers had been modified into permanent small storage sites. Vast warehouses and UN living quarters had been constructed. Bathrooms with hot-water showers had been built, and concrete foundations and walls had been poured for temporary tent structures that had been there for years. François Fille, the Belgian MSF head of mission, met me at the airstrip, and we drove to the MSF office. Loki was a busy place, with trucks moving cargo, and aid workers sitting behind computers in offices with the windows open. The heat was like a sauna as we walked along a carefully manicured path to François's desk on an open-air veranda. A Kenyan man from the village outside the perimeter fence watered flowers along the path. I was to leave the next morning for the village of Mapel. Over the next four hours I drank several Fantas as François explained the structure and politics of OLS and the main security risks of working in the south.

François took me to the canteen, for the daily mandatory security briefing for new arrivals. About fifteen of us—aid workers, journalists and OLS officials—stood in a semicircle around a former British Special Operations officer, a lean man about thirty-five years of age in safari shorts who was in charge of security for OLS. "Right, ladies and gentlemen. This is your security briefing." For the next half-hour he detailed the risks and the dos and don'ts of dealing with the rebels in South Sudan. "If anything goes wrong," he said, "we can evacuate you by air. But remember, ladies and gentlemen. Time. Airplanes take time. Four to six hours on a good day, days if there is more than one evacuation request. Right. Any questions? Good. Thank you. Off you go, then." Within a few minutes, the canteen was flooded with UN and aid workers coming for their scheduled meal and for the requisite beers afterwards at the bar. That night I slept in one of the guest tents and was reminded by the Kenyan staff that laundry pickup was before 10 a.m. It was like a safari camp, and I slept well.

The next morning I flew to Mapel, taking in the clear blue sky and the brown desert below. The vibration of the small propeller airplane was steady, and the constant engine hum was barely masked by the headphones the pilot had given me to wear. As we approached the dirt airstrip to land, I could see rebel soldiers gathered around pallets of food that had been air-dropped by OLS planes. Jean, the MSF co-coordinator in Mapel, met me and explained that the rebels took what they wanted, and what remained was then taken to the feeding centres to be distributed there. At night the soldiers went to the centres and took food back from the mothers. "They call it *tayeen*. It's a kind of protection tax imposed by the rebels," he told me. Jean had been working in Mapel for six months and had seen the worst of the famine. We sat in the shade in one of the few clusters of trees in the village. He explained the medical treatment proto-col we were using at the feeding centre, where at the time only 300 or so people were admitted. (During the peak months of the famine, there had been 2,300.) "We've revised the protocol so many times that now it's perfect," he said. As he talked, a thin girl with the swollen feet of marasmus stood by the trees with six other girls watching us. I smiled at them. Three of the six had swollen feet as well. I asked Jean about them. "The pro-tocol is perfect, but the food taxes are high," he said. "OLS turns a blind eye, and we can do nothing about it."

I went to several other villages before flying on to Khartoum, where I met with OLS directors and with Ambassador Tom Eric Vraalsen, the UN special representative for Sudan. I raised the concerns that MSF had, and after being assured by the ambassador that MSF was "an important partner," I was reminded that there was "a process for raising concerns." The broad frame-work of OLS was not up for discussion, which would "risk undo-ing what had been negotiated over the last ten years." I asked about the lack of access to the Equatoria region and said that all areas needed to be accessible for humanitarian assistance. The ambassador replied, "Ideally, that is true. But the needs in Equatoria are not as great as in, for example, Bar el Gazel. If we ask for too much we may not get anything."

Our own reviews were well under way. Over the next few months I flew back and forth from Europe to Sudan several times. I met with rebel leaders, officials from the government of Sudan, OLS and NGOs, and officials and ambassadors of OLS donor governments. But most important, I went to some of the villages and towns where MSF was working. After a six-hour flight over the desert from Loki, I arrived in the village of Ajiep late one afternoon. Nearly the whole village had come to the airstrip. I had brought some mail and medical supplies with me. Sudanese villagers unloaded the small plane as I met the MSF team. The co-coordinator, Marie-Anne, took me to the health post, a small mud-and-bamboo building with a few beds for overnight patients, and then on to the feeding centre. It was like all of the other MSF feeding centres I had seen over the past months. Several hundred people were there that day, and I examined one starving child with a hugely swollen abdomen. It was swollen not because of starvation but because of leishmaniasis, a fatal parasitic infection carried by sand flies. I explained to her mother that because of the fighting, we couldn't set up to give her daughter the four weeks of necessary intravenous drug treatment. "I will feed her and I will wait," she said.

We had a bonfire that night. The stars brightened a black

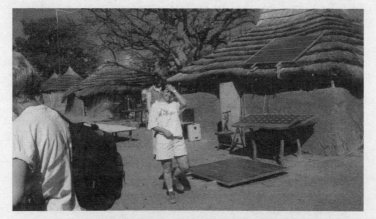

MSF health post in Ajiep

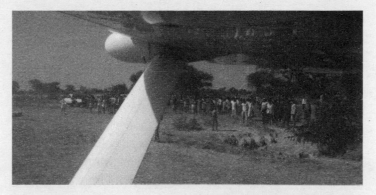

Sudanese villagers unload a small plane in Ajiep

sky. As I talked with Marie-Anne and some of the village elders, one of the expatriates played his guitar. Around eleven, two other elders joined us. They said that the Khartoum government militia had been spotted on horseback at a rail line a few kilometres away and that the MSF team should evacuate back to Loki until the militia had left the area. Marie-Anne was torn between the safety of the team and abandoning the village. But the elders were adamant. One old man said, "We will go to the bush. We cannot protect you. You are not soldiers or saints. You cannot help us if you are dead. And we will still need help once the militia have gone."

Early the next morning Marie-Anne gave the keys to the feeding centre and health post to the village chief. As we packed computers, radios and baggage, I watched groups of women, children and old people walk with small bundles along well-worn paths into the bush. We heard the OLS plane in the distance and we climbed into the flatbeds of several MSF pickup trucks. As men sang, the elders came with us to see us off, and naked children waved at us as we passed on our way to the airstrip. I stared back at a woman who stood silently with her child as we drove by. She looked at me with strong, resigned eyes. I had examined her child in the feeding centre the day before. She turned and walked towards the bush. She would keep waiting.

Another village near Ajiep had also faced the threat of a militia attack. The OLS plane was late, and the MSF team had fled to the desert bush with the villagers. They had a portable radio and were calling in every two hours. Militia had come into the village and burned, raped and killed. They were now searching the outlying bush. François was frantic with yet another evacuation from another village, and we were taking turns on radio standby. I was on duty from 11 p.m. to 2 a.m. I did not know what I would say if they did call from the bush, but I remembered from my time in Somalia how important it was that someone was waiting at the other end of a radio. No one called. The next morning the team was picked up, and I met them that afternoon as they arrived in Loki. Peter, a twenty-five-year-old Dutch logistician, got off the plane with Sylvie, a Belgian nurse, also about twenty-five.

"If they catch them, the women will be raped. I was afraid of being raped," said Sylvie.

"We left them behind," said Peter, his eyes bloodshot.

We walked without talking to the truck in the baking heat. In Ajiep, the militia had come to fight the rebels. But the OLS security officer said it had only been "a small attack." Only a few men were killed, only a few women were raped, and only a few women and children were taken to be sold as slaves in North Sudan. By the end of the week, six of seven MSF teams had been evacuated, and four of the seven villages where they had been working had been attacked.

I had a beer with Xavier, a French MSF logistician. We sat on the porch of his office. Pounding the plywood table, he said, "The government blocks aid flights and attacks at will. The rebels take what they want at will. OLS has no will. The mothers and children die, and we are silent! This is humanitarian? It is intolerable to know this and say nothing. I feel it in my gut like a cri de coeur. I want to scream!"

Two days later, early in February 1999, I was back in

Brussels, going over the final draft of our review of OLS with
Jean-Marie Kindermans. I had been told by OLS officials several
times in "unofficially official terms" that if MSF caused "a stink"
we would be expelled from OLS. And yet it was clear that if we
said nothing, nothing would change. We had prepared op-eds
to run in key international newspapers and had organized
meetings with officials in Sudan and Nairobi and at the EU. I
was to go to the United States with Marie-Christine for meetings with the head of UNICEF, the president of the UN Security
Council, UN agency officials, the editorial board of the
Washington Post, other journalists and the National Security
Council at the White House. A senior official from UNICEF in
New York called me in Brussels the night before we left. "There
are obviously some difficulties with OLS, but I am sure we can
work them out between us. There is no need to bring this to the
press." After a year of private protests, the failure of OLS had not
been addressed. I checked in at my Brussels office before flying
to New York. I had an email from a Dutch MSF logistician at
Loki. He was a quiet, determined worker and had never had
much to say when I had met him before. His email was simple:
"When you get to NY and the White House, forget all the political bullshit and just tell the fucking truth."

After our meetings in New York, Marie-Christine and I
flew to Washington. Our flight had been late. We quickly passed
through security at the White House and went into a side
building of the complex. John Prendergast, the Clinton administration's National Security Council adviser on Africa, was
waiting with his team. I poured myself a coffee, then gave a
detailed presentation on the history of OLS, its failures during
the 1998 Bar el Gazel famine, and the humanitarian implications of the U.S. government's support of the rebels through
OLS. I spoke for half an hour, and then the youngest staffer
politely suggested that MSF had gone too far in criticizing OLS
publicly. I started to reply, but Marie-Christine interrupted. In a

thick French accent she said, "But you are not understanding. The rebels are taking the food from the mothers and their babies. The rebels are making a theft, and the mothers are burying their children. It is like this."

No one spoke. I took a sip of my lukewarm coffee. I looked around at the cream-coloured panelled walls and wondered how many times this room had fallen silent. Finally, a more senior aide turned to me and began to respond to my analysis. Again, Marie-Christine leaned forward. "No. It is a theft, and the children are hungry. This is not—how do you say—correct. OLS knows it is not correct. We know it is not correct. You know it is not correct. Only you can fix it. You must fix it." There was nothing more to say.

OLS's initial response to our public challenge was, predictably, defensive. However, even as our analysis was called "inaccurate and unbalanced," we were not expelled. A few months later, Jean-Hervé Bradol, the operations director for the Paris office of MSF, and I were in Nairobi to meet with OLS officials. Our luggage had been lost, and after we apologized to Dr. Shaw, the director of OLS, for our T-shirts, he reassured us that MSF was a valuable partner, "with or without a T-shirt." He explained that OLS was being restructured, that the rebels had acknowledged a problem with "corruption leading to food diversion" in certain areas, and that a system to better monitor distributed food was being implemented. "Let's forget the past and move on to the future," he said. Jean-Hervé and I left the meeting and agreed that, although OLS had left the distribution of the food aid in the hands of the rebels, overall the changes were an improvement.

In Sudan we had provoked changes in humanitarian practice. We would soon face a crisis about the meaning of independent humanitarian action. It would involve NATO, the greatest military and political alliance in world history, in one of the most complex regions of the world, the Balkans.

On March 24, 1999, I was in London visiting the MSF office. I took the night off to share a few too many drinks with my cousin Bernadette and other family members. The next morning, Jean-Marie called me on my mobile phone. NATO had started bombing Serb military positions in Kosovo and Serbia. Russia and China had blocked an earlier effort at the UN Security Council to authorize a NATO use of force. Now NATO was acting without the UN's authorization. The night the bombing started, British prime minister Tony Blair went on television and announced that the bombing was "in the name of humanity." NATO declared it was going to war to "prevent a humanitarian disaster." Whatever the reason, for the first time in fifty years, NATO and NATO member states were at war, and they were at war in Europe. As soon as the bombing started, Yugoslav president Slobodan Milošević accelerated his "Operation Horseshoe" inside the province of Kosovo, using his forty-thousand-strong police, militia and military forces to expel ethnic Albanians across the border to neighbouring states.

In the months before, under threat of NATO air strikes, the six-member Contact Group of Britain, France, Germany, Italy, Russia and the United States had been negotiating with Milošević to resolve the Kosovo question. Civil war in Kosovo had started in February 1998, when Kosovo Liberation Army (KLA) insurgents, backed by the Americans, took up arms against Milošević's Serbian forces, who had massacred dozens of Albanians in the Drenica region of the province. MSF had had teams in Kosovo since 1992, and in the six months prior to the NATO bombings, we drew attention to the crisis and frequently called for international observers. We denounced the Serbian forces' campaign of violence and intimidation against ethnic Albanians, who constituted 90 percent of Kosovo's population of two million. We had been offering medical care for the more than 200,000 people displaced or otherwise affected by the fighting. Fifty thousand of these people were constantly on the move, living in the mountains and valleys after fleeing Serbian attacks during which wells were poisoned and houses were burned. Snipers remained in the villages after people had fled. Families had been separated as children ran faster than adults. Terrified people had left without winter clothes, and many families had only one blanket to share as they slept in forests and valleys littered with land mines. As diplomatic initiatives pressed on, MSF, like UN and other aid agencies, expected the civil war to get worse before it got better.

The Dayton Peace Accords signed in December 1995 had focused on Bosnia and had not dealt with Kosovo. Milošević blocked further negotiations by refusing to issue exit visas to KLA representatives who planned to attend talks on Kosovo at Rambouillet Castle, outside Paris. On March 18, Milošević walked away from the Paris talks and escalated the buildup of his forces in Kosovo. Unarmed monitors for the Organization for Security and Co-operation in Europe withdrew from Kosovo. After months of threatening air strikes, NATO now found its credibility at stake. It had been severely damaged by the failure to prevent Serbian atrocities against Muslims in Bosnia. On March 24, NATO began bombing Serbian military targets in Kosovo and Serbia. Now NATO was a belligerent in war, and MSF had to be independent of its member states, as well as of the Serbian and KLA combatants. After Jean-Marie called me in London, he and I spent the next eighteen hours calling others to ensure that no MSF section would take money from NATO member states for humanitarian assistance in Kosovo. We established a series of agreements whereby MSF sections would underwrite each other. Particular attention was given to the cash needs of the Belgian section, which supported our largest operations both internationally and in Kosovo. With our financial arrangements secured, we declared MSF's humanitarian independence from all participants in the conflict.

Instead of breaking Milošević's resolve, the NATO bombings strengthened it. His response was swift and brutal. He intensified his months-long campaign of terror that was forcing hundreds of thousands of Kosovo's Muslim Albanians across the borders. It was the largest and fastest movement of refugees in Europe since the end World War II. Milošević expelled the press, and our MSF team—the last NGO to remain—was forced to withdraw on March 29 because of perilous security. In the months before, like diplomats, NATO and other aid agencies, we had expected the crisis to worsen inside Kosovo, not outside its borders. We had stockpiled food and other aid supplies inside Kosovo, and we and other aid agencies had limited aid resources outside Kosovo. In the days since the bombing had started, we had flown nineteen cargo planes of supplies and mobilized a massive expansion of our teams to the region.

The Canadian NATO ambassador called me on March 31 to say that Russian prime minister Yevgeny Primakov's diplomatic mission to Belgrade had failed and that NATO was going to continue the bombing. An American Stealth bomber had been shot down over Serbia, and NATO had launched a massive search for the missing pilot. In Macedonia, Slav nationalists launched violent protests outside the American embassy in reaction to Kosovo refugees flooding into the country. There was a real risk that Greece, Bulgaria and Turkey could be drawn into the tensions in Macedonia. Three American servicemen became "unwilling actors in a propaganda war" after being taken hostage in Macedonia by Serbian forces, beaten and displayed on Serbian national television. In Montenegro, which was still a part of Serbia but was led by a pro-Western government, civil war threatened to break out as Serbian anti-aircraft guns there fired on NATO warplanes. The NATO alliance was beginning to fray, with the hard-liners, the United States and Britain, on one side and Italy and Greece on the other. I knew the situation was tense even for MSF when the president of the board of MSF Greece called me to urge that MSF publicly take a position against the NATO bombing.

Early on the morning of April 4, I was once again in London, and once again Jean-Marie called me on my cellphone. More than fifty thousand Kosovar refugees were stranded in a no man's land after Macedonia closed its borders to them. Jean-Marie organized a teleconference of the general directors, including Lex Winkler, who was at the Kosovo–Macedonia border. "It's unbelievable," Lex told us. "Thousands are trapped here in the mud surrounded by a fence. Women and children are screaming and crying. The authorities will not let us help them." We emailed the directors a press release for immediate comment by telephone. An hour later we issued a statement around the world demanding direct and unhindered access to refugees at the Macedonian border. NATO had lost control of the military campaign. It had not anticipated the forced exodus of more than 300,000 Kosovars. "We are guilty of a failure of imagination," said the British Foreign Office in conceding that no plans had been made before the NATO air strikes to help refugees, and that NATO was not prepared for the "speed, savagery, and scale" of the Serbian response. *The Economist* and newspapers around the world said that the bombing was making ethnic cleansing worse, and that the war had gone horribly wrong. It was a public relations disaster for NATO.

I flew to the region to see the situation for myself. On the morning of April 5, Chris Stokes, the Belgian MSF coordinator, and I drove ten hours from Tirana, Albania, to the border town of Kukës. We were driving against the current of thousands of refugees in cars, tractors, caravans and on foot, making their way to reception centres MSF had set up in the south of Albania. At Kukës, another 100,000 Kosovar Albanians waited with little or no assistance. The majority were being housed in the farmhouses and apartments of Albanians who shared their meagre resources with the deportees. Populations of entire Kosovo villages had set up "wild tractor camps" in farmers' fields with plastic tarps draped over the vehicles for shelter. One group of about four hundred people had taken shelter in a chicken hatchery. The smell and living conditions were deplorable. The medical needs were not great, but people needed food, blankets and shelter. We were organizing a measles vaccination campaign, as many Kosovars had refused vaccination in the previous year, fearing that Serbian authorities would try to poison them. The KLA were recruiting from the refugees and launching cross-border attacks into Kosovo.

Christopher and I met with the MSF team that night to go over who would do what in the morning to expand shelter, transit clinics, water and sanitation, epidemic prevention and food and blanket distribution. Later we went to the town centre. It was cold and raining. The town square was packed with mothers in headscarves cradling their children in wet blankets under dripping plastic sheeting. Children cried, old men smoked, and younger men tore branches off trees to fuel small, smoking fires.

I stood at the border the next morning. An orderly line of vehicles and people on foot stretched back from the border for at least fifteen kilometres. In the distance, smoke clouded upwards from farmhouses that had been torched by Serb forces. NATO bombers flew overhead. Serbian soldiers looked out from guard towers about half a kilometre away and from hastily dug foxholes not far from the border. A hundred metres from the border, MSF and other aid agencies had set up transit medical clinics for the refugees as they poured across. One old man cried inconsolably into his hands as I bandaged a six-inch laceration on his forehead. He had been hit with the butt of a rifle when he left the deportation line to urinate in the bushes. He was terrified for his son, who had been taken away by

Serbian forces, some of whom he recognized as local police.

That day, April 6, Milošević offered a unilateral ceasefire with a return of the refugees. NATO refused, demanding full compliance with the Rambouillet agreements, and stepped up its bombing campaign. The UN Security Council was still dead-locked. Russia threatened to support Milošević militarily against NATO. The United States warned that Russian support would have grave consequences. Milošević closed the borders. By the time he reopened them, 300,000 refugees had been forced into Macedonia, Montenegro and Albania—three of the poorest regions of Europe. Fearing that thousands would storm through barbed-wire fencing, Macedonia surrounded refugees with sol-diers and riot police. At the same time, "fearing an explosive influx," Germany said that Kosovo's Albanian outcasts should remain in the Balkans, while Tony Blair ruled out the possibility of allowing any to settle in the U.K. The next day, NATO allies announced they would airlift up to 100,000 refugees out of the Balkans for temporary shelter in their countries.

Media attention remained focused on the refugees, and NATO was losing the propaganda war badly. NATO Command set up Operation Allied Harbor to provide humanitarian assistance. British foreign secretary Robin Cook said NATO would act as "a humanitarian agency, providing security and safety to refugees while prosecuting military action." NATO airlifts were used to bring in aid supplies. President Clinton set up a committee to raise funds and coordinate military logistical support for an American humanitarian NGO network that was working in Kosovo. Many in the NGO network were openly supporting the NATO action, but MSF had to remain independent, and we immediately withdrew our American office from the network. NATO member states held meetings with the Albanian, Montenegrin and Macedonian governments without involv-ing the UN agencies on the management of refugees. The UN High Commissioner for refugees was sidelined. Only half of its funding needs for the region had been met, its funding coming primarily from states that were also members of NATO. At the Albania–Kosovo border, eight thousand NATO troops poured in as Italian forces set up a mobile field hospital while other troops dug in artillery and started building refugee camps. Deeper in Albania, French, German and eight other NATO member-state forces were building camps and moving refugees in. NATO drew media attention to what was now being done to assist the refugees. It blamed aid agencies for having "been caught off the hop," for "not expecting so many refugees" and for "reacting slowly to this human catastrophe."

At the borders, Serbian forces had stripped more than half of the refugees of their identity papers. Consequently they were not being registered by UNHCR—an essential first step to their legal status as refugees—and some were being forcibly moved by NATO forces from transit reception sites to other locations in the region and in Europe. Registration was not merely an administrative issue. In places like the south of Albania, organized-crime gangs preyed on refugees, kidnapping them for prostitution rings in central Europe and elsewhere. In several press conferences I and others in MSF acknowledged that getting aid into the region required the logistical capacity of NATO, but asserted that the UNHCR absolutely must lead the humanitarian effort. Otherwise, there was a risk that humanitarian aid would be seen as part of NATO's military campaign. We reminded NATO forces that refugee rights and international law needed to be respected, and warned that NATO relief efforts could put refugees at risk. In the face of crisis, it was a difficult argument to make without looking needlessly territorial, but the safety of the refugees demanded that we make it. Several days later, Serb forces shelled refugee camps established by NATO in Kukës, Albania, and in Macedonia and Montenegro.

Milošević was a known—and soon to be indicted—war criminal, and there was no doubt he was committing crimes against humanity in Kosovo. In the three weeks that the bombing had continued, we had been taking the testimonies of refugees throughout the region. A fifteen-year-old girl told us that her village had been surrounded by policemen: "We were at home. There were soldiers everywhere, as far as the forest. A hand grenade was thrown in the direction of our house, and it landed just in front of me. My hand was wounded and I lost a lot of blood. We managed to escape along the river, through the forest and then along the road. Soldiers were posted every ten metres along the road. Once we had crossed the border, I was taken to the Italian camp and from there to the Kukës hospital to get some X-rays done. My identification papers were confiscated at the border."

By April 12, more than half a million people had been forced out of Kosovo. Hundreds of thousands more were trapped in the mountains inside Kosovo. Much of our aid in the region was blocked at customs. Civilian airspace was restricted by the NATO bombing, which limited our capacity to bring in the supplies we needed. There was a lack of relief coordination, the role that, under international law, the UN was meant to assume. I felt a near-explosive frustration. I wasn't alone. One MSF doctor wept as he watched Kosovars waiting in the rain across the border.

As NATO continued its bombings, commentators demanded ground troops. Clinton and Blair feared NATO casualties and publicly refused this option, though NATO undertook preparations for a wider offensive. While Blair proclaimed that the war was a "conflict of good versus evil" and that NATO had to keep bombing "to save the refugees," Richard Holbrooke, the American diplomat whose Yugoslav shuttle diplomacy had culminated in the NATO attack, maintained a hard *realpolitik* view. He argued that humanitarian concerns came last on his list of priorities for the war—after restoring stability in southeastern Europe and safeguarding the reputation of the United States.

Throughout the region, NATO brought in Apache helicopters for low-level attacks on Serbian ground forces. NATO forces dug in artillery at the Kosovo–Albania border and thousands of troops were moved in.

Most other aid agencies had continued to receive funding from NATO member states and cooperated publicly with NATO's aid efforts. Now, with nearly 600,000 refugees in the region and thousands more being forced over the border or trapped in the mountains, MSF couldn't just sit, watch and wait. Our silence would speak volumes. Humanitarianism had already been co-opted, and we had to struggle to regain some measure of independence. If humanitarian concerns were last on Holbrooke's list, they were first on ours. As I prepared for a press conference, I thought of the web of political motives behind the interventions in Somalia, Rwanda, Zaire and elsewhere. I knew that weeks before, UN peacekeepers had quietly withdrawn from Angola, where humanitarian assistance had been tied to a UN peace framework. When the framework collapsed, so too did humanitarian assistance to the victims of Angola's civil war. What if NATO ground troops came and succeeded in Kosovo? What if they came and failed? What if they didn't come at all? The needs of refugees and civilians across the border—Kosovars and Serbs alike—were real and immediate. With or without ground troops, we still had to struggle for an independent humanitarian space to try to meet those needs. I had called various MSF leaders to canvass their opinions on the question of whether MSF should support the call for ground troops. Rony Brauman, a former president of MSF France, said to me, "Remember, NATO is not a fascist army." Before the conversation could go any further, the battery on my cellphone went dead, and the press was waiting.

At the press conference, we condemned Milošević's ethnic cleansing campaign and said that up to one million ethnic Albanians had been forced from their homes in Kosovo but remained unaccounted for. World attention was focused on the fighting between Yugoslavia and NATO and on the effort to feed and settle refugees who had fled Kosovo—but what of those who remained? "Where are these one million people? What is happening to them?" I asked. I accused NATO of withholding satellite imagery and other information that would shed light on the location and condition of people still remaining in Kosovo and insisted on a humanitarian space inside and outside Kosovo that was independent of the belligerents.

The inevitable question of whether or not MSF would support NATO ground troops came from David Rieff. I knew and respected David as a journalist and as one of the leading thinkers on humanitarianism. I refused to answer, saying that NATO didn't need our assent for a unilateral intervention that was happening anyway. Rieff pushed hard, arguing that it was intellectually incoherent not to call for ground troops to stop Milošević while at the same time highlighting the plight of people still in Kosovo. For Rieff, it was "only in the Balkan wars, where, uniquely in [his] experience of such conflicts, [he] believed that it was . . . imperative to take sides."[2] Mine wasn't the best argument, but for us it was not a question of intellectual coherence but rather one of pragmatism. If we provided moral cover for a NATO-led "humanitarian war" today, there would be no turning back to a morally coherent claim for an independent humanitarian space tomorrow. For more than an hour, Rieff and other journalists pushed for an answer: "Yes or no?" It was the toughest press conference of my life, but I refused to be drawn in.

A few days later we released the refugee testimonies we had gathered, evidence to support our public accusation that Milošević was committing war crimes. I flew back to Brussels.

In the weeks that followed, MSF faced our own internal crisis. The Greek section became caught up in the partisan politics of its own country and the politics of war in the region. Greece was a NATO member, and yet 90 percent of its population opposed the NATO bombing of Kosovo and Serbia. Inside Greece was a strong pro-Serbian majority, and the Greek government struggled to find a way to assuage pro-Serb domestic sentiment while remaining a member of NATO. The Greek government worked out an agreement with the Serb government to allow Greek NGOs to enter Kosovo and Belgrade. But where they could and could not go—and therefore what they could and could not see—would be determined by the Serb government. Greece also obtained an agreement with NATO that Greek NGOs would have access to humanitarian corridors free from air strikes. One Greek NGO had already made good on the arrangement, to public acclaim in Greece and Serbia, and the Greek MSF section was under enormous domestic pressure to do the same. Its board secretly agreed to participate, and de facto to accept Serb restrictions on its movements. Yet the board knew that because we were worried that an MSF presence in Serbia could give a humanitarian legitimacy to a government we were publicly accusing of crimes against humanity in Kosovo, we wanted to first send a highly experienced non-partisan international team into the country to freely and independently evaluate the humanitarian needs. The Greek MSF board also knew that the Serb government had consistently denied MSF re-entry visas into Serbia on these terms.

On May 7 the president of the Greek board led a convoy of MSF vehicles carrying medical supplies and bearing Greek flags into Kosovo and Belgrade. By the terms of the secret arrangement, the supplies were delivered to a Serb government hospital. The head of the Greek board publicly accused NATO of attempting to bomb the vehicles and of having no respect for humanitarian corridors, and raised doubts about the reality of ethnic cleansing.

The actions of MSF Greece went against everything MSF stood for and the careful path MSF was treading in the region.

We managed to stop the mission. Weeks of intense debate, phone calls and emergency meetings of boards and the International Council followed. The Greek board claimed it had had "no choice," as it had to meet the demands of the pro-Serb majority in Greece. It had shown little regard for the manipulations of war, had actively or at best naively played into these, and had broken the trust vital to membership in any organization. The Greek MSF board refused to acknowledge the position of the rest of the MSF movement. On June 12, the other eighteen members of the International Council voted unanimously to expel the Greek section. We had to protect the independent humanitarian character of the organization. We could not succumb to the passions that war can inflame inside civil society. We had to maintain the legitimacy of our voice in speaking out against crimes against humanity. And we had to ensure that humanitarian action not be used as political fodder in war. As far as I know, it was the first time an international organization had taken such an action. It felt like we had lost a member of the family. I was not proud of it. None of us were. (In early 2005, the Greek section was reintegrated as a member of the MSF movement after agreeing to share MSF's operational and humanitarian principles.)

By May 24, Milošević was formally indicted for war crimes committed in Bosnia. By mid-June Russia and the United States had reached an agreement on a political solution to the crisis. After seventy-eight days of bombing, Milošević conceded. The Clinton administration had been within days of mobilizing a ground invasion of 175,000 troops. A UN-mandated peace-keeping force known as KFOR entered Kosovo on June 13, and within weeks, the majority of refugees were able to return. Bernard Kouchner was selected by Kofi Annan, the UN secretary-general, to be his special representative in Kosovo and to head up the UN mission there. For Kouchner, Kosovo was a front-line test of what he and others called the "right of states to intervene."

Kouchner declared, "I don't care about world government . . . We must always be on the minority side, the suffering side . . . Now there is an increasingly recognized right to intervene. You say in advance, 'Mr. Dictator, you have no right to threaten or kill a minority. And if you insist, we have a huge army, all the countries of the world, that will prevent you from doing that.' The idea is prevention. Deterrence. Maybe it will take only one bomb, or none at all. But you say, 'We are here. Do not kill these people.' This is the new way to be a world militant."

The "humanitarian war" was hailed as a NATO victory, and for some, like David Rieff, it portended the end of humanitarianism as a neutral and independent action. For Tony Blair, military intervention "for righting humanitarian distress" would "spread the values of liberty, the rule of law, human rights and an open society." For him, Kosovo was the first step in a "New Doctrine of International Community" where "values and interests merge."

MSF had a different analysis. We denounced war crimes in Kosovo, but at the same time we had confronted NATO's direct involvement in humanitarian action, an uncertain role for UNHCR, the lack of humanitarian protection inside Kosovo and the implications of NGOs' being funded by states that were at war. These were key questions in a crisis during which humanitarian action had become a justification for a military and political intervention. Despite the presence of thousands of UN-mandated troops, retribution killings of Kosovar Serbs began. By the end of June 1999, tens of thousands of Serbs had left Kosovo. With a massive reconstruction effort under way inside Kosovo, we continued to be present, giving and supporting direct medical care and monitoring the humanitarian situation for both ethnic Albanians and Serbs.

On October 15, 1999, I was in Paris opening the first conference of our Campaign for Access to Essential Medicines. I was just leaving the podium when my cellphone rang. A man claiming to be Geir Lundestad, the chair of the Nobel Peace Prize Committee, told me that MSF had been awarded the Nobel Peace Prize. He said that the public announcement would be made in fifteen minutes. We had been scammed before, so I politely took his name and number and asked my assistant to call the Nobel committee to verify what I had been told. It was true. I went to a stall in the bathroom and had a smoke. I wrote down a few notes on what we would say and returned to the conference room to tell Bernard Pécoul, the French director of the Access campaign. "Ce n'est pas vrai?" he asked.

"Oui, c'est certain," I replied.

He interrupted the speaker and proudly proclaimed, "MSF has been nominated for the Nobel Peace Prize!" The audience clapped and smiled politely.

I stood up and said, "Now that Bernard has announced the nomination, I would like to announce that MSF has been awarded this year's Nobel Peace Prize."

Within minutes of the official announcement, hundreds of journalists and scores of satellite-news trucks descended on our Paris office. Staff sang and danced in the hallways, and others rushed out to buy crates of champagne. In MSF offices and four hundred projects all over the world, the scene was the same. The Nobel committee noted MSF's commitment to "independent medical humanitarian action," and to "speaking out which helps to form bodies of public opinion opposed to violations and abuses of power." At a hastily called press conference, Philippe Biberson, the president of MSF France, said, "We are not sure that speaking out saves people but we are certain that silence kills."

After eighteen hours of solid interviews, I began to worry that the prize might turn MSF into a "Nobelized" institution that offered solemn slogans but was divorced from the reality of the people we were trying to help. Before the announcement, I had planned to go to Mariinsk, Siberia, to investigate access to tuberculosis treatments for Russian prisoners. I decided to stick with my plan. I travelled to Moscow's airport, where, as I had done in 1987, I drank too much vodka with a man who wanted to go to the West. I flew to Kemerovo, Siberia, and then drove through the bleak hinterland to Mariinsk, home to several high-security prisons known as Colony 33 that held 29,000 men. The prisons had been gulags during the Soviet era.

I spent two weeks working with the MSF team. We were treating hundreds of prisoners with TB and trying to introduce treatment for some who had multi-drug-resistant TB (MDR-TB). More than three million people were being held in Russian prisons. More than one-tenth were sick with active TB, and one-quarter of those had MDR-TB. The prison and public health authorities had been using unscientific and disproved treatment methods developed during the Soviet era, and prisoners were released only to spread the diseases into their home commu-

Russian prisoners in exercise pen

nities. There, inexpert private practitioners replaced a public health system that had collapsed. MDR-TB was spreading beyond Russia's borders, with more than 100,000 cases identified worldwide, many of which could be traced through DNA bio-typing to Russian prisons.

The MSF team in the prisons was isolated, and the work wasn't easy. In cells designed for twelve there were sometimes as many as fifty prisoners. In nearly lightless rooms with poor ventilation, the air was cloudy with constant cigarette smoke. Thin, sallow men with TB received treatment sporadically, and none were getting enough food. A prison mafia controlled everything, from sex slaves and access to cigarettes and food to a black-market trade in illegal and medical drugs. We needed—and got—the assent of the mafia boss to implement the nine-month TB treatment program. Even under the best conditions it was a complicated medical protocol, involving several different drugs and sputum testing. I examined one man in the solitary-confinement wing whose entire body except for his hands and face was covered in tattoos. The guards gave him his daily TB tablets. "Thanks for these," he said to me in terse Russian, as the guards translated. "Prison is a shithole. But even I want to live."

I flew back to Moscow to meet several Ministry of Health officials and Mumar, our head of mission. We were running a clinic program for some of the 100,000 Muscovites—mostly men known as bomji, or bums—made homeless after the collapse of the Soviet empire and the introduction of market-oriented economic reforms. I sat in the clinic for a few hours and just watched. Then I went outside for a smoke with Sergi, a hard-faced fifty-year-old engineer working with us, and my translator and driver. Another man was smoking outside too. He asked me for a cigarette, which he put in his coat pocket. "Out here I am a bomji," he said. "I come to the clinic because they treat me like I am normal. It's only for a while, but I feel normal." Sergi bought him a pack of smokes from a nearby street vendor. Sergi started to weep as we drove to the MSF office. "He could be me, he could be any of us," he said.

At the office, Chechnya, not TB or homelessness, was Mumar's main concern. Following public demands from MSF, the Russian government had finally allowed some 160,000 refugees fleeing the fighting in the breakaway North Caucasus republic to cross into neighbouring Ingushetia. Mumar reminded me—as I knew well—that only three years before, unknown assailants had assassinated six Red Cross workers. Mumar and our national staff feared reprisals from the Russian secret police for the public demands we were making. Now, as the Russian army moved more than a thousand armoured vehicles into northern Chechnya, and pilots continued an aerial bombing campaign, new media restrictions were imposed on reporting from the republic. Since the start of the civil war in 1994, Russian forces had shown a near contempt for civilians. Intensive, indiscriminate bombing, gunship helicopter attacks and land assaults by Russian forces had killed more than seventy thousand of Chechnya's one million people. For five years, fearful for Russia's stability, the international community had found it expedient to remain silent on what it considered Russia's "internal" affair. The West was supporting Boris Yeltsin diplomatically and financially, rescheduling some $70 billion in debt. The lack of firm reaction against clear violations of the rules of war sent a green light to the Kremlin to continue its offensive in Chechnya. I sat with Mumar going over the careful wording of our next press release, one that would again insist on respect for and access to suffering civilians.

When I got back to my office in Brussels, waiting for me was a note from my good friend Paul Hogan, an artist working in Sri Lanka with Tamil and Muslim children affected by that country's civil war. "I have learned that fear is the mother of fearlessness, and the beginning of possibility," he wrote.

"Somehow, I think that strange little group called MSF discovered this a long time ago." I emailed David Rieff in New York, discussing some of the UN failures that were already evident in Kosovo. In his reply to me Rieff referred to MSF's refusal to be drawn in on the question of ground troops. "You were right, I was wrong," he wrote. I was in New York a few days later for a meeting on tuberculosis, and Rieff and I met at his favourite restaurant. We talked about organized humanitarianism in the face of what was now the first overtly humanitarian war. MSF was struggling with its implications for East Timor, Sierra Leone, Angola, Burundi and Chechnya. Rieff and I agreed that MSF had to fight as a civil-society organization to reclaim an independent humanitarian space. But after three bottles of wine, I wasn't sure I knew what that meant.

On December 8, a small MSF swarm descended on the Grand Hotel in Oslo, Norway. Amidst media interviews and phone calls, I struggled to complete the acceptance speech. I had been working on it for weeks, meeting with key people in MSF and canvassing others for ideas and support. I wanted to get it right, but the night before the ceremony, the speech remained unfinished. Philippe Biberson and Françoise Bouchet-Saulnier, an MSF specialist in humanitarian law, and I worked into the small hours of the morning to get it done. In hard-hitting language we referred to the crises in North Korea, Kosovo, Rwanda and Goma, and asserted the necessity of our independence. For years I had struggled to find the right words to describe how I understood the relationship between humanitarianism and politics. In the course of that long night, Philippe said that humanitarianism was not about ending or justifying war; it was the struggle to create human spaces in the midst of what is profoundly abnormal. In that moment I understood that to allow that space to exist, we had to be willing to confront political power. It's an imperfect struggle, and it never ends. In the acceptance speech I wrote: "The humanitarian act is the most apolitical of all acts, but if its actions and its morality are taken seriously, it has the most profound of political implications."

Before the ceremony, I met the king and queen of Norway. The protocol officer had wanted me to turn off my cellphone, but with the kidnapping of two MSF staff in Sierra Leone that day, the crisis in Chechnya and the former Greek section of MSF demonstrating outside the ceremony hall, I couldn't. As we talked, my phone rang. The king was not pleased. I answered and, leaning over to him, explained that it was my future mother-in-law. "Oh god, I understand, I understand. Take the call, take the call," the king said, waving away his protocol officer.

That afternoon, on deep blue carpets and with scores of trumpets blaring, Marie-Eve Raguenaud—an MSF field doctor who, as she put it, felt like she "had been plucked from a hospital in Burundi"—and I accepted MSF's Nobel Prize. What was most important to MSF was that we demonstrate our commitment to speaking out clearly and unambiguously in our refusal to accept the unacceptable. With the world's media and ambassadors present, I opened the acceptance speech by saying: "The people of Chechnya—and the people of Groznyy—today and for more

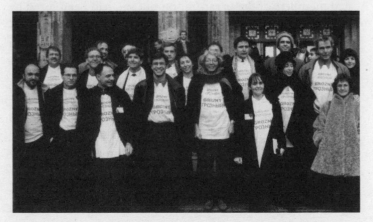

Outside the Nobel ceremony

than three months have endured indiscriminate bombing by the Russian army. For them humanitarian assistance is virtually unknown. It is the sick, the old and the infirm who cannot escape Groznyy. While the dignity of people in crisis is so central to the honour you give today, what you acknowledge in us is our particular response to it. I appeal here today to His Excellency the Ambassador of Russia, and through him to President Yeltsin, to stop the bombing of defenceless civilians in Chechnya. If conflicts and wars are an affair of the state, violations of humanitarian law, war crimes and crimes against humanity apply to us all—as civil society, as citizens, and as human beings." The Russian ambassador shifted uncomfortably in his seat. He was surrounded by the MSF horde wearing T-shirts that read "Stop the Bombing of Civilians in Groznyy!"

A few weeks after the Nobel ceremony, MSF was invited to the UN to address the Security Council on the protection of civilians in conflict. It was an important opportunity to distinguish between humanitarian assistance and political protection. Again I asked Françoise Bouchet-Saulnier to help me with the presentation. Not only was she one of the brightest and most dedicated members of the organization but she had been hired by Rony Brauman shortly after MSF's split with Kouchner, and if anyone understood the difference and relationship between humanitarian and political responsibilities, it was her. I met with several MSF people in Europe to discuss ideas, and then flew to New York with a suitcase of files and papers I had collected over the years. Françoise and I sat together for a few days in a small back room of the MSF office in New York, drinking too much coffee and eating too many doughnuts, while we hammered out MSF's presentation.

We had worked so late the night before that on the morning of the presentation, I overslept. I arrived just in time. A UN staffer cleared me through security and all but swept me into a blue leather chair in an anteroom to the Security Council chamber itself. I spoke for my allotted thirty minutes, emphasizing the necessity of a political response to political problems, a humanitarian response to humanitarian problems, and for robust and credible peacekeeping forces for security and protection concerns. I referred to Somalia and highlighted the danger of mixing protection with humanitarian assistance; to places like Zaire where war crimes had taken place or were taking place with impunity and where the UN had not intervened militarily or in any meaningful political way; and to Kosovo and the negative impact the "humanitarian war" had had on independent humanitarian action. I suggested that if the distinctions between short-term relief of suffering and the longer-term political responsibility for protection and security were blurred, the lack of clarity would ultimately be to the detriment of the victims of conflict. Language matters, I said: it determines how a problem is framed and defines the range of possible solutions. I referred to Rwanda, about which no member of the Security Council had been able to use the word *genocide*, and where the political crime of genocide erased the possibility of humanitarianism. The Security Council authorized a humanitarian intervention as a solution—one that obscured or sanitized the problem, and thus erased the UN's political responsibility to intervene to stop genocide. An intervention that used force to stop the massacres would have been the right response. I referred to the inability of the Security Council to even discuss violations of the laws of war in Chechnya because of Russia's veto in the council and the lack of transparency around voting. Visibly upset, the Russian ambassador dismissed my comment as preposterous and insisted that Chechnya was an internal matter and of no concern to the Security Council. I countered that while states should be able to abstain, they should not be allowed to exercise their veto on matters that involved the protection of civilians in conflict, and that the rationale for each Security Council vote should be public.

—

By August of 2000, more than a year after the victory of NATO's humanitarian war, with more than 43,000 KFOR troops present, upwards of 200,000 minority Serbs and Roma Gypsies had left Kosovo. Small enclaves of Serbs remained inside southern Kosovo surrounded by Albanians, and small enclaves of Albanians remained in the northern Mitrovica region surrounded by Serbs. I flew to Priština, Kosovo, with Alex Parisel, the general director of MSF Belgium. That night over beers, one MSF doctor told me, "I don't believe in what I am doing any more." I stayed for nearly two weeks, listening, talking and trying to understand.

Around both Serb and Albanian enclaves, there were organized campaigns of violence that included drive-by shootings, hand-grenade attacks, verbal abuse, robbery, blackmail and arson. More than 500 people had been killed and many more wounded since June 1999. We were supporting medical care for about 750,000 people in Kosovo. Some MSF teams were running mental health programs, and had started to go to the homes of people too frightened to go out. Outside one Albanian enclave, a Serb man had punched one of our doctors in the face, and the lives of some of our Albanian staff were repeatedly threatened. It was often too dangerous to move sick or wounded patients to the hospital. We pressed for better security, calls that were usually answered by a symbolic increase of KFOR patrols for a few days. KFOR was not backing up civilian police. In the past year, only 3,100 of the 6,000 necessary international police officers had arrived, and some had to be sent home because they couldn't drive or handle a weapon. There had been no integrated effort to stop the violence, and not one perpetrator had been convicted since the start of the UN mission. Indeed, after a year in Kosovo, Dennis

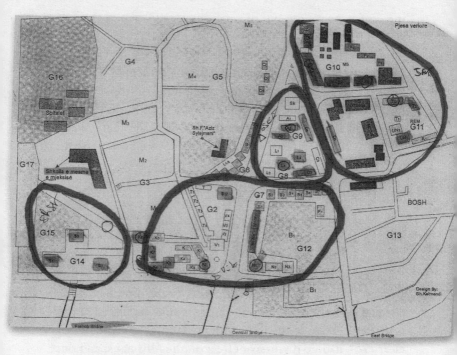

Map of Priština, Kosovo, indicating Shkolla Serb enclave

McNamara, the UN special envoy for humanitarian affairs, had been caustic in admitting there was an "implicit tolerance for intolerance," and that there should have been a wide use of emergency powers by the military at the beginning to prevent this culture of impunity.

Early one afternoon, I drove with our team through a heavily guarded KFOR checkpoint over the bridge to the Shkolla Serb enclave. It was nearly empty of Serbs. Since June 1999, most had fled to Serbia, but some, especially the old, remained. Three tall apartment buildings surrounded a small square with an outdoor café on one side. Albanian men sat smoking and drinking coffee. Across from them, French soldiers atop a KFOR armed vehicle were also smoking and drinking coffee. As we got out of our vehicle, the men in the café started jeering at us; one gave us the universal single-finger salute. We walked up three flights of stairs to a metal apartment door. It was spraypainted and heavily dented. Some of its sheet metal was cut through, and pieces of fire-retardant insulation from inside the door were on the floor. Else, the MSF nurse, knocked in code, telling the occupant that it was a friend. Inside, shattered window glass covered the floor. An old woman walked slowly in her nightgown to sit in her thickly padded armchair. She was about seventy years old. Even with two televisions and a radio turned on, we could still hear the men taunting her from the café below. She wanted diazepam and "something" for her "nerves" because she couldn't sleep. "All night they beat the door," she said, "all day they scream at me." Else took her blood pressure. The woman's family had all left for Serbia in the months before. She had refused to go, hoping things would get better. "I was born here. I want to die here with my family," she said. It was clear KFOR had no dissuasive effect on the Albanians, and our requests for better security had no effect on KFOR. It was also clear that we were helping to maintain the delusion that this woman was safe, and that by giving her "something for her nerves" we were making her clouded judgment worse.

In a Serb enclave just south of the city, I went inside the candlelit Orthodox church and watched three women praying to hand-painted icons. I walked outside, past a tent used as a school for Serb children, and through an opening in the barbed wire surrounding the church. A group of Albanian teenagers jeered and spat at me. I wiped the saliva of one boy off my sleeve. I went up the stairs of a small building to a clinic on the second floor. The Serb doctor smoked constantly as we talked in the dark room. We were supporting his clinic with medicines and other equipment. "Our people's biggest problem is fear," he told me. "We give them medicine for their anxiety, but this medical act collides with their liberty. It immobilizes them. But what am I to do? It is the destiny of our people."

I asked him about protection under the KFOR forces. "KFOR tells us they will help us if we cooperate with them," he explained. In fact, KFOR had been making humanitarian assistance conditional on that cooperation. Only weeks before, KFOR had denied an escort to a convoy from Štrpce, a Serb enclave. As the KFOR commander explained it, sanctions had been placed on the enclave "for the recent vandalism of the UN building and aggression toward KFOR peacekeepers in the municipality." KFOR had also imposed sanctions on and suspended "all humanitarian assistance projects . . . in the [Albanian] Kamenica municipality . . . because of hostile actions against KFOR soldiers that included violent demonstrations, rock throwing and a grenade attack." Humanitarian assistance was to be "redistributed to villages supporting UN and KFOR . . . until the residents of Štrpce and Kamenica demonstrate an earnest interest in cooperating with UNMIK"—the UN Mission in Kosovo—"and KFOR." I had a final cigarette with the Serb doctor, whose parting words to me were, "You must speak so that a situation that is hopeless may change."

I wanted to discuss the situation with Bernard Kouchner, but despite my repeated efforts to arrange a meeting, his office said he was unavailable. There were rumours that the hatred between Serbs and Albanians had plunged Kouchner and his colleagues into a depression. Weeks before my visit, his officials admitted that the unwillingness of KFOR forces to take risks that might cause harm to themselves would mean that the informal partitioning of Kosovo would not be challenged, only managed.

While we continued medical work elsewhere in Kosovo, we decided to stop our mental health program in certain Serb and Albanian enclaves and we asked community groups to move people like the old woman in the apartment, if they wanted to go. And we spoke out. At a press conference we accused the UN and KFOR of a "failure to protect minorities." I said that people in the enclaves were facing an increasingly fearful and hopeless situation. "The solution is not to give diazepam for legitimate fear. The solution is pro-active security." One reporter asked me if our response would provoke Bernard Kouchner. "MSF and Bernard Kouchner split over differences of approach to humanitarian action," I answered. "He's taken a political path, we've taken a humanitarian one." The paths were very different. Humanitarian assistance could not provide for the physical protection of people. NATO had intervened ostensibly on humanitarian grounds, but now the UN was failing to protect minorities. Worse still, KFOR was making humanitarian assistance conditional on cooperation with a political agenda. But the people of Kosovo had a right to humanitarian assistance, and the international community had a duty to allow the space for that assistance. As humanitarians we had a responsibility to make sure that our actions relieved suffering—rather than masking or anesthetizing it— so that the people we were helping could make free and autonomous decisions.

In late 2000, I returned to Khartoum with two others from our European headquarters. In the months before, villages I had visited on previous trips, like Ajiep and Mapel, had been directly and in some cases repeatedly bombed by the government air force. Sudanese Antonov aircraft were dropping high-altitude and cluster bombs, and possibly bombs containing chemical weapons. Their impact was devastating. There had been many casualties, and many of our feeding centres, clinics and hospitals had been destroyed. The Red Cross had suffered a similar fate elsewhere in the south, despite its well-marked airplanes and aid-delivery sites. We were working in other rebel-held areas near government-controlled oil fields where Western and Chinese oil corporations were based. Our facilities there had also been bombed. Operation Lifeline Sudan was about to start yet another internal review, and although it had lodged its usual protests to the government of Sudan, the bombing continued. We were there to demand that the bombings stop. I was just back from Cambodia, and with my jet lag, I hadn't slept well. I was up before sunrise, going over my notes in the small garden of the Khartoum MSF compound. I listened to the Muslim call to

Dinka people in Sudan

prayer from loudspeakers at a nearby mosque and paused to listen to the long-tailed birds starting to sing just before sunrise. That day the temperature reached 35 degrees Celsius.

We met with several officials, including the minister of foreign affairs and the minister of humanitarian affairs. I said that we could accept that mistakes happen in war, but that these bombings were not mistakes. The government had accused MSF of smuggling weapons to rebels in the south, a completely baseless and false accusation. The three days of meetings were at first tense and formal. One minister told me, "The rebels choose to move among civilians; the airstrips do not belong to MSF, they are part of our sovereign country, we are in a war, and while the rebels are there, they will be bombed in a war." However, Sudan was vying to occupy the African seat for non-permanent members of the Security Council and it had to be seen to be respectful of international humanitarian law. I reminded the minister that all countries were bound by humanitarian law. Over the following days, as the meetings progressed, the tone shifted. We had lunch with the minister of foreign affairs at a private restaurant overlooking Tuti Island, where the Blue and White Nile rivers meet. The minister drank a large glass of clear water and poured a glass for me. "From the Nile itself—the life of Sudan!" he said. He talked of the "great collaboration" that existed between the government and MSF. I took another sip of water. "Do you collaborate with the Americans?" he asked.

"We work to deliver humanitarian assistance," I said. "Sometimes that means dealing with all sorts of interesting characters and governments." By the end of our meetings, the minister of foreign affairs observed that while "the rebels only hit and run, we are the government and have a duty to respect humanitarian assistance, and we will." The government retracted its allegation of weapons smuggling, and on our last day in Khartoum, the minister arranged for an article to run in the national newspaper: "The Government of Sudan welcomes MSF in Sudan, and will cooperate together to facilitate MSF's humanitarian work in the North and South Sudan."

How long our new "cooperation" would last, I did not know. At one point during one of our meetings the minister had expressed his fascination with "you MSF fellows and ladies. Why do you do it?" he asked.

I replied immediately, "Because we can."

MEDICINES SHOULDN'T BE A LUXURY.

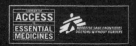

CREATING A WORLD OF POSSIBILITY: THE FIGHT FOR ESSENTIAL MEDICINES

When I gave MSF's Nobel Prize address in December 1999, I spoke of an injustice outside of the context of war. Ninety percent of all death and suffering from infectious diseases occurred in the developing world. As doctors we witnessed our patients dying from diseases like AIDS, TB and sleeping sickness and other tropical diseases because life-saving medicines were too expensive, and sometimes not available at all. The fight for access to essential medicines would be MSF's next challenge.

In 1998 I had been in the loosely controlled free-trade border zone between Cambodia and Thailand, where casinos, drug-smuggling rings and the sex trade thrive. HIV/AIDS was rampant there, especially among the "beer girls" who worked the bars and brothels. MSF offered the girls AIDS education, condoms, medical care and treatment for other sexually transmitted diseases. I went with Maurits van Pelt, the MSF head of mission, to a house behind a brothel, where I met a girl of about sixteen. She lay in her bed covered in skin sores, but I could tell she had once been beautiful. She had a fever and asked me to help her. She was dying of AIDS. She was being supported by her friends, who continued to work the bars. At the International HIV/AIDS Conference in Vancouver, only two years before, researchers had announced that a new treatment had converted AIDS into a disease as treatable as diabetes. Antiretroviral, or ARV, drugs had been developed with largely publicly funded research, and the rights to them had then been sold to the pharmaceutical industry. The lifelong ARV treatments were now patented, and the monopoly allowed the companies to charge whatever they wanted, which was usually the highest price the market would bear. In 1998 the average cost of the patented drugs was $15,000 a year. One of the girl's friends had heard about the new ARVs and said in broken English, "She no more good for bar. No medicine for her. Impossible. But we still see her." Her friend was right. There wasn't a hope in hell that we could offer this young girl anything more than comfort.

Ten years before, when I had worked in Rwanda as an HIV researcher, the WHO estimated that there were 150,000 cases of AIDS in the world and predicted that by the late 1990s there could be as many as two to three million AIDS cases, a prediction that proved to be optimistic. By 1999, HIV/AIDS had become a global catastrophe. Worldwide, 19 million people had already died of the disease, and nearly 3 million more were dying every year. Thirty-three million were infected with the virus, and millions of infections were added to the toll each year. Prevention strategies had been implemented, but the disease continued its relentless march. It moved primarily among poor people and people forced to the margins of society. It spread like wildfire through the Caribbean, South America, Russia and the former Soviet republics, China and India. But nowhere did it hit as hard as it did in Africa. There, the virus had migrated from the margins to affect the entire population. Teachers, soldiers, civil servants and doctors and other health care professionals all over sub-Saharan

Africa were now dying of AIDS. Countries like Botswana, with more than 39 percent of its people infected, were teetering on the verge of collapse. In sub-Saharan Africa, more than half of the people infected were—and still are—women. In 1999, across the continent, 11 million children were orphaned because of AIDS. That same year, new life-saving ARV drugs were being used to treat 400,000 people, 99 percent of whom lived in Europe and North America, where mortality dropped by 70 percent. Less than 1 percent of all ARV drugs were sold in Africa, where two million people died of AIDS every single year.

Individual pharmaceutical corporations and the industry's lobby group, PhRMA (a group of 100 of the biggest drug companies in the world, with seven lobbyists for every congressman in Washington, and hundreds more lobbyists in Europe as well), had lobbied Western governments to oppose measures that would make HIV drugs cheaper and more available in the poorer regions of the world. PhRMA feared that if patented drugs were sold at lower prices in the developing world, people in wealthy countries would demand the same, and profits would be driven down. In 1999, with global pharmaceutical sales at $337 billion, profits were massive. PhRMA companies were among the largest and most profitable of all Fortune 500 corporations, positions they had held for nearly thirty years. For years, the pharmaceutical industry had spent millions of dollars carefully cultivating its public image, emphasizing its commitment to research and development and to health. It had also spent millions lobbying Washington and other Western capitals to strengthen patent protection and to extend it internationally through the Agreement on Trade-Related Aspects of Intellectual Property Rights, TRIPS, an agreement that was all but written by PhRMA for implementation through the World Trade Organization (WTO).

Like the doctors and nurses MSF worked with all over the developing world, we were watching our patients die of treatable or neglected diseases. We were with our patients,

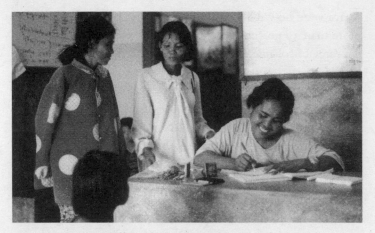

MSF national staff at a clinic in Cambodia

but the drug treatments weren't. Around the world, two billion people had no access to essential medicines. Poverty is a driving force behind poor health, and that was not a problem we could solve. But as doctors the lack of access to medicines was an injustice we could do something about. On the day it was announced that MSF had won the 1999 Nobel Peace Prize, we launched our Campaign for Access to Essential Medicines. The campaign was led by Dr. Bernard Pécoul, the former general director of our Paris office; trade lawyer Ellen 't Hoen; former pharmaceutical industry marketing executive Daniel Berman; and me. We sent a team of about twenty MSF people to work with local NGOs all over the world. Throughout 1998 and 1999 we organized a global coalition of more than a hundred NGOs and civil society organizations, among them CPTech, Health GAP, ACT UP and Oxfam in the North; global NGO networks like Health Action International; and smaller NGO networks in such places as India, Brazil, Guatemala and Cambodia, among them ACCESS, in Thailand, and the Treatment Action Campaign, in South Africa, where the Access coalition would first take on the drug companies.

As well as 45 percent of its army, more than five million of South Africa's 39 million people were infected with HIV/AIDS. And yet in the face of this crisis, pharmaceutical companies refused to lower prices for patented ARVs. In 1997, Nelson Mandela passed legislation that would permit two actions that are fully legal under international trade law. The first, known as compulsory licensing, allows a government to force a drug company to license its patent to a local generic producer, which then must pay a royalty to the patent holder. A government is allowed to issue a compulsory licence only after price negotiations with the patent holder have failed. The second provision, known as parallel importation, allows a government to shop the international market for the lowest price on a patented drug. Both provisions would lower the cost of ARVs in South Africa by at least 80 percent and enable the country to tackle an epidemic that some were calling South Africa's "holocaust plague."

PhRMA immediately labelled the South African legislation "piracy." The lobby group judged that the law would weaken the patent regime and undermine the profits on which, it argued, research depended. Thirty-nine PhRMA companies launched a court challenge in South Africa against the government and lobbied the European Union and the U.S. government to keep pressure on South Africa until the offending law was repealed. "The U.S. government . . . will defend the legitimate interests and rights of U.S. pharmaceutical firms," wrote State Department Assistant Secretary Barbara Larkin in a letter to Congress. The United States imposed trade sanctions on South Africa, and Vice-President Al Gore went to South Africa to tell Mandela in person that the United States would not tolerate the legislation. The vice-president of the EU, the French and Swiss presidents and the German chancellor all levied similar trade pressure during visits to South Africa. At the same time, PhRMA lobbied Western governments and the WTO to impose new limitations on compulsory licensing and to outlaw parallel importation, and they pushed for even tougher intellectual property provisions that would further restrict access to medicines in the developing world.

All over the world, the story was the same: PhRMA companies refused to lower their prices while millions were dying. In 1999, more than half a million people in Brazil were infected with HIV. Despite enormous political pressure from the EU and the United States, Brazil defied the PhRMA companies by producing its own generic ARVs and distributing them without charge to people with AIDS. Within months, hospitalization rates and treatment costs were cut by at least two-thirds. As the government continued its aggressive prevention campaign, AIDS mortality and the number of new HIV infections were cut in half. Thailand was eager to follow the same public health policies as Brazil but, like South Africa, felt the weight of intense political pressure from the U.S. and the EU.

For MSF and the Access coalition, the PhRMA companies' court challenge in South Africa was a line in the sand, a test case with global implications. Al Gore was running for president in the United States and was receiving campaign contributions from PhRMA companies. ACT UP activists chained themselves to his office door in Washington and disrupted his campaign speeches to protest the pressure he was putting on South Africa. The coalition supported these actions with simultaneous street demonstrations against PhRMA companies in South Africa and around the world, drawing international media attention. Ralph Nader, MSF and others published open letters to the White House demanding that it drop its threats against South Africa. Within days of these coordinated efforts, Al Gore reversed his position, insisting that he "was not afraid to stand up to the pharmaceutical industry." Soon after, President Clinton issued a statement saying that no African country would be sanctioned for using compulsory licensing or parallel importation provisions. For their part, the PhRMA companies backed a new presidential candidate.

In November 1999, we held a meeting in Amsterdam, which brought together over a hundred NGO members of the Access coalition, as well as EU and government officials, representatives from the WHO and other UN agencies, and some representatives of PhRMA. We were in search of alternatives to the WTO trade practices that impeded access to medicines in the developing world. The WTO meeting in Seattle was only weeks away, and in Amsterdam the EU and the WHO made their positions clear. The EU said that offering technical advice on trade issues to developing countries was an adequate solution to the access problem. The WHO representative, Michael Scholtz, said that in Seattle the WHO would support the view that "health" must not be a "barrier to trade." For most at the meeting, it was a shocking statement. The WHO is the only intergovernmental institution whose singular mandate is to protect and promote health internationally. I closed the meeting by publicly insisting that the organization fulfill its responsibility to ensure that "trade is not a barrier to health." A few days later, I spoke at the European Parliament in Brussels. While I made it clear that MSF was not anti-globalization, anti–free market nor anti-patent, we strongly protested the official EU trade position. We called on the EU to recognize its responsibility to guarantee that public health took priority over trade. A week later Dr. Bernard Pécoul went to the world trade talks in Seattle to lobby for "health exceptions to trade rules." The Seattle talks were reeling towards collapse because of disputes over textiles, agriculture and intellectual property. Outside, the building was surrounded by protesters, and inside, Bernard's appeal fell on deaf ears.

Beyond the fine rhetoric of speeches, the Access campaign took pragmatic action to provoke change. We pooled MSF's enormous purchasing power to drive down generic drug prices. At the same time, we researched the difference in prices between patented and generic ARVs and other HIV/AIDS-related drugs in various countries and posted these on the Internet for all to see. We found, for example, that fluconazole, a drug used to treat AIDS-related meningitis, cost 70 cents U.S. a day in Thailand, but $20 a day in Kenya. The drug was patented in Kenya, which meant only one company had the right to produce it and could charge whatever it wanted. Needless to say, more people were dying of AIDS-related meningitis in Kenya than in Thailand. But in Thailand, too many were dying of AIDS, period. MSF, together with groups like ACCESS, launched a legal challenge to Bristol-Myers Squibb's twenty-year monopoly patent on the sale of the antiretroviral didanosine in Thailand so that generic production of the drug might be permitted. All over the developing world, we educated governments about compulsory licensing and parallel importation and encouraged them to use these provisions in order to provide cheaper drugs. We also pushed a reluctant WHO to adopt a resolution supporting these measures, and at meetings of the WTO, UN and G8, lobbied them to do the same.

We met numerous times with representatives of PhRMA companies. On one occasion, at an exclusive restaurant in Brussels, Bernard Pécoul, Daniel Berman and I had dinner with Sir Richard Sykes, a short, tense, bespectacled man who was then the CEO of SmithKline Beecham. Over the course of the meal, we proposed a tiered pricing scheme, with 95 percent price reductions for essential patented drugs in the developing world. Sykes rejected the proposal outright, but offered to pay for dinner. We declined the offer and paid for our share of the meal. We met with representatives from Bristol-Myers Squibb, Eli Lilly and Merck, and with World Bank officials in Washington, but we were unable to reach a workable agreement.

The pressure was building on the international community to allow national governments to take on the AIDS crisis. In May 2000, as part of the Joint United Nations Programme on

HIV/AIDS (UNAIDS), five pharmaceutical companies announced their intent to reduce prices of their patented ARVs for some African countries to an average price of approximately $2,000 per patient a year. The United States offered the countries loans at 7 percent interest to buy the patented drugs. However, more debt would not solve the problem but only make it worse. As Bernard Pécoul said, "The fact that a serious discussion has begun among drug companies on dramatically reducing the price of AIDS drugs is a victory. But a small one, much like an elephant giving birth to a mouse." We urged the African governments to reject the proposals, which they did.

As the campaign coalition gained public profile and political ground, PhRMA began to argue that until South Africa and other developing nations had the necessary infrastructure— "clocks, running water, and refrigerators"—to support HIV/AIDS drug treatments, it made little sense for governments to "sink resources into such medicines." Even after the EU and the Americans had dropped their trade threats against South Africa, the PhRMA companies steadfastly pursued their legal challenge against the South African legislation. In response, activists continued to hold street demonstrations and the Treatment Action Campaign, or TAC, filed its own legal challenge against the PhRMA companies. MSF and others in the campaign coalition publicly pressured governments around the world to support South Africa against PhRMA. Jamie Love, who played solitaire on his laptop constantly, even as he talked, was a man obsessed with compulsory licensing. His group, CPTech, brought together legal scholars and academics from every continent and submitted a legal briefing to the South African court, adding its weight to the global campaign against PhRMA.

Early in January 2001, I went to South Africa with Eric Goemaere, MSF's head of mission in the Khayelitsha shanty outside of Cape Town. Together with TAC, we were about to illegally and publicly import generic versions of ARVs. Khayelitsha sits hidden behind the Lion's Head Mountain that overlooks Cape Town, and in 2001 it was home to at least 450,000 people, more than half under the age of thirty, living in brick or corrugated-iron shacks, with raw sewage streaming alongside dusty dirt roads. Eric estimated that in Khayelitsha at least 50,000 people were HIV-positive. The MSF clinic was crowded that day. Nearly everyone had heard rumours that MSF and TAC were about to start offering people ARVs. They had also heard that for now only 150 people would receive the drugs. Some were angry that it had taken so long to get to this point; some tried to convince Eric and me that they should be treated before others; some sat with open Bibles, praying that they would be among those selected; most just sat and waited, too sick to move. At the clinic were many who had come to be tested for the virus. Like everywhere else in the developing world, people in Khayelitsha had been reluctant to be tested. As one man had explained to me in Thailand a few months before, "What's the point? Without treatment, it is a death sentence." Now, even the rumour of treatment was drawing people in to be tested.

That night Eric and I had a beer with Zackie Achmat, a very calm, openly gay, HIV-positive man, and the leader of TAC. We wanted to demonstrate that people had a right to the ARV treatment and that wide-scale treatment was possible even in the poorest of conditions in the developing world. We were also determined to break the false dichotomy between treatment and prevention, and, as they had in Brazil, make sure the two went hand in hand. April 19, 2001, was the date set for the hearing of the PhRMA companies' court case, and until then it remained illegal to import ARVs. Zackie argued that unjust laws had to be broken and that non-violent civil disobedience was the best way to do so. We agreed that MSF would purchase ARV drugs from a Brazilian producer, TAC would import the drugs, and MSF would prescribe them free of charge for sick patients in the Khayelitsha clinic.

The following morning, Eric and I met with John Kearney, the South African CEO of GlaxoSmithKline, the world's largest pharmaceutical company and a leader among the PhRMA companies in South Africa. As we had done many times before, I asked for a 95 percent reduction in the price of ARVs and for the 39 PhRMA companies to drop their court challenge against the South African government. Kearney calmly told us that Glaxo would "aggressively protect" its right to patent protection.

Eric and I went back to Khayelitsha and met with the committee that would choose from among the thousands of medically eligible patients the 150 who would go on the life-saving treatment. In a hot back room behind the clinic, I explained to the committee that in the coming weeks the whole world would be watching them. Outsiders would try to discredit the initiative, and in this instance, deciding who would get treatment was

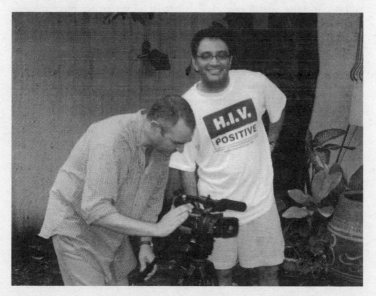

Zackie Achmat of South Africa's Treatment Access Campaign (TAC)

not a medical decision but a community one. Some committee members were people living with AIDS or HIV; none were doctors or nurses. Among them were social workers, women's rights advocates and advocates for workers' and children's rights, and all were advocates for access to treatment. The group would have to be prepared to publicly defend its decisions to the community and to the world at large.

Within days of our meeting with Glaxo, MSF's Ellen 't Hoen launched a Web-based "Drop the Case" petition. The Access coalition organized street demonstrations in New York, Copenhagen, Bangkok, Pretoria, Manila and other cities around the world. The European Parliament passed a resolution urging the PhRMA companies to drop their case, and many high-level politicians expressed their support for South Africa. At the Khayelitsha clinic, patients were selected without public protest, the illegal drugs were imported, and we started treating people with AIDS. The campaign coalition had sparked global public outrage at the rapacious pursuit of profit by pharmaceutical companies as million died of AIDS. On April 19, before the hearing was scheduled to start, the PhRMA companies unconditionally withdrew their case against the South African government. Audaciously, it declared that it was glad South Africa was prepared to respect international trade law. Quietly, it agreed to pay TAC's legal costs. Ellen 't Hoen, who had worked tirelessly to mobilize the campaign coalition, said, "We don't think the drug companies will be taking another developing country to court anytime soon."

By the end of the year, the per-patient price of ARVs had fallen from $15,000 a year for patented drugs to less than $200 for generic versions of the same drugs. A year after starting treatment, the majority of the 150 AIDS patients in Khayelitsha had gained at least 10 kilograms of weight, and 84 percent of patients were alive and well. We expanded the Khayelitsha program and started similar programs all over the world to demonstrate that it was possible to treat AIDS, even in what had earlier been considered by others to be impossible conditions.

For MSF, ARVs were the thin edge of the access wedge. In 2000, worldwide, 16 million people lived with active tuberculosis— half of whom were contagious. Annually, more than one and a half million people died of the disease, and more than 8 million new cases of TB were diagnosed each year. The treatment then was—and still is—complicated; it involves four to six drugs taken every day over six to nine months. In practice, while this standard therapy was effective, only one in six people with active tuberculosis had access to treatment. And those people who were receiving the drugs would often stop taking them once they began to feel better, as they could not afford to stay away from work—work that too often earned them less than $2 a day. Incomplete treatments accelerated drug resistance and led to the emergence of multidrug-resistant TB (MDR-TB). By 2000, MDR-TB had been identified in more than a hundred countries. Under the leadership of Jim Yong Kim and Paul Farmer from the Harvard-based Partners in Health, MSF and the Access coalition pushed the WHO to take more aggressive steps to deal with all forms of TB globally. Jim Yong Kim was instrumental in establishing a plan to increase equitable access to treatment and curb the spread of TB and MDR-TB. MDR-TB drugs cost about $8,000 per patient. We needed to bring down the price of cycloserine, the most expensive of them. In Geneva, I met with representatives of Eli Lilly and started a negotiation that eventually led to a 95 percent price reduction. MSF guaranteed the purchase and stocking of the drug for other NGOs and the WHO. We needed to be sure that the drugs were used properly. Again, with Jim Yong Kim, we pushed the WHO to create an oversight committee that would approve programs to administer the treatments.

Better and shorter TB treatments were still needed. There had been no new drugs for TB since 1967. Ninety-five percent of tuberculosis occurred in the developing world, and even when new drugs were identified, the pharmaceutical industry invested little if any research in them as the market was not deemed lucrative enough. But with a recent outbreak of TB in New York City, and elsewhere in the West, there was now a potentially profitable market. Ariel Pablo-Mendez at the Rockefeller Foundation thought that by bringing public funding and researchers to work with the pharmaceutical industry, new TB drugs could be developed and made available to patients in an equitable way. Ariel was obsessed with his idea, though it wasn't clear if it could work. MSF questioned, debated, but finally participated in an experimental public-private partnership. In November 2000 the Global Alliance for TB Drug Development was launched, and I joined as a founding board member for MSF. Giorgio Roscigno, an impeccably dressed, former PhRMA-company executive who, as he put it, "had defected to civil society," was its first acting CEO.

In October 2000, the WHO had come up with its Massive Effort campaign against AIDS, TB and malaria. It aimed to promote the distribution of bed nets for malaria, condoms for HIV prevention and drug donations for AIDS treatment, and to expand what were inadequate TB treatment programs. It said nothing about the need for new treatments. It said nothing about the responsibility of governments to address market failures to guarantee access to health care. For MSF, Massive Effort was not enough. A senior member of the WHO cabinet had heard that MSF was critical of the new campaign and called me on my cell as I was about to go on stage to speak at the conference that would launch the WHO campaign. He shouted into the phone, "You had better not be critical! If you are, WHO will cut off all relations with MSF!" I quickly called a few key people in MSF to ensure their support. I went to the lectern and said that the WHO campaign oversimplified complexities, accepted the status quo and failed to identify the need for new medicines and better public health strategies. Nobody cut off relations with MSF.

Late in 2000, my partner, Rolie, and I met in the Brussels airport. I had arrived from Thailand only three hours before and I had to go on to an urgent meeting in Sudan. Rolie had brought me a suitcase of fresh clothes, and we had dinner in a fluorescent-lit airport restaurant. I had been MSF's international president for almost three years. The pace was gruelling—I travelled constantly, sometimes to three continents in a week. It seemed I was always entering or exiting a crisis. There were some on the MSF International Council who wanted to rewrite the statutes to allow me another term as president. I had reached a threshold. I felt in some ways that I had become the struggle itself. I was afraid that if I kept going I would no longer know what I was struggling for. When I returned from Sudan, I taped a note on our fridge in Brussels: "I will not renew! I choose love!" Dr. Morten Rostrup took over as president, and Rolie and I returned to Toronto late in January 2001. A few months later we were married.

But I couldn't leave MSF completely. The Access campaign had won many battles over ARVs and better TB treatments, but

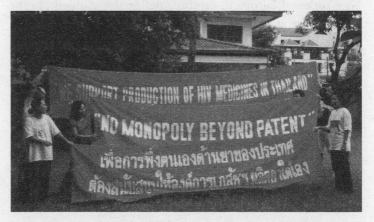

Preparing for protest marches for access to medicines in Thailand

still too many of our patients were dying of diseases for which there were no new treatments. Profit margins, and not global health needs, determine how pharmaceutical companies allocate their research and development budgets. And their R&D budgets are small, relative to profits and marketing. In 2001, PhRMA companies spent 14 cents per dollar of revenue on R&D, but spent 31 cents per dollar on marketing and advertising. When MSF had won the Nobel Prize, I had provocatively suggested a tax on global pharmaceutical sales to fund R&D for priority health needs. In Oslo we had announced that the Nobel Prize money would go towards researching new treatments for neglected diseases. Now, I wanted to focus pragmatically on this possibility.

Based in Toronto, I worked full time with Bernard Pécoul and the MSF Access team in Europe. With Els Torreele, a former Belgian biochemistry professor who fell in love with MSF, I became the co-chair of the Neglected Diseases Working Group. Together we led the group in examining how to stimulate drug R&D for neglected diseases. Some forty scientists, drug policy analysts and drug development specialists from the pharmaceutical industry and the WHO were part of the group. Over the next two years, we held meetings in India, Malaysia, Brazil, New York and Europe to carefully define the problem. In the first instance, it was clear that a fatal imbalance existed between the health needs of poor people in developing countries and the lack of R&D to develop medicines to treat them. In Zaire I had seen patients with African sleeping sickness, a disease that infects 300,000 people a year. Untreated, it leaves patients psychotic, and every year more than 60,000 die of from it. Many die because they do not get any treatment. Others die because the existing treatment, a drug called melarsoprol, is, when taken over time, less and less effective and sometimes toxic. Melarsoprol is an arsenic-based drug. It burns the veins as it is injected, causing excruciating pain during each of its ten required intravenous doses. I had heard patients scream and seen them restrained as the drug was injected. Melarsoprol causes swelling of the brain and sometimes seizures. Eight out of twenty who get the drug die: one dies of the treatment itself, while the other seven die of a strain of sleeping sickness that is resistant to the drug.

With Harvard University, we surveyed the twenty top-grossing pharmaceutical companies in the world and found that among the eleven companies that responded, eight spent nothing on R&D for diseases like African sleeping sickness. We also found that only 0.2 percent of the $60 billion spent globally every year on drug R&D went towards tuberculosis, malaria and acute respiratory infections, diseases that account for 18 percent of global mortality from all diseases. We found too that of 1,393 newly patented medicines marketed between 1975 and 1999, only 13 were for tropical diseases. Of these, 6 resulted from veterinary research and 4 from military research. Our investigation also revealed that patent protection often drove research that was far less innovative than PhRMA claimed. Most innovations were relatively inexpensive, minor molecular modifications that did not improve a drug's effectiveness but met the legal criteria for a new patent and thus generated increased profits. These so-called me-too drugs had become the primary focus of research and development, so much so that they represented 68 percent of all of the PhRMA companies' supposedly innovative drugs. In the United States, between 1981 and 2000, less than 5 percent of the drugs introduced by the top twenty-five pharmaceutical companies represented therapeutic advances, and of these, some 70 percent were developed with government funding. Indeed, many government policy initiatives compounded the inequities of the market. Government-supported research generated chemical compounds that represented drug leads. These were then bought up by PhRMA companies. Governments offered tax breaks and other monetary incentives for further research, but without the promise of blockbuster profits, leads for new drugs often sat undeveloped in company compound libraries. It was clear that market forces, aided by inadequate public policies, were completely failing the health needs of poor people in the developing world.

In 1998 I had been at an MSF clinic in the slum settlement of Kibera outside Nairobi. We were providing basic health care, offering treatment for illnesses like malaria and diarrhea and running an HIV/AIDS prevention program. I sat in the clinic office examining a listless five-year-old girl with malaria who, after three days of standard chloroquine treatment, was still vomiting and running a fever. Her malaria was clearly resistant to the medicine. Drug resistance is a natural phenomenon, and all infectious diseases will eventually develop resistance. New drugs must constantly be found. I was talking with the girl's mother when raw sewage started seeping in under the door. The hand-dug gutters alongside the dirt road had become blocked with garbage and were backing up, as they did about three times a week. As clinic staff mopped up the sewage, some of the thousands of people who live in the slum started cleaning out the gutters.

Every year, worldwide, almost two million people die of malaria. Ninety percent of these deaths occur in Africa, and because children have more delicate immune systems, 800,000 of those who die are children. With an eye to the potentially lucrative market of Western travellers, pharmaceutical companies were interested in developing drugs for malaria. The Special Programme for Research and Training in Tropical Diseases, the main international public body charged with research into tropical diseases, had, in 1999, set up a public-private partnership, the Medicines for Malaria Venture, or MMV, to develop completely new drugs. The process could take up to ten years, though, and some people thought it could take longer. More immediately, resistance to existing treatments was spreading. While we waited for the MMV to show results, experts in our Neglected Diseases Working Group thought that by combining two existing anti-malaria drugs into one tablet, we might be able to develop an effective treatment in the short term. The problem was real and immediate, but there seemed to be no way to get anyone to do anything about it.

With no viable alternatives on the landscape, we decided to do it ourselves. We set out to create our own not-for-profit drug development company to address the very practical problem of drugs for the most neglected diseases. We called it the Drugs for Neglected Diseases initiative, or the DNDi. Bernard, Els and I put together a group of experts led by Yves Champey, a recently retired and unassuming but determined pharmaceutical executive, to draft a business plan. Over the course of two years, we established a network of fifteen African research centres linked with MSF, the Pasteur Institute, and the medical research councils of India, Malaysia, Brazil and South Africa. We now had the capacity to do the research, but we needed money and access to compound libraries to make rapid progress. At the Kananaskis G8 Summit in 2002, I asked for money for the DNDi. Bernard, Ellen and Daniel did the same at other G8 meetings and at meetings with other potential donor governments. We all came up empty.

Bernard and Yves had persuaded the Japanese Pharmaceutical Association to give us access to some of its molecular compounds, but we needed more. I met with Jean-Paul Garnier, the CEO of GlaxoSmithKline, at the company's global headquarters in Philadelphia. Garnier was relaxed and tanned and agreed to work with us on a case-by-case basis. It was a short meeting, as he had to leave early for Washington. The next morning the New York Times reported that the largest political fundraising dinner in history had raised $30 million for George W. Bush's re-election campaign. The dinner had been hosted by Garnier.

The DNDi still needed $25 million and we were having trouble finding it. So much so that Bernard and I worked hard to persuade MSF to give the DNDi its start-up capital. It did, but only after an intense internal debate (read: battle) during which we argued that if MSF itself wouldn't put up the money, no one else would.

Since its start in 1999, MSF's Campaign for Access to Essential Medicines had achieved a lot, and in 2002 Richard Horton, the editor of the *Lancet*, one of the world's leading medical journals, wrote that "MSF and organizations like it are leading the global health policy process that the WHO is essentially following." The campaign coalition had become a global civil society movement. It had challenged the mystique of Big Pharma, pushed governments to meet their responsibilities and demonstrated that practical alternatives were possible. Within three years of initiating ARV treatment for 150 people at the Khayelitsha clinic in South Africa, MSF had over 40,000 people in thirty developing countries on treatment. In 2001, in response to pressure from the campaign coalition, the UN launched its Global Fund to fight AIDS, Tuberculosis and Malaria. In 2002 we pushed the WHO to launch a commission on public health, innovation and patents. It did, and it found that the current patent regime undermined R&D for priority health needs. The coalition had aggressively cajoled the WHO and UNAIDS to assume their responsibility to get people with HIV/AIDS on treatment. In 2003 the new director-general of the WHO, Lee Jong-wook, declared the lack of access to HIV/AIDS medicines "a global health emergency." With his announcement, both the WHO and UNAIDS started their ambitious plan to get three million people in the developing world on ARVs within two years.

The campaign coalition also spawned other global health initiatives, such as the effort to create an R&D treaty for priority health needs. It pushed for numerous concrete government initiatives, such as the French government's tax on international travel; the revenue now funds the development of drug formulations to be used for treating children in the developing world. In July 2003, the DNDi was launched as a not-for-profit drug company, with four development projects—for African sleeping sickness, chloroquine-resistant malaria, Chagas disease and leishmaniasis. The founding members signed the statutes in the same room of the Geneva city hall where the original charter for the Red Cross was signed in 1864.

But the Access campaign also achieved less than perfect outcomes and experienced clear failures. In the face of the South African court case, it was obvious that compulsory licensing and parallel importation safeguards would apply only when the powerful agreed they would. MSF's Ellen 't Hoen and CPTech's Jamie Love, among others, understood that it was crucial to get from the WTO a political interpretation of the laws as they applied to essential medicines. The campaign coalition stepped up the pressure in the court of public opinion and continued to lobby governments. PhRMA also fought long and hard in the backrooms of the WTO and Western capitals. It wanted to maintain its highly lucrative patent monopolies and limit use of the safeguards to epidemics like HIV/AIDS. At a meeting in May 2001 in Geneva, I talked with Mike Moore, then the director-general of the WTO. He told me that he was committed to finding the "right balance" among the issues and a "win-win" solution for use of the safeguards. I wasn't really sure what this meant. There is no right balance between life and death when life is possible. There is no right balance between justice and injustice when justice is possible. With active support from MSF and others in the campaign coalition, Brazil and a group of African countries took the official lead at the WTO, advancing the position that sovereign governments have a duty and a right to determine their public interest and to act to safeguard public health.

The battle lines were by now predictable, with the governments of developing countries and the campaign coalition on one side, and the pharmaceutical lobby, the United States, Canada and the EU governments on the other. (Switzerland, PhRMA's European home, took a particularly hard line.) With other trade disputes still unresolved, it was not clear which way things would go. Resolution came in the form of the old aphorism "What's good for the goose is good for the gander." Days after the October 2001 anthrax terrorist attacks in Washington and New York, during which five people died and seventeen others were infected, both Canada and the United States wanted to guarantee stockpiles of ciprofloxacin, the drug of choice to treat anthrax. Each negotiated with Bayer Pharmaceutical but could not reach price agreements, and both governments publicly threatened to issue compulsory licences for generic production. Around the world, the campaign coalition hammered home the hypocrisy of Western governments' invoking the threat of compulsory licensing in the face of anthrax while denying the same right to the developing world in the face of HIV and AIDS. Days later, on November 14, 2001, the WTO released its Doha Declaration: "We agree that the TRIPS Agreement [which governs use of compulsory licensing and parallel importation] does not and should not prevent [WTO] members from taking measures to protect public health. Accordingly, while reiterating our commitment to the TRIPS Agreement, we affirm that the Agreement can and should be interpreted and implemented in a manner supportive of WTO members' right to protect public health and, in particular, to promote access to medicines for all." The Doha Declaration was a great victory for the campaign coalition. As Ellen 't Hoen said, "Now it is up to governments to use these new powers to bring down the cost of medicines and increase access to life-saving treatments." PhRMA had been outmanoeuvred.

But PhRMA did win on one crucial point. As one *Wall Street Journal* reporter put it, PhRMA had managed to "fob off" to a WTO committee the question of how countries with no generic pharmaceutical manufacturers could legally get generic versions of patented medications. After nearly two years of concerted lobbying by both PhRMA and the campaign coalition, an agreement on the question was reached in late 2003. Presented as a gift to the poor, it created a maze of red tape and hurdles that, once passed, could in theory allow for export of generic versions of patented medicines to a requesting country. Canada was the first country to make changes in its patent legislation to meet the terms of the new agreement. Canada's legislation, first called the Pledge for Africa, was passed in May 2004. Like the legislation that soon followed in Norway and Switzerland, it has been an abject failure. In the capitals of these Western nations, PhRMA had worked out the terms of the rhetorically pleasing legislations, terms so restrictive, costly and bureaucratically onerous that by the end of 2007 not a single pill had legally crossed a border from Canada, Norway or Switzerland to the developing world. The campaign coalition had been outmanoeuvred by PhRMA.

Through the Access campaign, a coalition of diverse groups had acted in solidarity against injustice and collectively challenged existing arrangements of power among elites, opponents and authorities. We sought out partners among NGOs, among government and among industry. We found insiders that supported our goals, and we looked for potential defectors that we could convert. We were neither dogmatic nor ideological, but practical and principled. The highly flexible, decentralized network allowed for joiners and leavers, and could be highly opportunistic. This approach allowed the coalition to attack unjust policies and practices while negotiating specific agreements with the pharmaceutical industry and pushing governments to meet their responsibilities. We acted from a particular conception of our relationship to each other as human beings—one rooted in the dignity of the other in relation to the self. Dignity cannot be granted, but it can be recognized. As the dying beer girl's friend said in Cambodia, "No medicine for her . . . but we still see her."

In 2004, Rolie and I had our son, Rohin. After choosing to start a family, I knew that the constant travel and potential risks of my involvement with MSF would no longer be possible. With Rolie and our first child, I found a different way to live my questions. I formally left MSF and became a research scientist at St. Michael's Hospital in Toronto, and a professor at the University of Toronto. With access to medicines increasing, I wanted to focus on finding a way to harness the natural compassion of communities—compassion I had witnessed again and again in war and in situations of social crisis—to improve the treatment and prevention of HIV/AIDS. In 2004, James Fraser of MSF and I went to Malawi, a country already devastated by AIDS, the epidemic having killed 650,000 Malawians since 1985. Now, almost 1 million of 12 million people in the country carried the virus. The wards of the Zomba Central Hospital in south Malawi were full of people; most were thin, drawn, emaciated. Outside, parents lay in the grass sweating with fever, while their children begged for food to give their parents. Alice, the only nurse in the facility, told me that more than 90 percent of those at the hospital had an AIDS-related illness. It wasn't a hospital but a morgue, with the living waiting to die among the dead.

In a small hamlet of houses some forty kilometres away from the main hospital in Zomba, I talked with a woman who had AIDS and tuberculosis and who, unsurprisingly, wanted to live. As we sat on a small carpet outside her house, she was breathless, and embarrassed about an AIDS-induced tumour that had started to appear on her face. Her name was Charity and she had two children, a little girl aged six and a boy aged twelve. Her son's name, Mpwale, means "gift." And he was a gift to her. Without the dollar a day he earned for twelve hours of work tending the cornfields of neighbours, Charity's family would surely have starved. As we talked, three other women gathered, and within minutes a clutch of twenty-one smiling, giggling children also collected around us.

I asked about the absence of men in the village. "They are all dead," Charity said. "They have all died of AIDS. Many women have died too," she told me. In Malawi, like most of sub-Saharan Africa, 60 percent of people living with HIV are women. I asked the children to raise their hands if both their parents were dead. Seven of the twenty-one children raised their hands. One-third of the children in that small village were without parents, orphaned because of AIDS.

If Charity did not get treatment, then seven orphans would become nine orphans—that is, 42 percent of the children in the village—and how they would survive was anyone's guess. There were half a million other orphans in Malawi just like them, and 94,000 children actually infected with HIV. Most survived on the tenuous kindness of people like Charity and the three other women in her village—tenuous because two of these four women are HIV-positive and all four have their own children to feed, and there is never enough for them. In 2006, five million people needed food assistance in Malawi. In 2007 drought struck Malawi for the fifth year in a row. This is, according to the UN Food and Agriculture Organization, a result of an emerging pattern of severe droughts due to climate change that is affecting much of South America and Asia. Quite apart from drought, AIDS has wiped out 15 percent of Malawi's workforce that once planted and harvested crops. So many have died of AIDS in Malawi that 10 percent of all families are headed by a child and half of all families are headed by a person over sixty-five, most often a grandmother who has watched her own children die. In Malawi, because of AIDS, the average life expectancy is thirty-six years—which, as it happens, was Charity's age.

James and I met with the Malawian principal secretary for health, Wesley Sangala. In 2003, four thousand people had been started on ARVs. "We now have the possibility of cheaper drugs, but not the personnel to deliver them," Dr. Sangala said. AIDS had killed an inordinate number of health care professionals, and of those that remained, most had to care for family members dying of AIDS at home. And some were leaving for "greener pastures." Malawi struggles to care for its 12 million people with fewer than a hundred doctors working in the public sector, and only 3,800 nurses in the entire country. In 2004, more than 60 percent of nursing posts were vacant, and one-third of all health care positions remained unoccupied. The number of doctors was further dwindled by the "brain drain." Upwards of 28 percent of all doctors working in the United States, England, Canada and Australia are foreign-trained medical graduates, 75 percent of them trained in developing nations like Malawi. It is a standing joke, and a matter of fact, that there are more Malawian doctors in Manchester, England, than in all of Malawi.

Dr. Sangala also lamented the poor condition of the country's health care system. His government's entire social services budget was a meagre $15 per person a year. The figure represented total spending on health, education and other social services, and included all foreign aid. Health systems are vital in the fight against disease and poverty, but in Malawi, as elsewhere in the developing world, health systems are unable to hire new workers and have had their policy choices constrained by World Bank and International Monetary Fund loan conditions. Still, Dr. Sangala said he was committed to breaking the back of the HIV/AIDS epidemic in his country. "It seems impossible. But we have to," he said. "We have no other choice."

Dignitas International, a hybrid academic NGO, was born from what James Fraser and I had witnessed in Malawi and the experiences and conversations we had had there. From its conception, Dignitas committed to working with the Ministry of Health in the Zomba district to develop an infrastructure

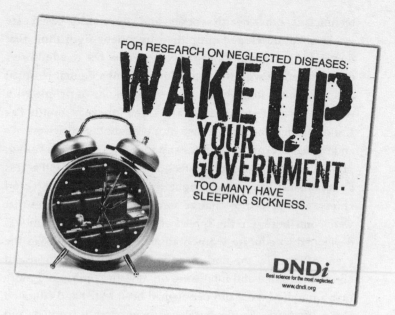

FOR RESEARCH ON NEGLECTED DISEASES:
WAKE UP YOUR GOVERNMENT.
TOO MANY HAVE SLEEPING SICKNESS.

DND*i*
Best science for the most neglected.
www.dndi.org

for community care of HIV/AIDS. We soon had the support of St. Michael's Hospital and the University of Toronto. James Fraser began building the practical elements of Dignitas, and within months we had assembled a team to design and test a model of community-based care. At the Zomba Central Hospital, we began caring for people with HIV/AIDS and training others to do the same. We joined people like Pax Chingwale, an accountant and a respected leader, who was living with HIV. He had already brought together a group of parents in Zomba to teach children—including his own—about HIV and AIDS. Pax was indomitable. "We cannot just lie down and watch our children die," he said. "We must stand up and show them how to live."

Over the next three years, working with the Ministry of Health in Malawi, Dignitas trained hundreds of nurses, lab technicians, other health workers and community-based care workers. We developed simplified treatment algorithms that nurses and community health workers now use to administer drugs to people with HIV/AIDS. In the Zomba Central Hospital and in remote village heath clinics, thousands of people with HIV or AIDS are tested, treated and cared for every month. Pax and other men and women like him brought together women's and orphans' groups. Dignitas supported them with training, prevention education, school fees, home-based care and access to treatment. Pax also brought together village elders and chiefs, who agreed to change some traditional practices that were contributing to the spread of HIV. A special program was developed to educate women about their legal rights in the event of rape. By the end of 2007, more than five thousand children, women and men were on ARVs in Zomba, and more than a hundred thousand people had been tested and educated about HIV/AIDS. The hospital had been freshly painted, and each week hundreds of healthy people went there or to village clinics to get their ARVs. (In the summer of 2007, on his way

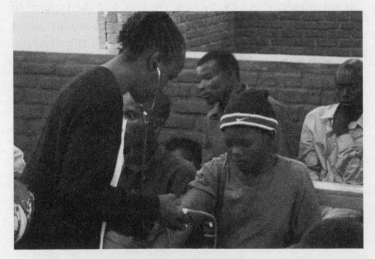

Nurse at Dignitas Clinic in Zomba, Malawi

home from a Dignitas meeting, Pax Chingwale died in a car accident. His funeral was one of the biggest Zomba had ever seen. Hundreds sang and danced as he was buried. Someone said, "Pax lived with courage. He has shown us it is the only way to live.")

By June 2007, across Malawi, the Ministry of Health, with support from organizations like Dignitas, had 100,000 people on ARVs. People from other parts of Africa continue to go to Zomba to learn about our approach to community-based care. We are working with other organizations in South Africa and with universities in Malawi and North America to further test and refine the model. As a community we have achieved living results and together we will achieve more.

The fight for access to essential medicines opened a world of possibility. By the end of 2007, around the world the WHO-UNAIDS program had nearly three million people on ARVs. Across Africa, for the first time in the epidemic's history, the number of deaths and new cases began to fall. In 2007, the Drugs for Neglected Diseases Initiative released its first drug, a combination medicine for chloroquine-resistant malaria. It has seventeen other drugs under development for the most neglected diseases. The campaign for access to essential medicines continues. How we approach global health has changed forever. While hurdles remain, the impossible is possible.

"There are means that cannot be excused.
And I should like to be able to love
my COUNTRY and still love justice.
I don't want just any greatness for it,
particularly a greatness born of blood
and FALSEHOOD. I want to keep it alive
by keeping JUSTICE alive."

— Albert Camus

UMMERA: ALWAYS WE BEGIN AGAIN

On September 11, 2001, at 8:20 a.m., I arrived at Newark Airport. On the plane from Toronto, I had been going over a presentation I was to make that morning in the UNICEF building across the street from the UN headquarters in Manhattan. The first slide of the presentation I never made read, "Today 24,000 people will die around the world of preventable or treatable neglected diseases."

In the cab from the airport, I looked up from my notes and saw smoke coming from one of the twin towers of the World Trade Center. The driver turned on the radio, and as I looked out at the slowing traffic, I heard him whisper "Oh my god." A commercial jet airliner had flown into the second tower. We didn't need the radio to tell us it was terrorism. From the cab, I watched the towers burn, and an hour later, from across the Hudson River, I watched them fall. I spent the next few hours doing what many New Yorkers did, and what thousands of MSF volunteers had done for more than thirty years all over the world: I tried to help the victims. I volunteered as a doctor at a triage site set up in Hoboken, New Jersey. In the hours that I was there, we waited for patients far more than we treated any. Those that were brought to us were mostly the walking wounded who could be ferried across the river to the triage site. One East Asian man with a broken wrist and dust and glass fragments in his eyes screamed from his stretcher, "I am American! Please, please . . . I can't see! Help me!" Beyond the smoke inhalation and respiratory distress, the broken hands and feet, the abrasions and cuts that we were treating, was the terror of what had happened. By eight in the evening, the flow of victims had stopped. The next morning I walked to the subway. American flags flapped from cars and windowsills; some had "It's War!" scrawled across them.

In New York City, at the Pentagon and in Pennsylvania, nearly three thousand people had died as a result of the al Qaeda terrorist attacks that comprised the first momentous event of the twenty-first century. For a brief time the world stood in solidarity with the United States. The French newspaper *Le Monde* declared in a front-page headline, "We Are All Americans," and in cities around the world, millions stood together in a moment of silence. The very real threat al Qaeda represented could not be denied.

But it was not long before the world rejected the American response to the attacks. Days after 9/11, President George W. Bush promised to lead a "crusade" against "evil." Even though he later retracted the word "crusade," he would use it again in the months to come. Some words evoke a visceral and historic meaning that cannot be forgotten—a meaning that certainly hasn't been forgotten in the Muslim world. The attacks of 9/11 were an effort by fundamentalist Muslim extremists to strike at the heart of Western economic and military power. They sparked a war in Afghanistan. They gave rise to the Bush administration's pre-emptive war policy that includes the preventative use of nuclear weapons and resulted in the illegal invasion of Iraq, an invasion that was first justified with claims about the presence of weapons of mass destruction and the material support Saddam Hussein had offered al Qaeda. When those claims were revealed as lies, the war was defended in the name of humanitarianism, human rights and democratic liberation. In just a few short years, the world has been remade into a place where the phrase "American exceptionalism" has become a euphemism for "you are either with us or against us" and has been used to explain the American withdrawal from the 1972 Nuclear Non-Proliferation Treaty, the failure of the U.S. Congress to even consider the legitimacy of the International Criminal Court, the pursuit of the weaponization of space, the imposition of a right-wing Christian ideology onto American foreign and international health policies, the rewriting of the rules of war to create non-status POWs, and the co-optation of traditional notions of humanitarianism as weapons of war itself.

On September 10, 2001, one million people in Afghanistan needed food aid from the UN World Food Programme, which, for years, had fallen short of its required donor funding. On September 12, the United States forced the closure of Afghanistan's borders, preventing people from fleeing and cutting off food supplies because the supplies "might help the Taliban." On October 7, an American-led coalition began bombing Afghanistan with the goal of unseating the Taliban and "hunting down" al Qaeda founder Osama bin Laden. By then, seven and a half million Afghan people needed food aid. George Bush said, "As we strike military targets, we will also drop food, medicine and supplies to the starving and suffering of Afghanistan." With borders still closed to food aid, Bush asked every American child to send "not a dime but a dollar" to the White House to provide relief for hungry Afghan children. Each day American bombs, medicine and 37,000 yellow daypack food rations fell from the sky to kill, to cure and to feed. The yellow food packets—meeting 0.005 percent of the population's food needs—were nearly indistinguishable in appearance from the yellow cluster bomblets dropped by bombers. Many children lost limbs or died picking up what they thought were food packs. Millions of Afghanis continued to starve. U.S. secretary of defense Donald Rumsfeld said, "It is quite true that 37,000 rations in a day do not feed millions of human beings. On the other hand, if you were one of the starving people who got one of the rations, you'd be appreciative." The Taliban saw the food and medicine as weapons of war and threatened to poison the airdropped food. UNICEF and UNHCR offices were attacked and burned by anti-Western demonstrators in Pakistan and Afghanistan. As demonstrations and threats against aid workers mounted, aid agencies in Kashmir, Bangladesh, Indonesia, Kenya and Somalia were forced to reduce or stop humanitarian work, depriving many people of much-needed assistance. While MSF protested the dropping of "bombs and bread," Secretary of State Colin Powell declared NGOs "a force multiplier" for the coalition and "an important part of our combat team."

Outside Jalalabad, where I had been in 1994, aid workers treated hundreds of civilians injured by the bombing. Across Afghanistan, the failure to discriminate between combatant and non-combatant targets meant that schools, hospitals, weddings and Red Cross warehouses were bombed. In the first nine weeks of the bombing, about three thousand civilians were killed collaterally as many cities and towns emptied. In the months that followed the fall of the Taliban in December 2001, coalition military personnel delivered food, medicine and blankets, and they started building schools and hospitals. In a battle for the hearts and minds of Afghanis, coalition forces tied their aid to intelligence gathering. One U.S. Army lieutenant said, "The more they help us find the bad guys, the more good stuff they get."

In early 2003, as the U.S. military finalized plans for invading Iraq, the U.S. Agency for International Development (USAID) recruited NGOs to work in the soon-to-be war zone.

The U.S. Department of Defense's Office of Reconstruction and Humanitarian Assistance was formed in January 2003 and insisted that all NGOs in Iraq receiving American funding fly the American flag. The invasion of Iraq proceeded with a "shock and awe" campaign, which, according to the author of the doctrine, Harlan Ullman, was inspired by the impact of the nuclear bombings of Hiroshima and Nagasaki. One week into the campaign, Ullman was not sure the strategy was going to work. "The question is will Baghdad give up without a fight, or will we have to go in and take it, or impose a siege and starve it?" The Red Cross and the UN secretary-general reminded the Americans that, under international humanitarian law, siege warfare against a city was illegal.

In Afghanistan, as Osama bin Laden evaded capture, the rhetoric of the war on terror shifted, and the mission became one to liberate Afghan women from their burqas and the Taliban regime. In Iraq, as the lies around weapons of mass destruction were explained away as "intelligence failures," the war became a civilizing mission to spread liberty, freedom and democracy. USAID then insisted that American NGOs working in Iraq and Afghanistan were "an arm of the U.S. government" and that they could speak to the media only with Washington's permission. In June 2004, even as MSF remained vigorously independent and outspoken, a team of five MSF aid workers was ambushed and brutally murdered in Badghis province, Afghanistan. The Taliban claimed responsibility for the assassinations: "We killed them because they work for the Americans against us using the cover of aid work. We will kill more foreign aid workers." With one warring party threatening MSF directly, and with the American-backed government of Hamid Karzai failing to investigate and prosecute those who carried out the assassinations, MSF decided to pull out of Afghanistan after more than twenty-four years of working there. It was criticized by some who argued that the rules of war had changed and that MSF should cooperate more, not less, with coalition forces. The criticisms were answered by Dr. Rowan Gilles, then international president of MSF, who said, "In the 'war on terror' all factions want us to choose sides. We refuse to choose sides, just as we refuse to accept a vision of a future where civilians trapped in the hell of war can only receive life-saving aid from the armies that wage it." By January 2008, tens of thousands of Afghan civilians had been killed and millions were still refugees. The inevitable casualties resulting from a reliance on air strikes has led to an alienation of the Afghan population from the occupying NATO force, and the harsh security environment has severely curtailed the ability of UN agencies and NGOs to deliver humanitarian assistance.

In Iraq, the militarization of aid by coalition forces, al Qaeda bombings of the UN and Red Cross headquarters, as well as numerous kidnappings of aid workers and the murder of British aid worker Margaret Hassan, forced MSF to pull out in early November 2004. Most other NGOs were forced to do the same. Days later, the coalition's all-out assault on the city of Fallujah began with an attack on a hospital. The hospital was seen as a centre of propaganda and a source of rumours about high civilian casualties. By 2006, an epidemiologic survey published in the *Lancet* estimated that at least 668,000 civilians had died in Iraq as a direct consequence of the invasion. A more recent survey, released in January 2008, suggested that upwards of one million civilians have died in Iraq. By early 2008, two million Iraqi people were displaced from their homes, and another two million are refugees in neighbouring states. Islamic NGOs operate publicly and with relative freedom, while, most often, the Red Cross and the handful of Western humanitarian NGOs that remain in Iraq operate in secrecy.

Since the end of the Cold War, humanitarianism and human rights have become a justification for military intervention by the world's strongest economic and military powers when their national interests are at stake. In the wake of 9/11, humanitarianism has become part of the spectacle of "shock and awe," a mere means to an end and a tool of war, a type of war fought by states that use torture in its conduct while they profess to champion human rights and humanitarian values. In 2004 a permissive, if not active, policy of sexual and religious humiliation and abuse and torture at the Abu Ghraib prison in Iraq revealed an occupying force bereft of moral restraint. In Afghanistan, Canadian and some other coalition troops handed over captured Taliban fighters to American forces or to the government in Kabul. Since 2002, when U.S. attorney-general Alberto Gonzales labelled the Geneva Conventions "quaint" and outdated, prisoners of war have been considered enemy combatants and therefore do not enjoy the protection of international humanitarian law. Many have been sent to and tortured in Guantánamo Bay or tortured in Afghan prisons.

The war on terror has been used to justify widespread, warrantless wiretapping in the United States and a deep erosion of civil liberties all over the world. It has resulted in the deportation of an unknown number of "persons of interest" to secret "black sites" in Europe and to states that are known to use torture. Five Canadian citizens have been classed "persons of interest." They are all of Middle Eastern origin with dual citizenship and have been deported to states that use torture. One of these men, Maher Arar, was "extraordinarily rendered" to Syria against his will by the United States after being detained during a flight stopover in New York. For ten months, he was held in a rat-infested cell three feet wide, six feet long and seven feet high, and was tortured. According to the findings of a lacerating public enquiry, the Royal Canadian Mounted Police and the Canadian Security Intelligence Service gave speculative, "inaccurate and unfair" information to the United States that led to Arar's deportation. The enquiry (during which some evidence was given in secret) found that "Canadian investigators made extensive efforts to find any information that could implicate Mr. Arar in terrorist activities" and "found none." What they did find was that Maher Arar was a passing acquaintance of another Canadian Muslim, Abdullah Almalki, suspected of terrorist links. Almalki, a truck driver, drove a company truck (one that many other drivers use) across the U.S. border on a delivery. While inspecting the truck, American customs officials found a map of a government research complex outside Ottawa. The map was one given out by the parking-lot attendant at the research park to guide deliveries to the complex. A photocopy of the map was shown to Maher Arar in Syria during his torture. Arar was seized by American authorities and sent away to be tortured because he is a Muslim who knew a Muslim who drove a truck that had a map in it given to another driver by a parking-lot attendant.

The Arar affair was a test case of civil liberties not just in Canada but also around the world. In Canada and internationally, the safeguards of democracy have been tossed out the window. The Canadian government has publicly cleared Maher Arar of any links to terrorism, apologized and paid compensation. The United States government, however, invoking its state secrets privilege, refuses to clear Arar's name and continues to have both him and his family on a secret terrorist watch list. In 2007, David Wilkins, the U.S. ambassador to Canada, said that the Canadian minister of public safety was "presumptuous" to question the United States on its treatment of Arar. When asked whether his government had any regrets about the Arar case, Ambassador Wilkins seemed puzzled by the question: "You talking about regrets by the United States? The U.S. made that decision [to deport] Arar based on the facts it had, in the best interests of the people of the U.S., and we stand behind it." Wilkins said that the United States, in fighting the war on terror, has to make "tough decisions," and that it would not "get second chances." There would probably be more deportations, and he suggested that Canadians with dual citizenship should consider themselves forewarned.

The law does not make us good and just, but it can protect us from what is not. The word *torture* derives from the Latin *tortura*, meaning twisting torment. The law itself can be twisted so that it is not clear what it means. In the words of U.S. House Majority Leader Steny Hoyer, "We have seen the line blurred—possibly deliberately—between legitimate, sanctioned interrogation tactics and torture." As well as national and international law, there is now the Third Law of the Bush administration. Under this law, what is illegal has been made *exceptionally* legal. The limits of interrogation have been redefined so that what is now permissible is not *really* torture, just techniques of "enhanced interrogation." These include waterboarding, cold cells, sexual and religious humiliation, hooding, sensory deprivation or overloading, and the infliction of pain to the point just before organ failure or death. All of this activity falls outside the web of international humanitarian and human rights law and judicial institutions that set limits on the use and abuse of state power in times of crisis. The Bush administration has made its own law by secret decree and it invokes state secrecy to avoid the constraints of public and political accountability. Presidential vetoes and signing statements are used against laws passed by a Congress that attempts to rein in the administration. How far will it go? As David Addington, legal counsel to Vice-President Dick Cheney from 2001 to 2005 and now his chief of staff, said, the Bush administration is "going to push and push until some larger force makes us stop."

As the war on terror is fought, "persons of interest" and prisoners of war are tortured, and the rights of non-combatant victims are ignored and abused. At the same time, humanitarian language and actions are used to justify and wage war, and Western citizens often find themselves condoning appalling acts for idealistic reasons. Samuel Moyn, a professor of human rights history, has observed that since 9/11 the United States has pursued "low-minded imperial ambitions in high-minded humanitarian tones. The effect on human rights as a public language and political cause has been staggering, and it is not yet clear whether they can recover."[1] Little wonder, then, that those who call themselves humanitarians are met with skepticism and in some cases an outright antipathy and even violence. This is not to say that the idea and practice of humanitarianism is worthy of such a reaction. It is not. But humanitarians need to reclaim its language and practice—and thus its political and human meaning. Humanitarianism is very much at a crossroads, and those who practise the humanitarianism I describe here must refuse to participate in an abuse of compassion.

"Refugee" once meant one who has refuge. In the opening years of the twenty-first century, Australia turned thousands of Afghan refugees away at sea, and interned others in walled camps for the unwanted. There, men commit suicide in despair, or sew their lips shut in protest against the silence imposed on them. In North Korea, famine and a virtual absence of humanitarian space continues at the hands of a totalitarian regime supported by external food aid. In China, the actions of aid workers and Chinese citizens who help North Korean refugees have been made criminal. In Darfur, war crimes, if not a genocide, continue in the presence of woefully understaffed and underfunded peacekeepers. In the shadow of impunity for the massacres of 1996 and 1997, war spread across the Democratic Republic of Congo, with seven regional states— some backed by France, others by the United States—vying for profit and control of the country's vast natural resources. Since 1997, between three and four million people have died there from the direct and indirect effects of war, and tens of thousands of children have been forcibly recruited as soldiers or sex slaves to militia armies. By 2008, the war had almost burned itself out, save for its original flashpoint in Goma, Kivu.

I was in Goma in 2007 and spoke with women who had been the victims of rape as a weapon of war and subjugation. Many of them felt shame for what they had suffered, but insisted that I listen to their stories and that I tell others. One fifteen-year-old girl waiting for gynecological surgery told me how she had been gang raped by militias. An old woman showed me her crippled knees, destroyed by the chains that had held her as she was raped over several days. Rape is so pervasive in Goma that the resultant gynecological wounds and destruction are considered combat injuries. A few NGOs like MSF and UN peacekeepers work in and around Goma, where 400,000 people are displaced from their homes and villages.

In Rwanda, meanwhile, the UN war crimes tribunal in neighbouring Arusha continues to try those accused of genocide. In November 2007, thirteen years after the genocide, Amnesty International called on states not to transfer people suspected of crimes during the 1994 genocide to Rwanda, where it alleged that suspects might not receive a fair and impartial trial, where they might be tortured to extract confessions in secret detention sites, where victims and witnesses are not adequately protected and where prison conditions are horrific, the buildings still holding some sixty thousand people suspected of genocide.

In 2007, I returned to Baidoa. Somalia has become the third front in the war on terror, as American and Ethiopian forces backing the transitional federal government, headquartered in Baidoa, battle the Islamic Courts Union in Mogadishu and elsewhere in the country. Also in Baidoa, Adan Hussein's orphanage is still running, having cared for more than ten thousand children since 1993 with little or no support from the outside world. Lesto Mohamed Idris had left the city in 1993 for Europe and the United States, but returned in 1995 to take his place as a clan elder. "This is my land, my country. I make my life here, I strug-gle here, and I will die here," he said to me. By early 2008 over a million people had fled the fighting in Mogadishu, millions are without enough food, and the potential for a famine worse than that of 1992–93 looms as the war on terror continues.

In this miasma of forgotten wars, torture and the war on terror, there are no easy answers, especially in the face of a very real terrorism. But I can live my questions. As a humanitarian, I can act from a feeling of shared vulnerability with the victims of preventable suffering. I have a responsibility to bear witness publicly to the plight of those I seek to assist and to insist on independent humanitarian action and respect for international humanitarian law. As a citizen, I can assume my responsibility for the public world—the world of politics—not as a spectator, but as a participant who engages and shapes it. The larger force that can push back against the wrong use of power can be the force of a citizen's politics that openly debates the right use of power and the reasoned pursuit of justice. Catherine Lu, a politi-cal philosopher and my friend, has described justice as a bound-ary over which we must not go, a bond of common humanity between us, and a balance among people of equal worth and dignity. It is also a choice. I fight not for a utopian ideal, but each day I make a choice, against nihilism and towards justice.

In the summer of 2006, I struggled to begin writing this book. I was canoeing on Big Hawk Lake in Haliburton, Ontario, and I watched two birds on the shore gathering twigs for their nests. I felt tears coming. I remembered the black-crowned finch in the window of the King Faisal Hospital morgue where I had sat with the dead infant and the waiting rats during the 1994 genocide. The finch looked at me then, and twelve years later, I still wondered what she saw.

I had returned to Rwanda in 2004 for a commemoration ceremony on the tenth anniversary of the genocide. I was ambivalent about going, especially in light of what Paul Kagame had done and was now doing in Congo. In the end I decided to go, to honour the dead, to expiate, to somehow begin again. I wanted to find Lulu, the four-year-old boy who had lived with his mother and sister in the broom closet beside my room at the hospital. He would be a teenager now. We had managed to stay in touch for a few years after the genocide, but we had since lost contact. I did find Lulu, and my wife, Rolie, was able to join us for our reunion. The day before Rolie and I left Rwanda, after a two-week stay, we attended the national ceremony commemorating the genocide at the Amahoro stadium in Kigali.

People had been streaming in—at least thirty thousand—since mid-morning. Slowly, silently, they walked. They came from all over the country but mostly from Kigali, wearing their best clothes, castoffs from used clothing bins in the West. There was no chatter as they sat on rows of cement benches. They adjusted umbrellas against the sun, passed water back and forth, waiting. Journalists and TV crews in T-shirts and jeans jostled for the best vantage points on the playing field below. Some smoked, some lay in the grass listening to music on their headphones, some talked on cellphones as they waited for the ceremony to begin.

I had worn sunscreen and remembered my sunglasses but had forgotten a hat. Rolie found a newspaper on the floor of the stands, and I occasionally put it on top of my head. My blue blazer was too hot, but I wouldn't take it off, not here, not today. The diplomats arrived in a convoy of bulletproof SUVs. Security men were everywhere, and soldiers were strategically placed around the stadium. The military band arrived in an uneven march, slightly out of tune. Kagame followed in his presidential vehicle, his wife beside him. All stood as he arrived and the national anthem was played. He read from a long, carefully prepared text. He chastised the French government, while diplomats shifted uncomfortably in their seats. The Belgian prime minister spoke, offering his mea culpa, sincerely, honestly. I couldn't help but notice his old-man teeth in a young man's face. "We failed you," he said, and then in Kinyarwanda, "We will not fail you again."

No one stood for him, but the crowd applauded respectfully. Then another diplomat spoke, then another, and then another. Their empty words were received with rote, empty applause. Rwandans, if nothing else, are polite. *Too polite*, I thought. Then came traditional Rwandan singers and dancers. There were the testimonies of genocide survivors—some prepared, some not, some short, some not. The crowd applauded for each, then fell into silence for the next singer, diplomat or witness. It went on for hours. Polite.

I noticed a few birds circling over the stands across the stadium. Below them, a woman caught my attention. She was twisting and rocking as the ceremony droned on. Her eyes were closed, her faced turned towards the sky. The woman beside her tried to hold her shoulders—consoling her, containing her. I watched her as she rocked. Then she started to turn, to sway. Then she rolled, her torso swivelling in circles. "Ah-wee! Ah-wee! Ah-wee!" she screamed, her head thrown back behind her shoulders. "Mama-we? Mama-we? Mama-we?" (Mother, where are you?) She collapsed back into the crowd and was passed, limp, unconscious, down to the playing field below. Security men took her and laid her gently on the grass. She didn't move at first, but then she rolled over and over, again and again. Each time her back was to the ground she reached towards the sky.

I looked down on the stadium field. Journalists and camera crews ran over to the woman. Some pushed hard against the others to get the closest shot. A security man in a black suit scuffled with a cameraman. The camera fell to the ground. A ripple of movement passed through the crowd as attention shifted from the podium to the woman on the playing field. She lay on her back now, her arms still pulling something to her from the sky. And then, from somewhere in the stadium, another woman's cry: "Ah-wee! Ah-wee! Ah-wee!" She too collapsed and was passed to the field below. And then another woman's cry. And then another. A diplomat struggled to be heard, his voice breaking to a stutter as he looked to the field. Through my tears, I watched the birds circling overhead. Rolie reached to hold my hand. I opened my fingers to hers.

Why do we remember? Perhaps it is because our answers are not yet right. Better the right question than the wrong answer. In Camus's The Plague, Tarrou says, "One can't forget everything, however great one's wish to do so: the plague was bound to leave traces, anyhow, in people's hearts." I remember the touch on my forearm of the woman who was one among many, and her slow whispered words. "Allez, allez . . . Ummera, ummera-sha." Hers is still the clearest voice I have ever heard.

I have a growing collection of sacred places. I find them wherever I go. Some are corners of parks, others are abandoned lots, and one is my wild garden at home. They are usually places where I can sit anonymously among old trees, grass, the earth. Sometimes I feel mournful, but then for a moment I feel free, as though a sadness I have collected somewhere along the way is spent. I often get up in the morning before dawn, drawn to a still presence in the space between night and day. I go to our garden to listen to the first call of the birds before the sunrise. I feel myself full again. Inevitably, before the birds, before the sun, our children have come into our bed. When I look at them sleeping, pulled into us for warmth, I know what they will face. I know why the struggle is right and good, and why always we can begin again.

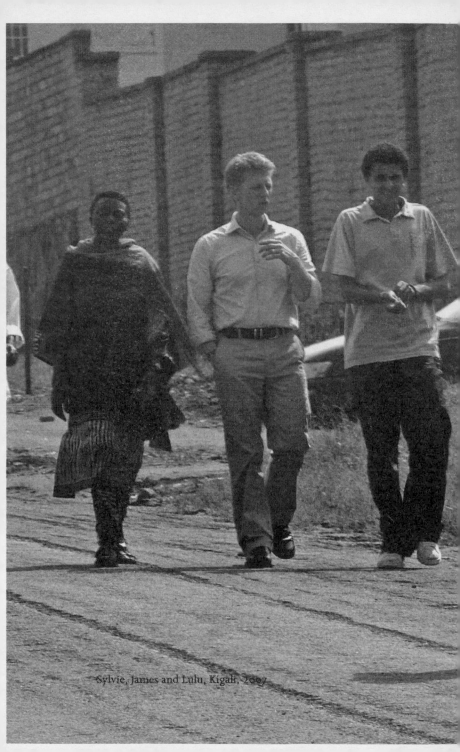

Sylvie, James and Lulu, Kigali, 2007

EPILOGUE
WHAT YOU CAN DO

The most important thing any of us can do is to actively and pragmatically assume our responsibilities as citizens for the world we live in. In the first instance, we can each support independent humanitarian action, and insist that in war governments and belligerents respect international humanitarian law, refugee law and the conventions prohibiting the use of torture. Beyond this, no one can do everything, but everyone can do something. Choose the issue that concerns you most. You may want to start by learning more about it and looking to see what others are saying and doing. Choose a political party or a non-governmental organization with which you feel an affinity, and through it, actively challenge relevant public policies, laws and practices both nationally and internationally. Making a donation, voting or writing to elected officials are easy first steps. But these are not enough. Join the organization. Bring your opinion to it, debate with others and get involved in its work as a volunteer or member. If you can't find an organization, then start one and let others join. Some of the organizations I support and have worked with or helped start are listed below.

Dignitas International   www.dignitasinternational.org

Dignitas International is testing and developing a community-based care approach to the HIV/AIDS epidemic in the developing world. It works with groups of vulnerable people, governments and researchers to increase access to prevention, treatment, care and support, including life-saving antiretroviral medications. It trains nurses, other health care professionals and community health workers in community-based care. Dignitas has more than eight thousand HIV-positive women, children and men under its care in Malawi, four thousand of whom are receiving ARV medicines for HIV/AIDS.

Médecins Sans Frontières / Doctors Without Borders   www.msf.ca

MSF is an independent medical humanitarian organization that delivers emergency aid to people affected by armed conflict, epidemics, natural or man-made disasters, or exclusion from health care. It is committed to publicly raising awareness of the plight of the people it helps.

Drugs for Neglected Diseases initiative   www.dndi.org

The DNDi uses an alternative not-for-profit public sector model to develop drugs for neglected diseases. It is committed to equitable access to new and field-relevant health tools to improve the quality of life and the health of people suffering from neglected diseases. It also works to raise awareness of the need to research and develop drugs for those neglected diseases that fall outside the scope of market-driven research and development, and to build public responsibility and leadership in addressing the needs of neglected patients.

Hope for Rwanda's Children Fund   www.hopefund.on.ca

Hope for Rwanda's Children Fund assists needy children and youth in Rwanda who cannot afford tuition, schoolbooks and school supplies.

SAFER *www.saferworld.ca*
Social Aid for the Elimination of Rape assists and supports women in the Democratic Republic of Congo who are victims of rape as a weapon of war.

War Child   *www.warchild.ca*
War Child helps children affected by war around the world by providing relief and by generating awareness, support and advocacy for children's rights everywhere.

The Global Alliance for TB Drug Development *www.tballiance.org*
The TB Alliance is researching and developing new treatments for tuberculosis.

Amnesty International   *www.amnesty.org*
Amnesty International is a worldwide movement of people who campaign for internationally recognized human rights for all.

Human Rights Watch   *www.hrw.org*
Human Rights Watch believes that international standards of human rights apply to all people equally and that progress can be made when people of good will organize themselves to make it happen.

NOTES AND SOURCES

References for the facts I include in the book are freely available through most public libraries or through an Internet search. Below I list the major sources I have drawn from for each of the chapters and those sources that are not easily obtainable on the Internet. In some places I have included a few additional comments on the chapter's content. I also offer some recommendations for further reading.

CHAPTER 1

Agamben, Giorgio. *Homo Sacer: Sovereign Power and Bare Life.* Translated by Daniel Heller-Roazen. Stanford, Calif.: Stanford University Press, 1998.

——. *State of Exception.* Translated by Kevin Attell. Chicago: Univeristy of Chicago Press, 2005.

Arendt, Hannah. *Between Past and Future: Eight Exercises in Political Thought.* New York: Penguin Books, 1954.

Debord, Guy. *The Society of the Spectacle.* Translated by Donald Nicholson-Smith. New York: Zone Books, 1994.

Dillard, Annie. *For the Time Being.* New York: Knopf, 1999.

Griffin, Susan. *A Chorus of Stones.* New York: Doubleday, 1992.

King, Thomas. *The Truth about Stories: A Native Narrative.* Toronto: House of Anansi Press, 2003.

Lévinas, Emmanuel. *Entre Nous: On Thinking of the Other.* Translated by Michael B. Smith and Barbara Harshav. New York: Columbia University Press, 1998.

Lu, Catherine. "Images of Justice: Justice as a Bond, a Boundary, and a Balance." *The Journal of Political Philosophy* 6, no. 1 (1998): 1–26.

CHAPTER 2 AND 3

Ascherson, Neal. *The King Incorporated: Leopold the Second and the Congo.* London: Allen and Unwin, 1963; London: Granta 2001. Citations are to the Granta edition.

Hochschild, Adam. *King Leopold's Ghost.* New York: Mariner Books, 1999. First published in 1998 by Houghton Mifflin.

Prunier, Gerard. *The Rwanda Crisis: History of a Genocide 1959–1994.* London: Hurst and Company, 1997.

Rittner, Carol, John K. Roth, and Wendy Whitworth, eds. *Genocide in Rwanda: Complicity of the Churches?* St. Paul, Minn.: Paragon House, 2004.

CHAPTER 4

A concise history of MSF is recounted in *Hard Choices: Moral Dilemmas in Humanitarian Intervention,* ed. by Jonathan Moore (Lanham, Md.: Rowman and Littlefield, 1998).

Other history described in the chapter is contained in *Populations in Danger, Médecins Sans Frontières,* ed. by François Jean (London: John Libby, 1992); *Life, Death and Aid: The Médecins Sans Frontières Report on World Crisis Intervention,* ed. by François Jean (New York: Routledge, 1993); *Populations in Danger 1995: A Médecins Sans Frontières Report* by François Jean (London: Editions La Découverte, 1995); *World in Crisis: The Politics of Survival at the End of the 20ᵗʰ Century,* ed. by Médecins Sans Frontières (London: Routledge, 1997); and *The Red Cross and the Holocaust* by Jean-Claud Favez, translated by John and Beryl Fletcher. Cambridge: Cambridge University Press, 1999.

Somalia

De Waal, Alex, *Famine Crimes: Politics & the Disaster Relief Industry in Africa.* Bloomington, Ind.: Indiana University Press, 1998.

Hirsch, John L. and Robert B. Oakley. *Somalia and Operation Restore Hope: Reflections on Peacemaking and Peacekeeping.* Washington D.C.: United States Institute of Peace Press, 1995.

Maren, Michael. *The Road to Hell: The Ravaging Effects of Foreign Aid and International Charity.* New York: The Free Press, 1997.

Netherlands Development and Cooperation. *Evaluation Report. Humanitarian Aid to Somalia. Chapter 8, Emergency Programme of Médecins Sans Frontières Holland.* Operations Review Unit, 1994.

Omaar, Rakiya. "Somalia: At War With Itself." *Current History,* May 1992: 230–234.

Patman, Robert G. "Disarming Somalia: The Contrasting Fortunes of United States and Australian Peacekeepers During United Nations Intervention, 1992–93." *African Affairs,* 96, no. 385 (October 1997): 521.

Razack, Sherene H. *Dark Threats & White Knights: The Somalia Affair, Peacekeeping and the New Imperialism.* Toronto: University of Toronto Press, 2004.

Somalia Operation Restore Hope: A Preliminary Assessment. London: African Rights, 1993.

CHAPTER 5

Coll, Steve. *Ghost Wars: The Secret History of the CIA, Afghanistan and bin Laden from the Soviet Invasion to September 10, 2001.* New York: Penguin Books, 2004.

Chaliand, Gérard. *Report from Afghanistan.* New York: Viking Press, 1982.

Rashid, Ahmed. *Taliban: The Story of the Afghan Warlords.* London: Pan Books, 2001.

Sreedhar, Rakesh Sinha, Nilesh Bhaget, O.N. Mehrotra, and Mahendra Ved. *Taliban and the Afghan Turmoil.* New Delhi: Himalayan Books, 1997.

CHAPTER 6

The MSF expatriates in Rwanda with me during the 1994 genocide were: Efke Bakker, Ilse Bijkerk, Pepijn Boot, Madeline Boyer, Jonathan Brock, Giovani Gabrini, Gilbert Hassouet, Patrick Henaux, Isabelle Lemasson, Sidney Maddison, Steve Manion, Jacques Ramsey, Fred Stahle, Jennifer Staples, Dana Toredada, Wayne Ulrich, Paul Van't Wout and Eric Vreede. Books and reports by Linda Melevern, Gerry Caplan, Roméo Dallaire and

Human Rights Watch, listed below, were indispensable to the background to this chapter.

Adelman, Howard, and Astri Suhrke. "Early Warning and Conflict Management: Genocide in Rwanda." CHR Michelson Institute, September 1995: 19, http://129.194.252.80/catfiles/2050.pdf (accessed February 27, 2003).

Barnett, Michael. *Eyewitness to a Genocide*. Ithaca, N.Y.: Cornell University Press, 2002.

Burkhalter, Holly. Congressional Testimony, Physicians for Human Rights Subcommittee on Human Rights and International Operations, "The 1994 Rwandan Genocide and U.S. Policy," May 5 1998. http://www.globalpolicy.org/security/issues/rwanda6.htm (accessed March 3, 2003).

Callamard, Agnès. "French Policy on Rwanda." In *The Path of a Genocide: The Rwanda Crisis from Uganda to Zaire*, edited by Howard Adelman and Astri Suhrke. New Brunswick, N.J.: Transaction Publishers, 1999.

Caplan, Gerry and the Organization of African Unity International Panel of Eminent Personalities. *Rwanda: The Preventable Genocide*. Report to the OAU, May 29, 2000.

Dallaire, Roméo. *Shake Hands with the Devil*. Toronto: Random House, 2003.

Human Rights Watch. *Choosing War. Leave None to Tell the Story*. http://www.hrw.org/reports/1999/Rwanda/Geno1-3-11.htm (accessed March 12, 2005).

Melvern, Linda. *Conspiracy to Murder: The Rwandan Genocide*. London: Verso, 2004.

——. *A People Betrayed: The Role of the West in Rwanda's Genocide*. New York: Zed Books, 2000.

——. "Missing the Story: The Media and the Rwandan Genocide." *Contemporary Security Policy*, 2001: 22(3). http://www.idrc.ca/en/ev 108204–201–1-DO_TOPIC.html (accessed December 12, 2006).

ODI. "The International Response to Conflict and Genocide: Lessons from the Rwanda Experience," Study 3, "Humanitarian Aid and Effects." London, 1997. http://www.um.dk/danida/evalueringsrapporter/ 1997_rwanda/b3/es.asp (accessed February 27, 2003).

Power, Samantha. *A Problem from Hell: America and the Age of Genocide*. New York: Basic Books, 2002.

Rwanda: Death, Despair and Defiance. London: African Rights, 1994.

United Nations. *The United Nations and Rwanda: 1999*. http://www.hrw.org/reports/1999/rwanda/Gen04–7–01.htm#P9_461 (accessed December 12, 2003).

UN Secretary General. *Report of the Secretary General on the Situation in Rwanda* (May 31, 1994). http://ods-dds-ny.un.org/doc/UNDOC/GEN/N94/234/12/IMG/N9423412.pdf?OpenElement (accessed March 1, 2003).

CHAPTER 7

1. Afsani Bassir Pour, "The Tragedy of the Zairean Refugees Shakes Washington Out of Its Passivity," *Le Monde*, April 27, 1997.

2. Agence France Press, "Emma Bonino Accuses Kabila of Transforming Eastern Zaire into a 'Slaughterhouse,'" May 6, 1997.

3. Guy Merineau, "Scenes of Massacres in the Former Zaire," *Le Monde*, July 12, 1997.

The Kivu region is the poorest and most densely populated region of the Democratic Republic of Congo (previously known as Zaire). Kivu is made up of indigenous communities and others known as Banyarwandans (the word *banya* means "from"). The indigenous communities are made up of Hunde, Nande, Tembo and Nyanga peoples. The Banyarwandans speak Kinyarwanda, have been in the Kivu region for more than 300 years and are made up of Hutus known as Bahutus and Tutsis known as Banyamulenge. The Banyarwandans existed in a centuries-old alliance that included intermarriage between its two sub-groups. President Mobutu came to power in a military coup in 1961 following the American CIA- and Belgian-backed assassination of Patrice Lumumba, the first elected prime minister of Congo/Zaire after Belgium granted the country independence. Once in power in 1961, the U.S.-backed President Mobutu stoked differences in the Kivu region and then played the role of arbitrator, thus maintaining his political power. In 1982 Mobutu revoked the citizenship rights of the Banyarwandans (both Bahutus and Banyamulenge), and officially branded them as strangers who could not hold public office. This pitted the Banyarwandans against the indigenous Hunde and Nyanga communities. The centuries-old alliance between Zaire-based Hutus and Tutsis within the Banyarwandans was broken with the 1994 influx of the powerful and militarized Hutu Ex-FAR and Interahamwe from Rwanda who sought a Hutuland in Kivu. The influx pitted the Zaire-based Bahutus against the Zaire-based Banyamulenge. The Banyamulenge gained support of the RPF government in neighboring Rwanda and joined the ADFL Rebel Alliance led by Laurent Désiré Kabila. The ADFL was supported by Rwanda, Uganda and the United States.

The Alliance of Democratic Forces for the Liberation of Congo-Zaire (ADFL) began to form over the summer of 1996, and declared its formal existence in October 1996. Led by Laurent Désiré Kabila, it was a merger of the Popular Revolutionary Party of Shaba, the National Resistance Council for Democratic Kasaii, the Revolutionary Movement for the Liberation of Zaire, and the Democratic Alliance of the Banyamulenge People (the Zaire-based Tutsis). Its stated aim was to topple Mobutu, and it had Rwandan, Ugandan and American backing.

America Mineral Fields Inc., based in Hope, Arkansas, and owned by Jean-Raymond Boulle and his brother Max Boulle, was heavily involved in promoting Joseph Kabila's accession to power in 1996. The company had had an indirect link with the rebel leader since 1993; their Belgian representative was also a military adviser to Kabila. Jean-Raymond Boulle met personally with Kabila in Goma in March 1997, while Max, also the owner of American Diamond Buyers, received the right to open the first diamond brokerage in Kisangani in early April 1997. Max Boulle purchased $100 million worth of diamonds in Kisangani shortly after the capture of the city in March 1997, thereby injecting money into the local economy and the finances of the ADFL.

America Mineral Fields lent $1 million to the ADFL authorities during the war, and reportedly paid Kabila an advance of between

$20 and $50 million prior to Jean-Raymond Boulle's arrival in Lubumbashi on April 16, 1997—a month before the civil war had ended—to sign an $885 million agreement, giving America Mineral Fields the rights to refine the spoil heaps in Kolwezi, to rehabilitate the Kipushi mine and to construct a zinc smelting plant and refining factory. America Mineral Fields also lent Kabila the use of its corporate Lear jet while he was still head of a guerrilla movement and paid the hotel expenses of other members of the alliance. For more information, see *L'enjeu Congolais. L'Afrique centrale après Mobutu* by Colette Braeckman (Paris: Fayard, 1999); Wayne Madsen's testimony before the house Subcommittee on International Operations and Human Rights on May 17, 2001 (http://www.house.gov/international_relations/mads0517.htm); *L'odyssée Kabila. Trajectoire pour un Congo nouveau?* by Jean-Claude Willame (Paris: Édition Karthala) which on page 84, cites the May 27, 1998, edition of *La Lettre Afrique Énergies*; "U.S. Firms Stake Claims In Zaire's War; Investors Woo Rebels In Mineral-Rich Area" an article by Cindy Shiner in Goma on page A1 of the April 17, 1997, edition of the *Washington Post*; and "Zairian Rebels' New Allies: Men Armed With Briefcases," an article by James C. McKinley Jr. in Lubumbashi on page A10 of the April 17, 1997, edition of the *New York Times*.)

Gnamo, Abbas H. "The Rwandan Genocide and the Collapse of Mobutu's Kleptocracy." In *The Path of a Genocide: The Rwanda Crisis from Uganda to Zaire*, edited by Howard Adelman and Astri Suhrke. New Brunswick, N.J.: Transaction Publishers, 1999.

Gowing, Nik. *New Challenges and Problems for Information Management in Complex Emergencies: Ominous Lessons from the Great Lakes And Eastern Zaire in Late 1996 and Early 1997*. European Union ECHO Discussion Paper. 1998.

Ismi Asad. "The Western Heart of Darkness: Mineral-rich Congo Ravaged by Genocide and Western plunder." *Canadian Centre for Policy Alternatives. Monitor Issue*. October 1, 2001.

Jennings, Christian. *Across the Red River*. London: Orion Books, 2000.

Montague, Dena. "Stolen Goods: Coltan and Conflict in the Democratic Republic of the Congo." *SAIS Review* 22, no.1 (2002).

Moore, David. "From King Leopold to King Kabila in the Congo: The

Continuities and Contradictions of the Long Road from Warlordism to Democracy in the Heart of Africa." *Review of African Political Economy*, 28:87 (2001): 130–135.

Nabeth, Pierre, Alice Crosier, Midrad Peadri, Jean-Hervé Bradol, EpiCentre and Médecins Sans Frontières. "Were Acts of Violence Committed Against the Rwandan Refugees?" *The Lancet*. October 1997.

Rosenblum, Peter. "Kabila's Congo." *Current History.* May 1998: 193–200.

United Nations. *Report of the Panel on the Illegal Exploitation of Natural Resources and Other Forms of Wealth of the Democratic Republic of the Congo.* 12 April 2001.

CHAPTER 8

1. Barbara Crosette, "Hunger in North Korea: A Relief Aide's Stark Report," *International Herald Tribune*, June 11, 1997.

2. David Rieff, *A Bed for the Night: Humanitarianism in Crisis.* p. 3.

3. "A Man Who Fights the Savage War of Peace: For Bernard Kouchner, the Province is a Frontline Test of the World's Right to Intervene," *Newsweek Special Issue*, June 1999.

Becker, Jasper. *La Grande Famine de Mao: 30 à 50 millions de morts.* Paris: Editions Dagorono, 1998.

Conquest, Robert. *The Harvest of Sorrow.* Oxford: Oxford University Press, 1986.

Haggard, Stephen, and Marcus Noland. *Famine in North Korea: Markets, Aid and Reform.* New York: Columbia University Press, 2007.

Ogata, Sadako. *Briefing Notes by Mrs. Sadako Ogata, United Nations High Commissioner for Refugees, to the (United Nations) Security Council.* New York, May 5, 1999. p. 6.

Rieff, David. *A Bed for the Night: Humanitarianism in Crisis.* New York: Simon & Schuster, 2002.

MSF's 1999 Nobel Peace Prize Acceptance speech was written by James Orbinski, Phillipe Biberson, Françoise Bouchet-Saulnier, Rony Brauman, Jean-Marie Kindermans, Alex Parisel, Austen Davis and Eric Stobbaerts. Others who contributed are Samantha Bolton,

Fiona Terry, Kristina Torgeson and many MSF volunteers and national staff who sent me ideas and emails from the field. I also reviewed ideas and in some cases early drafts with David Rieff, Jim Graff, Ursula Franklin, Craig Scott and Janice Stein.

CHAPTER 9

PhARMA members have little interest in pricing drugs for the market in developing countries because they are seeking to maximize global, not national profits, and do not want to set a low-price precedent that would increase demand in wealthy countries for similarly low prices. See page 69 of the UNDP's 1999 Human Development Report, available at: http://hdr.undp.org/en/media/hdr_1999_en.pdf

As of November 2007, UNAIDS estimates that 33.2 million people worldwide are HIV-positive, and that 2.5 million people were newly infected with HIV in 2007. For the first time, in most of sub-Saharan Africa, national HIV prevalence has either stabilized or is showing signs of a decline. In Southeast Asia, the epidemics in Cambodia, Myanmar and Thailand all show declines in HIV prevalence. The estimated number of deaths due to AIDS in 2007 was 2.1 million [1.9–2.4 million] worldwide, of which 76 percent occurred in sub-Saharan Africa. This is the first time a decline in the number of AIDS deaths has been identified. Declines are partly attributable to the scaling up of antiretroviral treatment services. AIDS remains a leading cause of mortality worldwide and the primary cause of death in sub-Saharan Africa, illustrating the tremendous long-term challenge that lies ahead for provision of treatment services, with the hugely disproportionate impact on sub-Saharan Africa ever more clear. HIV incidence (the number of new HIV infections in a population per year) is the key parameter that prevention efforts aim to reduce, since newly infected persons contribute to the total number of persons living with HIV; they will progress to disease and death over time; and are a potential source of further transmission. Global HIV incidence likely peaked in the late 1990s at over 3 million new infections per year, and was estimated to be 2.5 million [1.8–4.1 million] new infections in 2007 of which over two-thirds (68 percent) occurred in sub-Saharan Africa. This reduction in HIV incidence likely reflects natural trends in the epidemic as well as the result of prevention programs resulting in behavioural change in different contexts. It is important to note that increased investments in interventions for HIV prevention, treatment and care are showing results but also greatly increase the complexity of the epidemic and analysis of its trends. The 2007 UNAIDS analysis cannot adequately define the impact of specific interventions or programs. This will require special studies in local areas, including direct assessments of HIV incidence, mortality, program effectiveness and the burden of HIV infection, disease and death in children. See: UNAIDS & WHO. 2007 AIDS Epidemic Update. Accessed November 24, 2007, at: http://data.unaids.org/pub/EPISlides/2007/2007_epiupdate_en.pdf

The team of Core Group Members who worked to create the DNDi are: Yves Champey, James Orbinski, Bernard Pécoul, Els Torreele, Visweswaran Navaratnam, Dyann Wirth, Hellen Gelband, George Tyler, Eloan Dos Santos Pinheiro, Piero Olliaro, Vasantha Muthuswamy, Nirmal Ganguly, Rob Ridley, Michèle Boccoz, Patrice Trouiller, Fawzia Rasheed, Bruce Mahin, Vasantha Muthuswamy, Dominique Legros, and Giorgio Roscigno.

Cheru, Fantu. "Debt, Adjustment, and the Politics of Effective Response to HIV/AIDS in Africa," Third World Quarterly 23, no. 2 (2002): 299–312.

Fitzhugh Mullan. "The Metrics of the Physician Brain Drain." The New England Journal of Medicine, no. 353; 17: 1810–8.

Chin, James and Jonathan Mann. "Global Surveillance and Forecasting of AIDS." Bulletin of the World Health Organization 67 (1989): 1–7.

Chowdhury, Zafrullah. The Politics of Essential Drugs. London: Zed Books, 1995.

Cohen-Kohler, J.C. "The Morally Uncomfortable Global Drug Gap." Nature 82, no. 5 (2007). Available at: www.nature.com.

Correa, Carlos. Intellectual Property Rights, the WTO and Developing Countries. London: Zed Books, 2000.

Dye, Chris. "Stopping TB: Weighing the Alternatives." Paper delivered at Rockefeller Foundation Conference on TB Drug Development, Cape Town, South Africa, February 6–8, 2000.

Holme C, Cranberg, L, Owen-Drife J. "Tuberculosis: story of medical failure." BMJ 317(1998): 1260.

Keck, Margaret and Kathyrn Sikkink. *Activists Beyond Borders: Advocacy Networks in International Politcs.* Ithaca, N.Y.: Cornell University Press, 1998.

Meyer, David S. and Sidney Tarrow. "A Movement Society: Contentious Politics for a New Century." In *The Social Movement Society: Contentious Politics for a New Century,* edited by D.S. Meyer and S. Tarrow. Lanham, Md.: Rowman and Littlefield, 1998

Orbinski, James. "Health, Equity and Trade: A Failure in Global Governance." In *The Role of the World Trade Organization in Global Governance,* edited by Gary Sampson. New York: United Nations University Press, 2001.

Pécoul, Bernard, James Orbinski and Els Torreele, eds. *Fatal Imbalance: The Crisis in Research and Development for Drugs for Neglected Diseases.* Geneva: Médecins Sans Frontières / Drugs for Neglected Diseases Working Group, 2001. Available at www.accessmed-msf.org

Pécoul, B., P. Chirac, P. Trouiller and J. Pinel. "Access to essential drugs in poor countries: a lost battle?" *JAMA* 281 (1999): 361–67.

Piot, Peter, Francis Plummer, Fred S. Mhalu, Jean-Louis Lamboray, James Chin, Jonathan M. Mann. "AIDS: An International Perspective." *Science* 239 (1988): 573–579.

Robinson, Jeffrey. *Prescription Games: Money, Ego and Power Inside the Global Pharmaceutical Industry.* London: Simon & Schuster, 2001.

Russell, Sabin. "New Crusade to Lower AIDS Drug Costs; Africa's needs at odds with firms' profit motive." *San Francisco Chronicle,* May 24, 1999.

Sachs, Jeffrey. "Macroeconomics and Health: Investing in Health for Economic Development." Report of the Commission on Macroeconomics and Health. World Health Organization. Geneva, 2001.

Troullier, P., P. Olliaro, E. Torreele, J. Orbinski, R. Laing and N. Ford. "Drug development for neglected diseases: a deficient market and a public health policy failure." *The Lancet* 359 (2002): 2188–2194.

Velasquez, German. "Drugs Should Be a Common Good: Unhealthy Profits, Le Monde diplomatique." July 2003. http://MondeDiplo.com/2003/07/10velasquez

CHAPTER 10

1. Samuel Moyn, "The Genealogy of Morals," *The Nation*, April 16, 2007, pp. 25–31.

With UN food aid stopped by the American bombing, 7.5 million Afghans starved. Early American airdrops delivered 37,500 HDRs (Humanitarian Daily Rations) per day, meeting 0.005% of the population's needs. In all, American forces dropped 2.4 million food daypack rations in 2001 in Afghanistan. "They were intended to ease Afghan food insecurity, demonstrate American sensitivity to non-combatants and reduce international criticism of U.S. conduct. . . . While some rations were genuinely targeted toward malnourished populations, others were clearly directed to civilians allied with American forces. In one instance, widely showcased by the military, the U.S. Air Force dropped 17,200 [food daypack rations] to villagers around the Arghanab River after they assisted a group of U.S. marines by building a stone bridge over a shallow point in the river to facilitate a vehicle crossing." (Ben Sklaver, "Humanitarian Daily Rations: The Need for Evaluation and Guidelines," *Disasters* 27, no. 3 (2003): 259–271. Available at: http://www.blackwell-synergy.com/doi/pdf/10.1111/1467-7717.00232)

"The thousands of Afghan civilians who perished did so because U.S. military and political elites chose to carry out a bombing campaign using extremely powerful weaponry in civilian-rich areas (the isolated training camps were largely destroyed during the first week). For political reasons, it has been necessary to hide the human carnage on Afghan soil as much as possible from the western public. Given that many of the bombing attacks—such as those on civilian infrastructure (cars, clinics, radio stations, bridges) and those during November and December on anything rolling on the roads of southern Afghanistan—violated the rules of war, there are war crimes that need to be investigated. An inadequate count will make it impossible for the families of those wrongfully killed to get the compensation to which they are entitled. It will also impede international justice." (Marc Herold, "Counting the Dead: Attempting to Hide the Number of Afghan Civilians Killed by U.S.

bombs Are an Affront to Justice," *The Guardian*. August 8, 2002. Available at: http://www.guardian.co.uk/afghanistan/comment/story/0,11447,77 0999,00.html

On 2 June 2004, five MSF colleagues were brutally murdered on the road between Khairkhana and Qala-i-Naw in Afghanistan's Badghis province. The five who were lost are: project coordinator Hélène de Beir, logistician Pim Kwint, physician Egil Tynaes, translator Fasil Ahmad, and Besmillah, the team's driver.

Arendt, Hannah. "Collective Responsibility: Contribution to Symposium 1968." In *Amor Mundi: Explorations in the Faith and Thought of Hannah Arendt*, edited by J.W. Bernauer, S.J, Boston: Martinus Nijhoff, 1987.

Camus, Albert. *The Plague*. New York: Knopf, 1948; New York: Vintage Books, 1991: p. 250. Reference is to the Vintage edition.

Canada. Commission of Inquiry into the Actions of Canadian Officials in Relation to Maher Arar. 2006. *Report of the Events Relating to Maher Arar: Factual Background, Volume 1* (available at http://www.ararcommission.ca/eng/Vol_1_English.pdf).

Cole, David. "The Man Behind the Torture." *The New York Review of Books*, 6 December 2007: 38–43. A review of *The Terror Presidency* by Jack Goldsmith.

Danner, Mark. "The Logic of Torture." *The New York Review of Books*. June 24, 2004 (available at: http://www.markdanner.com/articles/show/34).

——. "Torture and Truth." *The New York Review of Books*. June 10, 2004 (available at: http://www.markdanner.com/articles/show/35).

Goldsmith, Jack. *The Terror Presidency: Law and Judgment Inside the Bush Administration*. New York: W.W. Norton, 2007.

Lu, Catherine. "Images of Justice: Justice as a Bond, a Boundary, and a Balance." *The Journal of Political Philosophy* 6, no. 1 (1998): 1–26.

Marty, D. *Secret detentions and illegal transfers of detainees involving Council of Europe member states: Second report*. Committee on Legal Affairs and Human Rights. Parliamentary Assembly of the Council of Europe. June 8 2007 (available at: http://news.bbc.co.uk/2/shared/bsp/hi/pdfs/marty_08_06_07.pdf)

Moyn, Samuel. "The Genealogy of Morals." *The Nation*, 16 April 2007: 25–31.

Prunier, Gerard. *Darfur: The Ambiguous Genocide*. Ithaca, N.Y.: Cornell University Press, 2005.

Ullman, Harlan. *Shock and Awe: Achieving Rapid Dominance*. Washington, D.C.: NDU Press, 1996 (available at: http://ics.leeds.ac.uk/papers/pmt/exhibits/223/Shock_and_Awe,_Achieving_Rap%5B1%5D.pdf).

Yoo, John. *War by Other Means: An Insider's Account of the War on Terror*. New York: Atlantic Monthly Press, 2006.

FURTHER READING

Five very good contemporary books on the issues and dilemmas of humanitarianism are:

Barnett, Michael and Thomas Weiss, eds. *Humanitarianism in Question: Politics, Power and Ethics*. Ithaca, N.Y.: Cornell University Press, 2008.

Rieff, David. *A Bed for the Night: Humanitarianism in Crisis*. New York: Simon & Schuster, 2002.

Steiner, Henry J. and Paul Alston. *International Human Rights in Context: Law, Politics, Morals*. Second Edition. Oxford: Oxford University Press, 2000.

Terry, Fiona. *Condemned to Repeat? The Paradox of Humanitarian Action*. Cornell University Press, Ithaca. 2002.

Weissman, Fabrice, ed. *In the Shadow of "Just Wars": Violence, Politics and Humanitarian Action*. Ithaca, N.Y.: Cornell University Press, 2004.

PHOTO CREDITS

CAPTIONS FOR PART AND CHAPTER OPENERS

Part One: Rwanda, 1988

Chapter One: Somalia, 2007

Chapter Two: Kevin, Jacqui, Madge, Deirdre and James Orbinski in London, England, 1966

Chapter Three: Tutsi boy at Mundende Clinic, Rwanda

Chapter Four: MSF Medical Feeding Centre, Baidoa

Chapter Five: Refugee camp in Afghanistan

Part Two: Genocide Memorial, Rwanda

Chapter Six: Ste. Famille Cathedral, June 1994

Part Three: Hutu refugees in the jungle near Kisangani, Zaire, in early 1997

Chapter Seven: Mai-Mai on the road to Masisi

Chapter Eight: Entrance to the MSF office in Amsterdam

Acknowledgements: Rolie Srivastava with Rohin and Taidgh, May 2005

INDEX

Page numbers in italics refer to illustrations.

Abdul (Somali guard), 79–80, 80, 88, 90, 96, 109
Abdullah (Afghani translator), 8
ACCESS (Thailand), 354, 358
Achmat, Zackie, 360, 361
ACT UP, 354, 356
Addington, David, 389
Adventist University of Central Africa (Rwanda), 49
Afghanistan, 8, 11, 17, 77, 137–59, 164, 181, 312, 382, 383–84, 385–86, 387, 389; Badghis province, 385; Charikar, 139, 149; Jalalabad, 137, 138, 139, 140, 141, 143, 144–45, 147, 148, 149, 151, 152, 153–54, 384; Kabul, 8, 137, 138, 139, 140, 144, 145, 146, 149, 151, 153, 154, 387; Kunduz, 138, 151; Mazar-e Sharif, 138, 151; Ministry of Health, 147, 155; Nangarhar province, 141, 142; Sarshahi camp, 139, 143–44, 145, 146, 147, 147, 148–53, 150, 153, 154, 155–56, 157; Torkham, 139, 142
Aga Khan, 59

Aga Khan University Hospital (Nairobi, Kenya), 100
Agreement on Trade-Related Aspects of International Property Rights (TRIPS), 353, 372
AICF, 97, 99
Aidid, General Mohamed, 87–88, 92, 95, 104, 105, 106, 107, 111, 114, 119, 130–31
AIDS, *see* HIV/AIDS
Albania, 321, 326, 327, 329, 342, 344; Kukës, 324, 327, 328; Tirana, 324–25
Ali (Somali orphan), 83–84, 97
Alice (nurse, Malawi), 14
Allen, Susan, 48, 50, 52, 59, 181, 240
Alliance of Democratic Forces for the Liberation of Zaire (ADFL), 266–69, 271, 272–76, 278–80, 281, 283, 284, 285, 286, 287, 288, 290, 291, 292, 293–94, 296, 297, 298, 299, 303
al Qaeda, 311, 382, 383, 386
Amalki, Abdullah, 388
America Mineral Fields Incorporated, 294

American Diamond Buyers, 294
American Refugee Committee, 285
Amnesty International, 178, 218, 391, 399
Angola, 11, 133, 329, 338
Annan, Kofi, 170, 296, 332
Annie (MSF logistician), 141
Anyidoho, Henry, 245
Arar, Maher, 387–88
Argentina, 176
Arone, Shidane Omar, 129
Australia, 24, 105, 120, 124, 128, 376, 390
Aziz, Abdul, 146–47, 148, 149, 151, 152–53, 154, 155, 156, 157–59

Bakke, Efke, 181, 194
Balas, Father Laurent, 272
Bangladesh, 68, 221–22, 384
Baril, General Maurice, 277, 278, 285, 286, 293
Barre, Siad, 77, 84, 85, 90, 114, 123, 127
Barthes, Dr. Olivier, 140, 144, 144, 146
Bastos, Dr. José Antonio, 275–76, 290
Bayer Pharmaceutical, 372
Belgian Congo, see Zaire
Belgium, 7, 10, 40, 48, 59, 67, 127, 168, 169, 173, 190, 272, 279, 318, 393–94; Brussels, 177, 306, 318, 358, 365; and former Belgian Congo, 53; in Rwanda, 42, 56, 58, 165, 169, 171–72
Benedict, Brother, 29–30, 31–32, 34, 127, 238–39, 241, 258, 301
Berman, Daniel, 354, 358, 369
Biafra, 68, 70
Biberson, Philippe, 305, 334, 338
bin Laden, Osama, 312, 383, 385
Bizimanna, Thérèse, 48, 181, 194, 217, 240, 241
Blair, Tony, 321, 326, 328, 333
Blok, Lucie, 156
Bonino, Emma, 297
Boot, Pepijn, 185–86, 206, 209
Borel, Dr. Raymond, 68, 69
Bosnia, 107, 135, 175, 176, 178, 322,

332; and Dayton Peace Accords, 322; Sarajevo, 157; slaughter of Muslims in, 97, 106, 322, 332; see also Yugoslavia (former)
Botswana, 353
Bouchet-Saulnier, Françoise, 338, 340
Bowie, David, 95
Boyer, Madeline, 193
Bradol, Dr. Jean-Hervé, 180, 320
Brauman, Rony, 329, 340
Brazil, 135, 229, 354, 356, 360, 366, 369, 371
Bristol-Myers Squibb, 358
Britain, 17, 18, 22, 26, 53, 76, 146, 152, 159, 165, 179, 218, 273, 283, 292, 294, 321, 323, 324, 326, 376; London, 17, 76, 321, 322, 324; in Somalia, 90
Brock, Jonathan, 130, 181, 206, 243–44, 305
Bulgaria, 323
Burundi, 170, 171, 172, 174, 177, 178, 217, 250, 263, 292, 338, 339
Bush, Barbara, 124
Bush, George H. W., 75–76, 106, 113, 123, 130
Bush, George W., 12, 369, 382, 383; Bush administration, 389

Cambodia, 91, 135, 168, 347, 351–52, 354, 354; genocide in, 164, 168
Camus, Albert, 380, 395; The Plague, 395
Canada, 7, 13, 18, 20, 21, 59, 132, 84, 88, 129, 164, 168, 180, 181, 184, 257, 260, 267, 268, 271, 277, 285, 288, 293, 310, 323, 372, 373, 376, 387–89; and Bill C-9, 13; Calgary, 30–31; Medical Research Council (Canada), 37, 64; Montreal, 18, 19–21, 29; Orangeville (Ontario), 71; Ottawa, 388; and Pledge for Africa, 373; in Sudan, 310; Toronto, 75, 116, 124, 126, 164, 182, 257, 290, 301, 365, 366, 374, 381

Canadian International Development Agency (CIDA), 59, 260
Canadian Public Health Association, 259
Canadian Security Intelligence Service (CSIS), 387
Caravielle, René, 174
CARE, 83, 86, 87, 95, 96, 100, 101, 105, 107, 110, 111, 114, 116, 124, 127, 292
Carter, Jimmy, 137
Central Intelligence Agency (CIA), 8, 122, 137, 141, 165
Centre Hospitalier de Kigali (CHK), 40, 44–48, 49, 62, 166, 173, 174, 191, 199–200, 180, 240
Ceppi, Jean-Philippe, 176
Chad, 220
Champey, Yves, 369
Chanda, Dixon, 140, 141, 145, 146
Chapman, Ben, 71
Charity (Malawi woman), 374–75
Chechnya, 11, 287, 337, 338, 339–40, 341
Cheney, Dick, 389
Chile, 34
China, 59, 67, 136, 137, 138, 159, 164, 229, 277, 306, 307, 309, 321, 352, 390; in Sudan, 310, 347
Chingwale, Pax, 377, 378–79
Chrétien, Jean, 267
Citizens' Network (Rwanda), 260
Clark, Phil, 273
Clinton, Bill, 106, 130, 178, 268, 299, 311–12, 326, 328, 356; Clinton administration, 132, 178–79, 319, 332
Cold War, 6, 11, 58, 84, 90, 135, 136, 166, 263, 302, 306, 386
College St. André, 200–201, 202, 203, 214, 242–43
Colombia, 133
Committee Against Genocide in Biafra, 68
Concern (Ireland), 96, 101, 124, 128
Conoco, 84
Contact Group, 321
Cooder, Ry, 240

Cook, Robin, 326
CPTech, 354, 359, 371
Cross, James, 18
Cushing, Chris, 133
Cyprus, 135, 224
Cyusa, Léondre, 215–16
Czech Republic, 176

Dallaire, Major-General Roméo, 168, 169–70, 176–77, 187, 196, 198, 200, 208, 219, 220, 224, 228, 230, 242
Davis, Austen, 3–4
Democratic Republic of the Congo, 297, 304, 390–91, 399
Denmark: Copenhagen, 362
Derir, Chief Hussein Mohamed, 112–13, 114, 118, 121, 123
Devereux, Sean, 123, 124
Dignitas International, 15, 376–79, 378, 398
Diseases: acute respiratory infections, 367; cancrum oris, 89, 96; Chagas disease, 371; cholera, 72, 140, 144, 152, 154, 155, 250, 251, 263, 267, 270, 273, 276, 278; dengue fever, 88; diarrhea, 43, 46, 50, 64, 72, 88, 89, 140, 143, 152, 186, 194, 216, 246, 250, 275, 286, 368; dysentery, 76, 83, 94, 217, 250; elephantiasis, 45; hepatitis, 88; kwashiorkor, 53; leishmaniasis, 316, 371; malaria, 13, 14, 88, 89, 122, 194, 200, 235, 236, 246–47, 261, 286, 291, 298, 364, 367, 368–69, 371, 379; malnutrition, 26, 53, 54, 55, 85, 158, 194, 200, 247, 264, 267, 300; marasmus, 315; measles, 50, 94, 124, 140, 144, 151, 152, 154, 155, 156–58, meningitis, 313; pneumonia, 46, 94, 100, 112, 200, 261; polio, 44–45, 46, 47, 57–58; sleeping sickness (African), 13, 282, 351, 366–67, 371; tetanus, 196, 229–30, 232; tuberculosis (TB), 13, 26, 47, 54, 164, 217, 242, 335–36, 37, 338, 351, 363–64, 365,

367, 374, 399; *see also* HIV/AIDS
Doctors Without Borders, *see* Médecins
    Sans Frontières (MSF)
Doll, Chris, 71
Dostum (Afghani warlord), 138, 153
Douglas, Tommy, 20
Drugs for Neglected Diseases initiative
    (DNDi), 369–70, 371, 377, 379, 398

East Timor, 11, 338
Eli (hospital worker, Rwanda), 195,
    204, 205, 211, 212, 217, 238, 252,
    253
Eli Lilly, 358, 363
El Salvador, 28–29, 91, 135
Else (MSF nurse), 344
England, *see* Britain
Ethiopia, 27, 84, 90, 91, 114, 391
European Union, 297, 306, 319, 355,
    356, 357, 359–60; Commissioner for
    Humanitarian Affairs, 267; European
    Parliament (Brussels), 357, 362
Everts, Hans, 100, 101, 102, 103
Executive Outcomes, 286
Ex-FAR (ex-Rwandan Armed Forces),
    263, 265, 266, 267, 268, 269, 271,
    272, 274, 278, 279, 280, 281, 287,
    292, 299

Farmer, Paul, 363
Férier, Marie-Christine, 309–310, 312,
    319–20
Fille, François, 314, 318
France, 9, 10, 40, 53, 59, 68, 97, 113,
    119, 140, 175, 198, 243, 263, 268, 275,
    286, 288, 292, 296, 297, 321, 327,
    355, 370, 382, 390; and Foreign
    Legion, 119; and Operation Turquoise,
    229, 231; Paris, 19, 67, 333; in
    Rwanda, 165, 167–68, 169, 171, 179,
    180, 190, 218–21, 222, 224, 229, 230,
    231, 233, 235, 237, 242, 248, 251,
    261; in Sudan, 310; in Zaire, 274
Fraser, James, 14–15, 293–94, 374,
    376–77

Front de Libération du Québec (FLQ),
    18
Fujimori, President Alberto (Peru), 72
Fundira, Emile, 50–52, 51, 59

G8 (Group of Eight), 358; Kananaskis
    Summit (2002), 369
Gabrini, Dr. Giovanni, 187, 194, 203,
    204, 209, 236, 239, 240
Gaillard, Philippe, 192–93, 198, 225,
    228, 231, 232, 242
Garnier, Jean-Paul, 369
Gastellu-Etchegorry, Marc, 272–74, 275
Geneva Conventions, 236, 387
Genocide, 9–10, 11, 163–64, 175,
    177–78, 179, 196–98, 218, 229, 231,
    237, 251, 260, 292, 293, 341; of
    Armenians by Turks, 164; of Jews and
    others by Nazis, 21–25, 69, 164, 175,
    258, 293; of Tutsis by Hutus
    (Rwanda), 9–10, 163–64, 167–81,
    185–251, 257–58, 260–63, 264, 299,
    303, 305, 391, 392–93
Germany, 24, 26, 41–42, 53, 67, 197,
    321, 326, 327, 355; Berlin, 24;
    Stuttgart, 293
Ghana, 182, 196
Gilles, Dr. Rowan, 386
GlaxoSmithKline, 361, 362, 369
Global Alliance for TB Drug
    Development, 364, 399
GOAL (Ireland), 96, 116
Godain, Graziella, 275
Goemaere, Dr. Eric, 248, 309, 359–60
Gonzales, Alberto, 387
Gore, Al, 355, 356
Gowing, Nick, 299
Great Lakes region (Africa), 165, 260,
    276, 304, 305
Greece, 323, 330–31
Guantánamo Bay, 387
Guatemala, 354
Gulf War (1991), 75
Guptill, Dr. Joni, 71, 78, 79–80, 81–83,
    84, 88

Habyarimana, Agathe (wife of Rwandan president), 165, 171
Habyarimana, President Juvénal (Rwanda), 52–53, 58, 60, 165, 167, 168, 170, 172, 263, 291
Hagerty, Amy (author's aunt), 24, 25
Hagerty, Joe (author's uncle), 24, 25
Haiti, 11, 178
Hank (U.S. soldier), 78–79
Harald V, King (Norway), 339
Harvard University, 363, 367
Hascoet, Gilbert, 193, 214, 232–33
Hassan, Margaret, 386
Health Action International, 354
Health GAP, 354
Hehenkamp, Arjan, 100, 108, 108, 111, 114, 117, 118, 120, 121, 123, 270–72, 276, 277, 285, 288, 289, 290
Heinzl, John, 71
Heinzl, Richard, 67, 71
Hekmatyar (Afghani warlord), 138, 153
Hellmer, Colonel Werner, 119–20, 121, 122
Henaux, Patrick, 193
Hepburn, Audrey, 95
Hezb-e-Islami, 153
Hill, Declan, 71
HIV / AIDS, 12–13, 14–15, 28, 37, 40, 41, 42–43, 47, 48, 50, 63, 166, 261, 351–53, 355, 356, 358–59, 360–63, 364, 368, 370, 371, 372, 374–76, 377–79, 398; and antiretroviral (ARV) drugs, 352, 353, 355, 356, 358, 359, 360–61, 362, 363, 365, 367, 370, 398; and craniofacial dysmorphy, 41, 64; International HIV/AIDS conference (1996), 352; pediatric AIDS, 37, 40–42
Hogan, Paul, 337–38
Holbrooke, Richard, 328, 329
Holland, 67, 181, 288, 318; Amsterdam, 3, 76–77, 105, 106, 111, 114, 116, 124, 126, 132–33, 136, 158, 181, 182, 184, 194, 234, 260, 357
Homer, 9; The Iliad, 9

Hong Kong, 308
Hope for Rwanda's Children Fund, 398
Hopkins, Gerard Manley, 238–39
Horton, Richard, 370
Howe, Admiral Jonathan, 130, 131
Hoyer, Steny, 389
Human Rights Watch, 178, 218, 399
Hurzi (Somali driver), 79–80, 83, 84, 88, 89, 90, 93, 94, 96, 98, 99–100, 103–104, 105, 108, 109, 110, 113, 114, 115, 117, 120, 121, 126
Hussein, Abdulahi, 97
Hussein, Adan, 97, 108, 110, 117, 124, 391
Hussein, Saddam, 75–76, 383

Idris, Lesto Mohamed, 93, 93, 95, 98, 101, 102–103, 108, 109, 110–11, 113, 115, 116, 117, 119, 122, 126, 391–92
Ignatios, Andrew, 105
Iman, 95
India, 32, 72, 138, 352, 354, 366, 369
Indonesia, 70, 384
Ingushetia, 337
Interahamwe (Rwanda), 167, 169, 170–71, 173, 174, 187, 190–91, 193, 198, 200, 201, 204, 208, 215, 216, 221, 224, 225, 230, 232, 233, 236, 237, 241, 242, 248, 252, 262, 263, 264, 265, 266, 268, 269, 274, 278, 279, 281, 291, 292, 299; and Operation Insecticide, 263
International Criminal Court, 383
International Medical Committee (IMC), 90, 96, 101, 109, 110, 114, 119
International Monetary Fund, 60, 165–66, 376
Iran, 76, 138
Iraq, 11, 75–76, 77, 78, 382, 384–85, 387; Abu Ghraib prison, 387; factions in, 75–76, 78; Fallujah, 386; MSF mission in, 76, 77; and Operation Provide Comfort, 76
Ireland, 18, 26, 96; Dublin, 26; Tipperary, 26

Isaq (Somali man), 98, 99, 124
Islamic Courts Union, 391
Islamic Relief Agency, 147, 155
Italy, 7, 53, 90, 129, 171, 321, 323, 327

Jackson, Michael, 58
Jacques (peacekeeper), 214, 216–17
Japan, 67, 280, 308, 385; bombings of
    Hiroshima and Nagasaki, 385
Japanese Pharmaceutical Association,
    369
Jean (MSF co-ordinator, Sudan), 315
Jeremy (UNHCR, Afghanistan), 145
Jess, Colonel, 123, 124
Jesse, Colonel Omar, 114
Jimmy Carter (son of Suki, Rwanda), 60
Jong-wook, Lee, 370
Juliana (MSF co-ordinator), 182

Kaatsch, Nicola, 304
Kabila, Laurent, 266, 267, 268, 293,
    294, 296, 297, 298, 303
Kabongo, Colonel, 286, 287–88
Kadir, Haji, 153–54
Kagame, Paul, 167, 187, 220, 2411, 260,
    261, 297, 299, 393
Kalid, Dr., 141
Kamanzi, Major Frank, 196, 230,
    233–34, 235, 236, 245
Karzai, Hamid, 385
Kashmir, 384
Katherine (MSF nurse), 105
Katrina (MSF nurse), 89
Kearney, John, 361
Keating, Colin, 177, 179
Kennedy, Robert, 20
Kenya, 37–39, 50, 78, 88, 90, 91, 96,
    313, 358, 384; Kibera, 368; Mombasa,
    78, 123; Nairobi, 37–39, 85, 88, 92,
    95, 100, 103, 181–82, 198, 207, 219,
    222, 309, 311, 313, 319, 320, 368
Khmer Rouge, 164, 168
Khyber Pass, 8, 139, 143
Kim Il Sung (father of Kim Jong Il), 307
Kim Jong Il, 306

Kim, Jim Yong, 363
Kindermans, Jean-Marie, 304–305, 313,
    319, 321, 322, 324
King Faisal Hospital (Kigali), 177, 180,
    187, 188–89, 190, 192, 193, 194–96,
    195, 201, 202, 203, 204, 206, 208,
    209–14, 211, 219, 221, 222, 225, 229,
    231, 233, 235–36, 237–38, 239–40,
    242, 244, 247, 248–49, 252, 392;
    Committee of Intellectuals, 212–14
King, Martin Luther, Jr., 20
Kosovo, 11, 321–30, 331–33, 338, 341,
    342; Drenica, 321; and expulsion of
    ethnic Albanians, 321, 323, 329;
    Kamenica, 345; Mitrovica, 342;
    Operation Horseshoe, 321; Priština,
    342, 343, 343; and refugees, 323,
    324–25, 326–30; Shkolla enclave,
    343, 343; Štrpce, 345; see also Serbia
Kosovo Liberation Army (KLA), 321,
    322, 324
Kouchner, Dr. Bernard, 68, 69, 70, 113,
    218–20, 332–33, 340, 345, 346
Kuwait, 75
Kyler, Steven, 186
Kyzner, Dave, 281, 287, 289, 293

Lake, Anthony, 178
Lane, Jim, 71
Laporte, Pierre, 18
Larkin, Barbara, 355
Laughi (clinic staff, Somalia), 117, 120
Legault, André, 136
Le Guillouzic, Hervé, 171
Leiberman, Michael, 29, 30
Lemasson, Isabelle, 193
Lennon, John, 19
Leopold, King (Belgium), 53
Lepage, Dr. Philippe, 40, 48, 64
Lewinsky, Monica, 311
Liberia, 126, 181; Monrovia, 126
Little, Jane, 282–83
London School of Hygiene and Tropical
    Medicine, 76–77
Loren, Sophia, 95–96

Lotrowska, Michel, 126
Love, Jamie, 359, 371
Lu, Catherine, 12, 392
Lulu (Rwandan Métis boy), 190–90,
    189, 193–94, 210–11, 234, 252, 253,
    393, 396
Lundestad, Geir, 334
Luxembourg, 67
Luxen, Jean-Pierre, 177
Lynne, Brian, 39

Macedonia, 323, 324, 326, 327
MacNeil, Don, 184, 190–91, 192, 196,
    212–13, 214, 219, 221–22, 225, 233,
    236
Mahdi, Ali, 92, 95, 105, 106, 107, 111,
    114
Malawi, 14–15, 374–79, 398; Ministry
    of Health, 15, 376, 377, 379; Zomba,
    14, 15, 374, 376, 378, 379
Malaysia, 70, 366, 369
Mandela, Nelson, 175, 355
Marie-Anne (MSF co-ordinator, Ajiep),
    316–17
Marks, John, 122
Masoud (Afghani warlord), 138
Matthysen, Dirk, 101–102, 103
Mauritania, 220
McCarthy, Gerry, 205–206, 235
McCurry, Michael, 175, 268
McDougall, Barbara, 136
McHarg, Marilyn, 71
McMaster University School of
    Medicine, 32–33, 63; Hospital, 47,
    63, 67
McNamara, Dennis, 342–43
Medicines for Malaria Venture (MMV),
    368
Médicins du Monde, 219
Médicins Sans Frontières (MSF), 3, 5, 6,
    8, 9, 11, 12, 13–14, 67, 76, 127, 135,
    136, 159, 176, 177, 178, 179, 180, 181,
    190, 207–209, 229, 231, 260,
    262–63, 264–65, 267, 270–71, 278,
    292, 294, 296, 297, 302, 303,

    304–306, 310, 330–32, 333, 337–41,
    385–86, 391, 398; and Campaign for
    Access to Essential Medicines, 13,
    333–34, 350, 354, 356, 357–58, 362,
    363, 365–66, 370–73; and "Forced
    Flight," 297; International Council of,
    304, 332, 365; and Neglected
    Diseases Working Group, 13, 366–68;
    and Nobel Peace Prize, 334–35,
    338–41, 339, 351, 354, 366; origins
    of, 67–70; see also Drugs for Neglected
    Diseases initiative; Médicins Sans
    Frontières (MSF), international sec-
    tions; Médicins Sans Frontières
    (MSF), missions
Médicins Sans Frontières (MSF), inter-
    national sections: MSF Belgium, 67,
    138, 177, 260, 265, 309, 314, 322,
    324, 342; MSF Brussels (international
    office), 309–310, 319, 337; MSF
    Canada, 67, 71, 132, 258; MSF France
    (Paris), 138, 175, 180, 218, 232, 252,
    262, 265, 305, 320, 329, 334, 354;
    MSF Germany, 304; MSF Greece,
    323–24, 330–32, 339; MSF Holland
    (Amsterdam), 3, 67, 77, 89, 132–33,
    181, 182, 234, 260, 265, 319; MSF
    Luxembourg, 67; MSF Spain, 67; MSF
    Switzerland, 67; MSF United
    Kingdom (London), 321
Médicins Sans Frontières (MSF), mis-
    sions: in Afghanistan, 137–59,
    385–86; in Iraq, 76; in Kosovo,
    321–30, 342–46; in Mozambique,
    193; in North Korea, 306–309; in
    Peru, 74, 75; in Russia, 335–37; in
    Rwanda, 164, 171, 172–75, 177, 178,
    188–251, 262; in Sierra Leone, 305; in
    Somalia, 77–124, 128; in Sudan, 311,
    312–20, 346–49; in Tibet, 164; in
    Zaire, 272–99, 301
Médicos del Mundo (MDM), 290
Merck, 358
Merlin, 283
Merv (CARE co-ordinator), 87–88, 100

Michel, Dr. Jean-Marc, 39, 44, 49
Milošević, Slobodan, 97, 321, 322, 323,
    326, 327, 329, 330, 332
Mitterand, François, 168, 179, 180, 193
Mobuto (Sese Seko), President (Zaire),
    165, 263, 266, 267, 283, 285, 286,
    291, 293, 296, 297
Mohamed (cook, Somalia), 114, 115
Montenegro, 323, 326, 327
Moore, Mike, 371
Moreels, Reginald, 177
Morgan, General, 87, 114
Morocco, 131
Moyn, Samuel, 390
Mozambique, 133, 193
Mpwale (son of Charity), 374
Muckle, Thomas, 32–33
Mumar (MSF head of mission, Russia),
    336–37
Museveni, President Yoweri (Uganda),
    165, 167

Nader, Ralph, 356
Najibullah, Prime Minister Mohammad
    (Afghanistan), 137
Nazis, 9, 22, 23, 24, 34, 69, 293;
    and Auschwitz, 21, 258; and
    Bergen-Belsen, 21; and genocide
    of Jews and others, 21–25, 34, 69,
    164, 175, 258
Nepal, 11
Netherlands, see Holland
Neufeld, Dr. Vic, 33–34
New Zealand, 176, 177, 229
Niger, 220
Nigeria, 68, 70–71, 229
Nolle, Jos, 71, 133
Non-governmental organizations
    (NGOs), role of, 10, 45, 50, 53, 58,
    78, 81, 85, 90, 91, 92, 95, 96, 97,
    103, 106, 108, 109, 110, 111, 114, 115,
    116, 119, 122, 124, 127, 130, 136, 138,
    146, 155, 260, 264, 265, 266, 267,
    268, 275, 276, 280, 283, 285, 286,
    287, 294, 299, 302, 304, 305, 306,
    309, 310, 313, 316, 323, 326, 329,
    331, 333, 354, 357, 363, 373, 376,
    384–85, 386, 391
North Atlantic Treaty Organization
    (NATO), 157, 320, 321–24, 326–30,
    331, 333, 342, 346, 386; and
    Operation Allied Harbor, 326
North Caucasus republic, 337
North Korea, 11, 306–309, 338, 390;
    and 6/29 Camps, 307
Norway, 146, 273, 373; Oslo, 338–39,
    366
Nuclear Non-Proliferation Treaty
    (1972), 383

Oakley, Robert, 131
Oderwald, Willem, 85–86, 103
Ojukwu, General, 70–71
Oka Monastery, 29, 31, 34, 127
Okri, Ben, vii; A Way of Being Free, vii
Ono, Yoko, 19
Orbinski, Bernadette, 321
Orbinski, Deirdre, 18
Orbinski, Kevin, 17, 20–21, 22, 29, 71
Orbinski, Margaret (Madge), 18–19,
    20–21, 22–23, 24–25, 258
Orbinski, Rohin, 374
Orbinski, Stan, 18, 19, 20, 21, 22,
    24–27, 258
Organization for Security and
    Co-operation in Europe, 322
Oxfam, 70, 178, 218, 250, 292, 354

Pablo-Mendez, Ariel, 364
Pakistan, 8, 68, 131, 137, 138, 139, 140,
    141–42, 146, 147, 149, 151, 152–53,
    154, 229, 384; Islamabad, 154;
    Karachi, 140; Peshawar, 139, 140–41,
    151, 154
Parisel, Alex, 342
Partners in Health, 363
Pasteur Institute, 369
Paul (doctor, Rwanda), 62, 180–81
Pécoul, Dr. Bernard, 334, 354, 357, 358,
    359, 366, 369

Peru, 72–75; Carabamba, 72, 73;
  Caramarcos, 72; Lima, 74; MSF in,
  74, 75; and Shining Path guerrilla
  movement, 72–73
Peter (MSF logistician), 318
Philippines: Manila, 362
PhRMA, 353, 355–57, 358, 359, 360,
  361, 362, 364, 366, 367, 371, 372–73
Pictet, Jean, 303
Pieters, Jules, 77, 78, 97, 100, 103, 104,
  105, 106–107, 114, 126, 137, 138,
  140, 151, 164–65, 173, 175, 180, 181,
  194, 202, 218, 220, 225, 230, 231,
  234, 248, 251–52, 259–60, 269, 289
Pinard, Guy, 291
Portugal, 53, 56
Powell, Colin, 107, 384
Prendergast, John, 319
Prescott, Geoff, 151, 155
Price, Dr. Rick, 94, 101, 124
Primakov, Yevgeny, 323

Rabbani, Prime Minister Mohammed
  (Afghanistan), 138, 153
Racine, Luc, 200, 203
Raguenaud, Dr. Marie-Eve, 339
Ramsey, Dr. Jacques, 187, 194
Red Cross, 68–69, 70, 77–78, 79, 83,
  86, 90, 91, 92, 95, 96, 103, 104, 105,
  107, 110, 111, 116, 119, 123, 124, 128,
  148, 164, 171, 172, 173, 174, 176, 183,
  184, 188, 190, 192, 193, 196, 198,
  202, 206, 207, 208, 209, 214, 218,
  221, 225–29, 230–31, 232–33, 235,
  236, 237, 239, 252, 267, 276, 283,
  285, 287, 289, 291, 292, 296, 303,
  306, 309, 337, 346, 371, 384, 385,
  386
Republic of the Congo, 298, 299
Richardson, Bill, 296, 297, 308
Rieff, David, 330, 333, 338
Robinson, Mary, 96
Rockefeller Foundation, 364
Romania, 87, 136
Roscigno, Giorgio, 364

Rosenfeld, Jack, 32
Rostrup, Dr. Morten, 273, 365
Royal Canadian Mounted Police, 387
RPA (former Rwanda Patriotic Front),
  262, 266, 269, 271, 272, 291, 293
RTLM (Radio), 169, 179, 198, 208, 212,
  214, 218, 221, 224, 237
Rumsfeld, Donald, 384
Russia, 50, 137, 138, 140, 141, 144, 147,
  148, 158, 159, 221–22, 287, 306, 321,
  323, 326, 332, 335–37, 340, 341,
  352; Groznyy, 339–40; Ministry of
  Health, 336–37; Moscow, 37, 335,
  336–37; Secret Service, 287
Rwabugiri, King (Rwanda), 41
Rwanda, 9–10, 37, 39–65, 67, 72, 74,
  163–253, 257–58, 260–70, 265, 266,
  270–72, 273, 276, 279, 280, 283,
  284, 289, 292–93, 294, 296, 297,
  298, 299, 303–304, 329, 338, 341,
  352, 391, 392–95, 398; and the
  Akuza, 165, 166; and the Arusha
  Peace Agreement, 168, 169, 170, 187;
  ethnic tensions in, 41–42, 48–49,
  50–52, 51, 58, 59, 62–63, 165, 166,
  190, 197, 205, 210, 211, 214, 215,
  244, 248, 250, 251, 290; genocide of
  Tutsis by Hutus in, 9–10, 163–64,
  167–81, 185–251, 257–58, 260–63,
  264, 299, 303, 305, 391, 392–93; and
  Hutu Power, 166, 237, 242;
  Kayibanda government, 58; and the
  Mai-Mai, 279, 283, 284, 286, 287,
  288; Ministry of Health, 56, 62; prisons in, 261, 265; refugees in, 261–62,
  304; and war crimes tribunal in
  Arusha, 391
Rwanda, places in: Akagara region,
  182–83; Amahoro stadium, 177,
  185–86, 206, 209, 270, 393–95;
  Butare, 52, 170, 173, 174, 177, 180,
  237, 248; Cyngugu, 237; Gisenyi,
  237, 250, 277; Humanitarian
  Protection Zone, 242, 248; Kibeho
  camp, 262; Kibuye, 237; Kigali, 9,

39–40, 43, 44–45, 46, 47, 49, 59,
60–61, 169, 170, 171, 172, 173, 174,
177, 180, 181, 182, 183–84, 187, 188,
191, 195, 198–99, 200, 202, 205,
206, 207, 209, 210, 214, 216, 219,
220, 222, 224–25, 230, 231–34,
235–37, 241, 244, 245, 248, 249–50,
251, 253, 261, 262, 270, 273, 285,
286, 288, 290, 292, 297, 299, 305,
393; Kikuyu, 56; Kimihurura, 207,
241; Mugonero, 56, 245; Mundende,
49, 53–56, 59, 60, 166; Rhuengeri,
242, 250, 289–92

Rwanda Government Forces (RGF), 171,
172, 173, 187–88, 190–91, 193, 196,
197, 199, 200, 201, 202, 205–206,
208, 210, 216, 218, 219, 220–21, 222,
224, 225–26, 228, 230, 231–34,
235–37, 241, 242, 244, 248, 250–51

Rwanda Patriotic Front (RPF), 167–69,
171, 182, 184, 185, 187–88, 190, 191,
193, 196, 197, 199, 204, 205, 210,
211, 214, 216, 217–18, 222, 224–25,
228, 230, 231, 233–34, 235–37, 241,
242, 243–48, 250, 251, 260, 262, 303

Sabine (MSF nurse), 174
Sahnoun, Mohammed, 91, 101
Ste. Famille Cathedral (Rwanda), 202,
214–16
St. Michael's Hospital (Toronto), 374, 377
St. Paul's (Kigali), 202–203
Sangala, Dr. Wesley, 375–76
Sartre, Jean-Paul, 70
Saudi Arabia, 137
Schindler's List, 175
Scholtz, Michael, 357
Sealy, Brian, 32
Secours Médical Française, 68
Senegal, 220
Serbia, 286, 321–30, 331–33, 342–46;
Belgrade, 323, 331
Sergi (engineer, Russia), 336–37
Seventh-Day Adventists, 39, 44, 49–50,
56, 207

Shanks, Dr. Leslie, 272–73, 284, 285
Shaw, Dr. (Director of OLS), 320
Siberia, 335–36; Kemerovo, 335;
Mariinsk, 335–36; prisoners in,
335–37
Sierra Leone, 11, 338, 339
Simpson, O. J., 175
Sir George Williams University, 19–20
Sisters of Mercy (Zaire), 282
Sisters of Mother Teresa (Rwanda), 202;
Sisters of Charity Orphanage, 202
Slims disease, see HIV/AIDS
Small, Ian, 71, 75, 111
SmithKline Beecham, 358
Social Aid for the Elimination of Rape
(SAFER), 399
Somali National Association, 122
Somali Red Crescent Society, 91
Somalia, 5–7, 11, 77–126, 127–32, 136,
142, 170, 178, 181, 182, 270, 312,
318, 341, 329, 384, 391; Baidoa, 5,
77, 78, 80–81, 82, 83, 84–86, 85,
86–90, 93, 94–97, 98, 100–105, 106,
107–26, 118, 127–28, 133, 391;
Bardera, 87, 128; Bay Camp, 93–94,
117; Belet Weyne, 129; Burao, 90;
Buurhakaba, 97–99, 100, 105, 108,
120, 121, 124; Hargeisa, 90; Hawina,
80–84, 97, 108; Kandesere, 110;
Kismayo, 110, 114, 122, 123, 124,
127, 129; Mogadishu, 7, 90, 91, 92,
95, 96, 97, 101, 104, 105, 106, 109,
111, 113, 114, 115, 116, 124, 127, 128,
129, 130, 131, 132, 172, 178, 391,
392; MSF mission in, 77–126, 133;
and Reconciliation Conference, 132
South Africa, 12–13, 15, 175, 178, 286,
288, 354–55, 356, 359–60, 362, 369,
370, 371; Cape Town, 359–60;
Khayelitsha, 359–61, 362, 370;
Pretoria, 362
South Korea, 309
Soviet Union, 8, 84, 306; in
Afghanistan, 137, 138, 140, 141, 144,
146, 158–59

Spain, 67, 176, 275, 290
Special Programme for Research and Training in Tropical Diseases, 368
Sri Lanka, 337–38
Srivastava, Rolie, 259, 365, 374, 393
Stein, Janice, 301–302
Stokes, Chris, 324, 325
Sudan People's Liberation Movement, 310
Sudan, 3, 11, 77, 309–20, 346–49, 347, 365, 390; Ajiep, 311, 312, 316, 316–17, 317, 318, 346; Bar el Gazel, 310, 311, 315, 319; Darfur, 11, 390; Equatoria, 310, 315; Khartoum, 311, 346, 347; Loki, 313–14, 316, 317, 318, 319; Mapel, 314–15, 346
Suki (Zairean government employee), 60
Switzerland, 67, 182, 242, 261, 355, 372, 373; Geneva, 363, 371
Sykes, Sir Richard, 358
Sylvie (mother of Lulu), 194, 210–11, 234–35, 252, 253, 396
Sylvie (MSF nurse), 318
Syria, 388

Taliban, 8, 383, 384, 385, 387
Tanzania, 168, 175, 178, 197, 250; Arusha, 168, 170, 217, 391; Dar es Salaam, 311; refugee camps in, 263–65
Teitelbaum, Donald, 122
Terrorism, 11–12, 381–83; anthrax attacks, 372; and "war on terror," 11, 382–90, 392
Thailand, 70, 351–51, 358, 360, 365, 365; Bangkok, 362
Thérèse (child, Rwanda), 217
't Hoen, Ellen, 354, 362, 369, 371, 372; "Drop the Case" petition, 362
Tibet, 136–37, 158, 164
Togo, 220
Torreele, Els, 366, 369
Torture, 7, 11, 34–35, 129, 158, 387, 388, 389, 391, 392, 397

Tousignant, General Guy, 261
Treatment Action Campaign (TAC), 354, 359–61, 361, 362
Tunisia, 188, 204
Turati, Dana, 187
Turkey, 76, 323; and genocide of Armenians, 164
Turner, Dr. John, 71–72

Uganda, 39, 43, 58, 165–66, 167, 171, 182, 187, 197, 238, 266, 279, 292, 303; Entebbe, 285; Kabale, 182; Kampala, 235
Ullman, Harlan, 385
Ulrich, Wayne, 86, 101, 102, 137, 140, 142, 145–46, 149, 151
UNAIDS, see Joint United Nations Programme on HIV/AIDS (UNAIDS)
UNICEF, 92, 111, 122, 123, 124, 144, 205, 235, 309, 310, 319, 381, 384
United Arab Emirates, 67
United Nations, 5, 7, 10, 11, 13, 75, 78, 90, 91–92, 96, 101, 105–106, 107, 122, 129, 130, 135, 143, 157, 166, 168–70, 171, 172, 176, 177, 178, 179, 180, 182, 190, 193, 196–98, 213, 214, 215–16, 220, 224, 251, 263, 264, 265, 266, 267, 270, 278, 283, 291, 292, 293, 296, 303–304, 306, 308, 310, 311, 313, 314, 315, 319, 321, 329, 332, 338, 340–41, 346, 357, 358, 385, 386, Convention on the Prevention and Punishment of Genocide, 177; Department of Humanitarian Affairs, 92; Department of Peacekeeping Operations, 198; Development Programme, 92; Food and Agriculture Organization, 375; Global Fund to fight AIDS, Tuberculosis and Malaria, 370; High Commissioner for Refugees (UNHCR), 92, 138, 146, 264, 266, 267, 269, 270, 273, 276, 278, 280, 283, 285, 291, 293, 297, 326–27, 333, 384; Joint United Nations Programme on HIV/AIDS

(UNAIDS), 358–59, 370, 379;
Security Council, 76, 91–92, 107,
131, 132, 168, 169, 176, 177–78, 180,
196, 198, 218, 229, 230, 237, 261,
264, 267, 268, 292, 296, 303–304,
313, 319, 321, 326, 340–41, 348;
World Food Program, 92, 105, 146,
155, 158, 306–307, 309, 383; see also
UNICEF; World Health Organization
United Nations, and Afghanistan, 137,
138–39, 140, 145, 148, 149, 152
United Nations, and Iraq, 75, 76
United Nations, and Kosovo: KFOR,
332, 342, 343, 344, 345, 346; United
Nations Mission in Kosovo
(UNMIK), 345
United Nations, peacekeeping forces of,
92, 101, 105, 107, 120, 124, 126, 127,
128, 129, 130, 131, 135, 157, 164, 168,
169, 171–72, 176, 187, 188, 191, 202,
214, 221–22, 224, 225, 243, 261, 268,
277, 329, 332, 341, 345, 391
United Nations, and Rwanda: Advance
Humanitarian Team, 171; Human
Rights Commission on Rwanda, 180,
197; International Criminal Tribunal
for Rwanda, 261; United Nations
Assistance Mission in Rwanda
(UNAMIR), 168–70, 171, 172, 177,
179, 180, 182, 183, 184, 185, 186–87,
187–88, 189, 190, 191–92, 193, 194,
196–98, 200, 203, 204, 205, 206,
208, 217, 218–19, 220, 221, 222,
224, 225, 229, 235, 239, 241, 245,
251, 253, 261, 262
United Nations, and Somalia, 170, 172;
"100-Day Plan," 92, 105; UNITAF,
130; United Nations Operation in
Somalia (UNOSOM), 91, 107, 122,
124, 130, 131–32
United Nations, and Sudan: Operation
Lifeline Sudan (OLS), 310–11, 312,
313–20, 347
United Nations, and Zaire, 260, 277,
278

United States, 7, 10, 19, 46, 59, 72, 76,
91, 96, 165, 172, 177, 178–79,
196–97, 206, 218, 263, 268, 269, 270,
277, 281, 287, 288–89, 292, 293, 294,
296, 297, 299, 306, 308, 309,
319–20, 321, 323, 326, 328, 332, 348,
355, 356–57, 359, 367, 372, 376,
382–85, 387–90, 391; in Afghanistan,
137, 141, 383–84; Hoboken, New
Jersey, 382; in Iraq, 11, 75–76,
382–83, 384–85; National Security
Council, 319–20; New York City, 11,
41, 96, 294, 319, 338, 340, 362, 364,
366, 372, 381–82, 387; Office of
Reconstruction and Humanitarian
Assistance, 385; and Operation
Lifeline, 78; and Presidential Decision
Directive 25 (PDD 25), 178–79; in
Rwanda, 167, 169, 171, 251; in
Somalia, 78, 84–85, 106–108, 110,
111, 113, 114–16, 117–24, 118, 127–28,
130–31, 132, 172; in Sudan, 311; and
United International Task Force
(Operation Restore Hope), 107–108,
113, 127, 130, 131; and U.S. Agency for
International Development (USAID),
59, 105, 141, 384, 385; and "war on
terror," 11–12, 382–90, 392;
Washington, DC, 319, 356, 358, 369,
372, 382
University Hospital (Butare), 173
University of San Francisco, 48; Project
San Francisco, 50
University of Toronto, 302, 374, 377
Uwilingiyama, Agathe (Prime Minister,
Rwanda), 172
Uwimana (boy, Rwanda), 60–62

van Alphen, Dr. Dana, 87–88, 90, 91,
92–93, 93, 94–95, 97, 100, 103, 104,
105–106, 109
Van de Perre, Dr. Philippe, 40, 64
Van Empelen, Wouter, 106, 108, 109,
111, 113, 114, 118, 120, 121, 122, 123,
124, 174

van Pelt, Maurits, 351
Van Schoor, Vanessa, 71
Vanessa (sister of Lulu), 210, 234–35, 252, 253
Venturelli, Dr. José, 34–35
Vietnam, 69–70; "boat people," 69–70
Vraalsen, Tom Eric, 315
Vreede, Eric, 181, 182, 194, 203, 209, 221, 222, 225, 236, 239, 240

Wakali, Dr., 147, 155
War Child, 399
Weil, Simone, 9
Wenceslas, Father, 215–16
Wilkins, Carl, 206–207
Wilkins, David, 388–89
Winkler, Lex, 324
Woods, James, 178
World Bank, 60, 165, 260, 358, 376
World Health Organization (WHO), 13, 92, 145, 309, 352, 357, 358, 363, 364–65 366, 370, 379; Massive Effort campaign, 364–65
World Trade Center, attack on (2001), 11, 381–82, 387
World Trade Organization (WTO), 13, 353, 355, 357, 358, 371, 372; Doha Declaration, 372
World Vision, 96, 107, 114
World War I, 42
World War II, 21–26, 69, 90, 323

Xavier (MSF logistician), 318

Yaache, Colonel, 196, 219, 245
Yeltsin, Boris, 337, 340
Yemen, 91
Yugoslavia (former), 77, 91, 97, 105, 106, 107, 156–57, 164, 175, 176, 178, 261, 303, 321, 328, 330; Muslims in, 97, 106; Sarajevo, 133, 157; Serbs in, 97, 106; Vukovar, 157; see also Bosnia

Zablon (hospital manager, Rwanda), 56–57
Zachariah, Dr. Rony, 173–74, 177, 180
Zaire, 10, 53, 58, 59–60, 165, 169, 178, 217, 224, 233, 242, 250, 251, 260, 263–70, 271, 272–99, 301, 303, 304, 329, 341, 366; Bukavu, 231, 250, 274, 276, 291; Bunia, 274; Goma, 59–60, 231, 250, 260, 263, 266, 268, 272, 273, 274, 276, 281, 283, 285, 286, 287, 289–90, 292, 293, 294, 338, 391; Hombo, 278; Hutus in, 265; Kashusa, 298; Kinshasa, 297, 299; Kisangani, 294, 296, 298; Kivu, 250, 263, 265, 266, 267, 268, 271, 276, 278, 279, 283, 285, 286, 287, 288, 289, 290, 291, 293, 294, 297; Masisi district, 272, 274, 275, 276, 283, 284; Matanda, 284; Mugunga refugee camp, 266, 268, 274–75; Mweso, 281; refugees in, 260, 263–70, 272–99; Sake feeding centre, 273, 273, 276, 282–83, 288, 291, 293, 295; Shaha province, 291; Shabunda, 278, 292, 293, 298; Tingi-Tingi, 292, 298; Tutsis in, 265–66, 288; Walikali, 278; Wendji, 298, 299; Uvira city, 268; Zairean Presidential Guard, 285
Zaire Armed Forces (FAZ), 266, 271, 274, 279, 280, 283, 287, 293
Zambia, 140, 259, 259,
Zomba Central Hospital (Malawi), 374, 377, 378

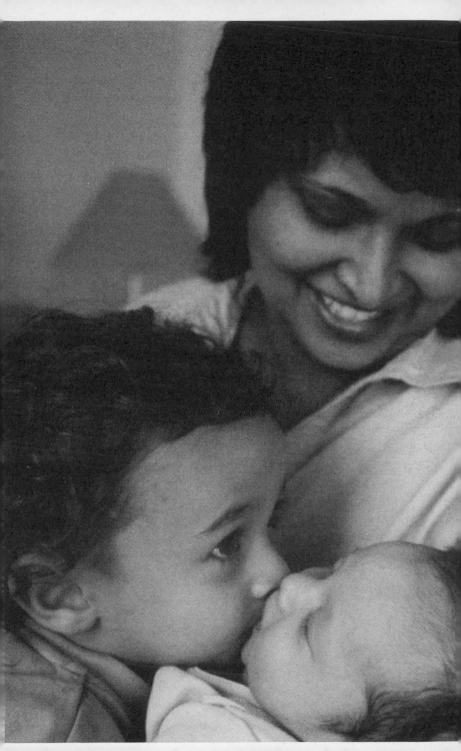

ACKNOWLEDGEMENTS

There would be no book without three important people. The first is Martha Kanya-Forstner, my editor on this project. She, more than anyone, has helped me tell this story—bringing it from a conversation between us to a book—and in this she is indeed a gifted editor. She has taught me something of the skill of writing and guided me on this journey. Thank you Martha for loving the people in the stories as much as the stories themselves and for all that you have brought to this project. It is richer for it and would not have happened without you. And thank you too for friendship—it is precious indeed. The second is Bruce Westwood, who attended a lecture I gave at the University of Toronto on the eve of the American invasion of Iraq in 2003 and who subsequently hounded me until I agreed to "think about writing a book." Thank you Bruce for your friendship and tenacity. The third is the most important. She is my partner and friend, Rolie. To her I owe everything, especially permission to use the letters R and L. Without these, this book would have been more difficult to write. Rolie lives daily with the travails of my heart and mind, with the passions and ideas that have possessed me for so long, and from which I now freely choose. She is the mother of our children, and shows me daily that love is the beginning of all that is meaningful, and my life is indeed full with meaning.

I would like to especially thank Jean-Marie Kindermans and Philippe Biberson, both of MSF, who will certainly disagree about much of what I have said in this book. Even still my thoughts have benefited beyond measure from my discussions and friendship with them. I would also like to acknowledge the many thousands of volunteers, national staff and headquarters staff who work with courage and determination to bring humanitarian assistance and protection to people in need. There are far too many to name from MSF, the Red Cross (ICRC), UN agencies, from among UN peacekeeping forces and from other organizations. Most especially I would like to thank Bernard Pécoul, Samantha Bolton, Winifred Simon, Rick Bedel, Jules Pieters, Kathleen Metcalfe, Carol Devine, Françoise Bouchet-Saulnier, Daniel Berman, Ellen t'Hoen, Els Torreele, Jacques DeMilliano, Jean-Hervé Bradol, Rony Brauman, Jos Nolle, Alex Parisel, Zackie Achmat, Jim Kim, Paul Farmer and Phil Clarke, each of whom has been a particular inspiration to me. I would also like to thank St. Michael's Hospital and the Munk Centre for International Studies, both at the University of Toronto, for their support for this writing project. For research assistance, I thank Barry Burciul, David Egan, Andrea Paras, Ankita Jauhari, and Joe Belliveau. Others, each in their own way—known and unknown and at different times—have helped me with this writing project. They include Michael Lieberman, Jacqui, Kevin, Deirdre and Bernadette Orbinski, Justin Reynolds, Carolynne Hew, Phil Playfair, Peter Scott, Patti Strong, Robbie Chase, Chris Romeike, Andrew Fedosov, Eric and Rhys Hoskins, Samantha Nutt, Ian Small, Michelle Oser, Vic Neufeld, John Frid, Ursula Franklin, Harriet Friedman, Gerry Caplan, Solly Benatar, Janice Stein, Lou Pauly, Gerry Helleiner, John and Elizabeth Fraser,

Vincent Tovel, Art Slutsky, Ron Diebert, David Welch, Melissa Williams, Jim Graff, Craig Scott, Peter Hajnal, Michael Barnett, Joanna Santa Barbara, Graeme MacQueen, Ed Mills, Stephen Lewis, Allan Rock, Bob Fowler, Lloyd Axworthy, Roger Lemoyne, David Rieff, Michael Young, Rene Fox, Jack Rosenfeld, John Westheuser, Steve Simon, Ao Loo, Peter Raymont, Michelle Latimer, Michèle Hozer and all at White Pine Pictures, and especially to Patrick Reed. To each and all, a full thank you.

The book's title is inspired by a line in the song-poem "Anthem" by Leonard Cohen. The book is for my children. I felt it important to tell this story now, while what remains is still fresh. I tell it in what has often been, since their birth, a sometimes desperate wish that I can make their own inevitable journey easier. In writing this book, I missed my children's first day of school. I hope it may have some use on their last. For my children: The world is as it has always been. It is a terrible and beautiful place, and a place of possibility. And it is more beautiful for me that you are in it.

ABOUT THE AUTHOR

Dr James Orbinski is a veteran of many of the world's most complex and disturbing humanitarian emergencies. In 1998, he received the Governor General's Meritorious Service Cross for his work as the Médecins Sans Frontières (MSF) Head of Mission to Rwanda during the 1994 civil war, and the following year he was the recipient of the 1999 Nobel Peace Prize on behalf of MSF.

Dr Orbinski is a founder of the Drugs for Neglected Diseases Initiative, a not-for-profit pharmaceutical research and development entity focused on the diseases of the South. He recently founded Dignitas, based in Malawi, an organization focused on community based treatment, care and prevention of HIV in the developing world. Currently, he is a Research Scientist and Associate Professor of Family and Community Medicine and Political Science at St. Michael's Hospital and the University of Toronto. He lives in Canada but travels widely.

Buy Rider Books

Order further Rider titles from your local bookshop, or have them delivered to your door by Bookpost.

Fighting the Banana Wars and Other Fairtrade Battles by Harriet Lamb	9781846040849	£7.99
Iran Awakening by Shirin Ebadi	9781846040146	£7.99
The Lucifer Effect by Philip Zimbardo	9781846041037	£8.99
The Voice of Hope by Aung San Suu Kyi	9781846041433	£7.99

FREE POSTAGE AND PACKING
Overseas customers allow £2.00 per paperback

By phone: 01624 677237

By post: Random House Books
C/o Bookpost
PO Box 29
Douglas, Isle of Man
IM99 1BQ

By fax: 01624 670923

By email: bookshop@enterprise.net

Cheques (payable to Bookpost) and credit cards accepted

Prices and availability subject to change without notice.
Allow 28 days for delivery.
When placing your order, please mention if you do not
wish to receive any additional information.

www.rbooks.co.uk